THE GLOSSARY OF FASHION DESIGN

Compiled & Edited By:

Dr. Padmaja Saha

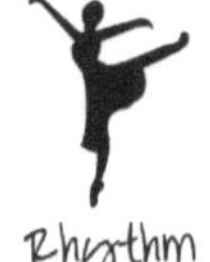

Rhythm

Independent
Publication

THE GLOSSARY OF FASHION DESIGN

Compiled & Edited By:
Dr. Padmaja Saha

ISBN:9798862078633

9798862078633

Published by:

Rhythm Independent Publication,

Jinkethimmanahalli, Varanasi, Bengaluru, Karnataka, India - 560036

For all types of correspondence, send your mails to the provided address above.

The information presented herein has been collated from a diverse range of sources, comprehensive perspective on the subject matter.

3D Printing In Fashion

3D Printing in Fashion is a cutting-edge technology that incorporates the process of creating three-dimensional objects by layering materials such as polymers, metals, or textiles. In the context of fashion design, it refers to the use of this innovative technique to produce custom-made garments, accessories, footwear, and even jewelry. By utilizing 3D printing technology, fashion designers can bring their imaginative concepts to life, pushing the boundaries of traditional manufacturing methods. It enables designers to produce intricate and highly detailed designs that would be challenging or impossible to achieve using conventional techniques.

A-Line Dress

A-line Dress An A-line dress is a type of dress that is characterized by its shape, which resembles the letter 'A'. It is a classic silhouette that is narrow at the top and gradually widens towards the bottom. The dress typically has a fitted bodice that skims over the waist and hips, flaring out into a wider skirt. The A-line dress is a versatile and timeless style that can be worn for various occasions. Its simple yet elegant design makes it suitable for both casual and formal events. This dress is a popular choice among women of all ages, as it flatters many different body types. One of the key features of the A-line dress is its flattering silhouette. The design of the dress helps to create the illusion of a narrower waist and elongated legs. This makes it a great choice for women who want to accentuate their curves or create the illusion of an hourglass figure. The A-line dress can be made from a variety of fabrics, including cotton, silk, and chiffon. The choice of fabric can greatly affect the overall look and feel of the dress. For a more casual look, a cotton or linen A-line dress can be worn with flat sandals or sneakers. On the other hand, a silk or chiffon A-line dress can be dressed up with heels and jewelry for a more formal occasion. The A-line dress can also be styled in different ways to suit individual preferences. It can be worn with a belt to cinch in the waist and add definition to the silhouette. A jacket or cardigan can be layered over the dress for added warmth or style. Additionally, accessories such as a statement necklace or scarf can be used to enhance the overall look of the dress. In summary, an A-line dress is a classic and versatile style that is characterized by its shape. It has a fitted bodice and a flared skirt, creating a flattering silhouette. The dress can be made from various fabrics and can be styled in different ways, making it a go-to choice for many women. Whether it's for a casual outing or a special occasion, the A-line dress is a timeless option in the world of fashion design.

A-Line Mini Skirt

An A-line mini skirt is a short, straight skirt that is fitted at the hips and gradually widens towards the hem, creating an "A" shape silhouette. It is a staple piece in fashion design, known for its versatility and timeless appeal. The A-line mini skirt is characterized by its flattering fit and length. It typically hits above the knee, emphasizing the legs and creating a youthful and playful look. The A-line shape of the skirt provides ease of movement and comfort, making it suitable for a variety of occasions. One of the key features of an A-line mini skirt is its high waistline. This design element accentuates the waist and creates a feminine and elongated silhouette. The skirt is often designed with a waistband or belt loops, allowing for the addition of a belt to further enhance the waistline. An A-line mini skirt can be crafted from various materials, including denim, cotton, suede, or leather, offering different textures and finishes. It can be styled in countless ways, making it a versatile piece that can seamlessly transition from daytime to evening wear. For a more casual look, an A-line mini skirt can be paired with a tucked-in graphic t-shirt and sneakers. This combination creates a laid-back and effortless outfit perfect for running errands or meeting friends for brunch. To elevate the A-line mini skirt for a more formal occasion, it can be paired with a blouse or a tailored blazer. Adding heels or ankle boots completes the polished look, making it suitable for a business meeting or a night out. In conclusion, an A-line mini skirt is a timeless and versatile piece in fashion design. Its flattering silhouette and length make it a go-to choice for women seeking to enhance their style. Whether dressed up or down, the A-line mini skirt is a wardrobe staple that can effortlessly elevate any ensemble.

A-Line Skirt

An A-line skirt is a type of skirt that is designed to have a shape resembling the letter A. It is narrower at the waist and gradually widens towards the hem, creating a silhouette that is flared and tapering. This design gives the skirt its distinctive A-line shape, hence the name. The A-line skirt is considered a classic and timeless style in fashion design. It was popularized by Christian Dior in the 1950s as part of his revolutionary "New Look" collection. Dior's A-line skirts were a departure from the more restrictive and structured styles of the wartime era, offering women a more feminine and flattering silhouette.

Accessory Design

Accessory design in the context of fashion design refers to the creation and development of decorative items that enhance and complete a fashion ensemble. These accessories can include a wide range of items such as jewelry, handbags, belts, scarves, hats, and shoes. The main goal of accessory design is to provide additional elements that complement and enhance the overall appearance of an outfit. Accessories can add personality, style, and uniqueness to an individual's fashion choices, allowing them to express their individuality and personal taste. They can also be used strategically to elevate a simple or plain outfit, turning it into a stylish and fashionable ensemble. Accessory designers typically work closely with fashion designers to create cohesive and harmonious collections. They consider factors such as color, texture, material, and shape to ensure that the accessories align with the overall aesthetic and concept of the fashion line. They also need to stay updated with the latest fashion trends and consumer preferences to create accessories that are relevant and appealing to the target market. In addition to aesthetic considerations, accessory designers also need to prioritize functionality and practicality. For instance, handbags should not only be visually appealing but also spacious and durable. Shoes should not only look stylish but also provide comfort and support. The balance between aesthetics and functionality is crucial in accessory design. Research and sketching are essential steps in accessory design. Designers often explore various sources of inspiration, including fashion history, art, nature, and cultural references. They then create detailed sketches, paying attention to details such as proportions, construction, and embellishments. Advanced technology may also be used, such as computer-aided design (CAD) software, to create digital representations of the accessories. Once the design is finalized, accessory designers collaborate with manufacturers and artisans to bring their creations to life. They provide detailed specifications and work closely with these professionals to ensure that the final products meet their vision and quality standards. All in all, accessory design plays a crucial role in the fashion industry, as it adds depth, variety, and individuality to fashion ensembles. Through careful consideration of aesthetics, functionality, and trends, accessory designers create items that enhance and complete a look, allowing individuals to express their personal style and make a fashion statement.

Advocacy In Fashion

Advocacy in fashion refers to the active promotion and support of certain causes, values, or beliefs within the fashion industry. It involves using the influence of fashion design, production, and consumption to raise awareness and bring about positive change. Advocacy in fashion can take various forms, depending on the specific cause or issue being addressed. It can involve using fashion as a platform to highlight social, environmental, or political issues and push for their improvement or resolution. For example, fashion designers may create collections that challenge societal norms or stereotypes, encourage body positivity, or promote sustainable and ethical practices in the industry. Advocacy in fashion also extends to the production and supply chains of fashion products. It involves advocating for fair labor practices, supporting artisans and craftsmen, and ensuring transparency and accountability in the manufacturing processes. This includes striving for safe working conditions, fair wages, and the elimination of child labor and exploitation in the fashion industry. Additionally, advocacy in fashion involves the responsible consumption and promotion of fashion products. It encourages consumers to make conscious and informed choices about their purchases, considering the social and environmental impact of fashion items. This may involve supporting brands and designers that align with their values, choosing sustainable and ethically-produced garments, or participating in clothing swaps and upcycling initiatives. In recent years, advocacy in fashion has gained momentum and become an integral part of the industry. Fashion designers, brands, and consumers are increasingly using their voices and platforms to advocate for change and promote a more inclusive, sustainable, and responsible fashion industry. Through collaboration, education, and awareness-raising campaigns, advocacy in fashion aims to shift the industry towards a more conscious and responsible future.

Ankle-Length Jeans

Ankle-length jeans refer to a style of pants that are designed to reach the ankle when worn. This type of jeans is popular in fashion design for its versatile and modern look. Ankle-length jeans are typically made of denim fabric, known for its durability and rugged appeal. The length of ankle-length jeans is specifically tailored to fall just above or slightly below the ankle bone. This unique cut is a staple in contemporary fashion and offers a stylish alternative to full-length or cropped jeans. Ankle-length jeans can be found in various silhouettes, including straight, skinny, or wide-leg, allowing individuals to choose a fit that flatters their body type and personal style.

Artistic Expression In Fashion

Artistic Expression in fashion refers to the creation of unique and aesthetically appealing designs that convey the designer's creative vision and evoke emotional responses from viewers. It is the process of using fashion as a medium of self-expression, allowing designers to communicate their ideas, concepts, and beliefs through their creations. In fashion design, artistic expression is achieved by combining various elements such as colors, textures, patterns, and silhouettes in innovative and thought-provoking ways. It involves experimenting with different materials, techniques, and styles to push the boundaries of conventional fashion and create something visually striking and conceptually meaningful.

Asymmetric Top

An asymmetric top in the context of fashion design is a garment that exhibits a distinct lack of symmetry or balance in its design. It is characterized by uneven or unequal proportions, lines, or elements that create an unconventional and dramatic aesthetic. Unlike traditionally symmetrical tops that have equal proportions on both sides, an asymmetric top incorporates elements that are deliberately designed to be unequal. This can include asymmetrical hemlines, varying sleeve lengths, off-center necklines, or unbalanced patterns or designs. These intentional irregularities contribute to the visual interest and uniqueness of the garment.

Atelier

An atelier is a term used in the context of fashion design to refer to a workshop or studio where clothing, accessories, or other fashion items are created. It is typically a space where fashion designers, pattern makers, tailors, and other craftspeople come together to bring designs to life. Within an atelier, the design process often begins with conceptualization and sketching. Fashion designers use their artistic skills to envision different garments or accessories and create detailed drawings or renderings of their ideas. These sketches serve as a blueprint for the creation of the final product. Once the design is finalized, pattern makers come into play. They take the designer's sketches and create the patterns, which serve as templates for cutting the fabric. Pattern making requires careful calculation and understanding of measurements, as each piece of fabric needs to fit together precisely to create the desired shape and silhouette. The next step in the atelier is the cutting and sewing of the fabric. Tailors and seamstresses use the patterns to cut the material and then stitch the pieces together to construct the garment. This process involves skilled craftsmanship and attention to detail to ensure the highest quality and durability of the finished product. In addition to garment construction, ateliers often focus on other aspects of fashion design, such as embroidery, beading, or appliqué work. These embellishments add intricate details and textures to the final product, making it unique and visually appealing. An atelier is not only a place where fashion items are created but also serves as a collaborative space for designers and artisans to exchange ideas, techniques, and expertise. It fosters creativity, innovation, and craftsmanship, ensuring that each fashion piece produced is a work of art. In conclusion, an atelier in the context of fashion design is a workshop or studio where designers, pattern makers, tailors, and other craftspeople come together to bring fashion ideas to life. It encompasses the entire design process, from conceptualization and pattern making to cutting, sewing, and embellishment. It is a space that promotes creativity, collaboration, and the highest standards of craftsmanship in the fashion industry.

Athletic Romper

An athletic romper is a one-piece garment designed for women that combines the functionality and comfort of athletic wear with the style and versatility of a romper. It is a popular choice for active women who want to look fashionable while participating in sports or engaging in other physical activities. The design of an athletic romper typically features a short or mid-length bottom half, which is similar to shorts or cropped pants, and a fitted or loose-fitting top half, which resembles a sleeveless or short-sleeved shirt. The combination of these elements allows for ease of movement and provides coverage and support in all the right places.

Avant-Garde Fashion

Avant-Garde fashion refers to a style of clothing and accessories that push the boundaries of conventional fashion design. It is characterized by its experimental and unconventional nature, often challenging traditional aesthetics, techniques, and materials. Avant-Garde fashion designers are known for their innovative and forward-thinking approach to clothing. They frequently incorporate unexpected elements, such as unconventional silhouettes, asymmetrical designs, and unique fabric manipulations. Avant-Garde fashion pieces often blur the line between clothing and art, serving as a form of self-expression and pushing the boundaries of what is considered wearable.

Babydoll Dress

A babydoll dress is a type of short, loose-fitting dress that is typically characterized by its empire waistline, short length, and flared skirt. This style of dress is inspired by the babydoll nightgown, which was popularized in the 1950s by the fashion designer Sylvia Pedlar. The babydoll dress is known for its youthful and feminine aesthetic, often featuring delicate details such as lace, ruffles, or bows. It is commonly made from lightweight and flowy materials, such as chiffon, silk, or cotton, which add to its airy and ethereal nature. The dress is designed to be comfortable and easy to wear, making it a popular choice for casual or summer occasions.

Baggy Jeans

Baggy jeans are a type of denim pants that have a loose and oversized fit. This style of jeans is characterized by its relaxed silhouette, which is achieved by incorporating extra fabric into the design. Baggy jeans are often associated with streetwear and hip-hop fashion, as they provide a comfortable and casual look. Typically, baggy jeans feature a high waist with loose-fitting hips and thighs, gradually tapering down towards the ankles. The excess fabric allows for greater freedom of movement and provides a more relaxed feel compared to other types of jeans. Baggy jeans are often styled with a rolled or cuffed hem, further accentuating their loose and laid-back look.

Ball Gown

A ball gown refers to a type of formal dress that is typically worn to formal events such as proms, galas, and black-tie affairs. It is known for its elegant and glamorous design, characterized by a floor-length skirt with a full, voluminous silhouette. The ball gown is designed to make the wearer feel like a princess or a queen, exuding grace and sophistication. It is often made from luxurious fabrics such as satin, silk, taffeta, or velvet, further enhancing its regal appeal. The bodice of the gown is usually fitted and accentuates the waist, while the skirt flares out dramatically, creating a dramatic and eye-catching effect.

Ballet Leotard

A ballet leotard is a form-fitting, one-piece garment that is specifically designed for ballet dancers. It is an essential component of a ballet dancer's wardrobe, as it provides both comfort and functionality while also highlighting the elegant lines of the dancer's body. The ballet leotard is typically made from a stretchy and breathable fabric, such as nylon or spandex, which allows for a full range of motion and helps to wick away moisture during intense rehearsals or performances. The fabric clings to the body, highlighting the dancer's muscles and form, while also providing support and protection. Ballet leotards come in a variety of styles, including tank, short-sleeved, cap-sleeved, and long-sleeved options, allowing dancers to choose the one that best suits their personal style and the requirements of their performance. The neckline of the leotard can also vary, ranging from high necks to low-cut scoop or V-necklines. This variety ensures that dancers can find a leotard that not only enhances their technical abilities but also reflects their individuality and aesthetic preferences. The design of the ballet leotard takes into consideration the specific movements and positions required in ballet. It typically features a high-cut leg line, which elongates the leg and creates a beautiful line from the hip to the ankle. The leotard also offers a secure fit, with a tight bodice that stays in place as the dancer moves and performs intricate movements. Some leotards include additional features, such as mesh panels or decorative embellishments, to add visual interest and enhance the overall design. In addition to its functional advantages, the ballet leotard has become a symbol of grace and elegance in the world of ballet. Its sleek and minimalist design allows the focus to remain on the dancer's movements and technique, rather than on the garment itself. The simplicity of the leotard also allows for easy layering with other ballet essentials, such as tights, leg warmers, and ballet skirts. In conclusion, the ballet leotard is a quintessential garment in the world of ballet. Its form-fitting design and stretchy fabric provide dancers with comfort, support, and freedom of movement, while also accentuating their physique. With its variety of styles and necklines, the ballet leotard allows dancers to showcase their individuality and personal style. Whether in the studio or on the stage, the ballet leotard remains an iconic and essential piece of attire for every ballet dancer.

Balloon Sleeve Blouse

A balloon sleeve blouse is a type of women's blouse that is characterized by its exaggerated, voluminous sleeves. The sleeves are designed to resemble the shape of a balloon, hence the name. This style of blouse has become increasingly popular in the fashion industry due to its unique and statement-making design. The balloon sleeve blouse typically features sleeves that start narrow at the shoulder and gradually widen as they extend down towards the wrist. The voluminous shape is achieved through pleating or gathering fabric at the shoulder or upper arm, creating a puffed effect. The sleeves often have a loose and billowy silhouette, adding a touch of drama and femininity to the overall look of the blouse.

Balloon-Sleeve Top

A balloon-sleeve top refers to a style of clothing commonly found in women's fashion. This design features exaggerated, voluminous sleeves that resemble the shape of a balloon, hence the name. The sleeves are typically gathered at the shoulders and gradually expand towards the cuffs, creating a dramatic and statement-making look. The balloon-sleeve top has become increasingly popular in recent years, as it offers a unique and fashion-forward twist to a traditional blouse or shirt. This style can be found in various types of tops, including t-shirts, blouses, sweaters, and dresses, allowing for versatility in different outfits and occasions. Balloon sleeves can also be found in different lengths, ranging from short sleeves to three-quarter or full-length sleeves, offering options for different seasons and personal preferences. One of the main advantages of the balloon-sleeve top is its ability to add visual interest and dimension to an outfit. The exaggerated sleeves create a sense of volume and drama, instantly elevating the overall look. This design element can make a simple and basic ensemble stand out, allowing individuals to make a fashion statement effortlessly. Additionally, the balloon-sleeve top is a versatile piece that can be styled in various ways to suit different aesthetics and occasions. For a more casual and laid-back look, it can be paired with jeans or leggings, creating a trendy and effortless outfit. On the other hand, when styled with tailored pants or a skirt, the balloon-sleeve top can be transformed into a chic and polished ensemble suitable for more formal settings. In terms of fabric choices, the balloon-sleeve top can be crafted from a wide range of materials. Lightweight fabrics such as cotton or chiffon are commonly used for summer versions of this design, offering breathability and ease of movement. For colder seasons, heavier materials like wool or knit can provide warmth and coziness while still maintaining the distinct balloon sleeve shape. In conclusion, the balloon-sleeve top is a fashion-forward and versatile clothing item that adds drama and visual interest to an outfit. With its exaggerated and voluminous sleeves, it offers a unique statement-making look that can be styled in various ways for different occasions. Whether worn casually or dressed up, the balloon-sleeve top is a trendy and fashionable choice in contemporary women's fashion.

Balmacaan Coat

A balmacaan coat is a type of coat that is known for its loose and relaxed silhouette. It is typically knee-length or longer and features a wide collar, raglan sleeves, and an A-line shape, creating an elegant and timeless look. The balmacaan coat originated in Scotland in the mid-19th century and was initially designed as a practical outerwear option for outdoor activities such as hunting and fishing. Named after the Balmacaan Estate in Inverness-shire, Scotland, where it was first popularized, this coat quickly gained popularity due to its functionality and versatile design. One of the key features of a balmacaan coat is its loose fit. The coat's roomy silhouette allows for layering underneath, making it an ideal choice for colder weather. The loose fit also provides ease of movement and adds a relaxed and effortless charm to the overall look. The wide collar of a balmacaan coat not only adds a touch of sophistication but also serves a practical purpose. It can be flipped up to provide extra protection against the elements, such as wind or rain. Additionally, the collar can be worn open or closed, allowing for different styling options. Raglan sleeves are another characteristic feature of a balmacaan coat. These sleeves extend from the collar to the underarm, creating a diagonal seam that gives the coat a distinctive and flattering shape. Raglan sleeves provide a comfortable and unrestricted fit, allowing the wearer to move their arms freely. Another defining element of a balmacaan coat is its A-line shape. The coat typically flares out gradually from the shoulders to the hem, resembling the letter "A." This design not only adds elegance to the coat but also allows for easy layering over various types of clothing, from sweaters to dresses. Overall, a balmacaan coat is a classic and versatile outerwear piece that combines functionality with timeless style. Its loose fit, wide collar, raglan sleeves, and A-line shape make it a go-to choice for those seeking a coat that is both practical and fashionable.

Bandeau Bikini

A bandeau bikini is a type of women's swimwear that consists of a strapless top and a bottom. It is characterized by a straight neckline that wraps around the chest area, providing minimal coverage and a simplistic design. The bandeau bikini is commonly used in fashion design to enhance a woman's silhouette, offering a more minimalist look compared to other bikini styles. The bandeau bikini top typically features a bandeau shape, which is a narrow strip of fabric that circles the bust area. This design allows the wearer to showcase their shoulders and collarbone, creating an elongating effect on the upper body. The lack of straps makes it an ideal option for sunbathing or lounging by the pool without worrying about tan lines or discomfort caused by straps digging into the skin.

Bandeau Swimsuit

A bandeau swimsuit is a type of swimwear designed to be worn by women. It is characterized by a strapless top that wraps around the bust, providing minimal coverage and support. The bandeau swimsuit is popular for its sleek and chic design, making it a stylish option for beach or poolside lounging. Unlike traditional swimsuits with shoulder straps, the bandeau swimsuit offers a more daring and shoulder-baring silhouette. It is often favored by individuals who want to showcase their shoulders and collarbone, creating a feminine and alluring look. The absence of straps also allows for minimal tan lines, making it ideal for sunbathing and tanning.

Basketball Shorts

Basketball shorts are a type of shorts specifically designed for the sport of basketball. They are part of the overall basketball uniform and are typically worn by players during games and practices. These shorts are characterized by their loose and baggy fit, allowing for ease of movement and maximum comfort on the basketball court. In terms of design, basketball shorts usually feature an elastic waistband with a drawstring, ensuring a secure and adjustable fit. The waistband is often adorned with the team's logo or additional embellishments to represent the sport or team identity. The shorts themselves are made from lightweight and breathable materials, such as polyester or mesh, to promote ventilation and evaporation of sweat. The length of basketball shorts varies, but they typically fall around or just above the knees. This length offers players a balance between mobility and coverage, allowing for ample leg movement while still providing some modesty and protection. Additionally, the loose fit of these shorts ensures that they do not restrict the range of motion for players, enabling them to jump, run, and pivot without hinderance. Basketball shorts are often characterized by their vibrant color schemes and bold designs. They frequently display team colors, logos, patterns, or graphic prints. This not only promotes team spirit and unity, but it also allows for easy identification of teammates on the court. Due to the popularity of basketball and its influence on streetwear fashion, basketball shorts have transcended their original purpose as sportswear. They have become a staple in casual and athleisure wear, commonly worn by people outside of basketball activities. Their loose and comfortable fit, along with their trendy and stylish designs, make them appealing for everyday wear. In conclusion, basketball shorts are a type of shorts designed specifically for players to wear during basketball games and practices. They feature a loose and baggy fit, an elastic waistband with a drawstring, lightweight and breathable materials, a length that falls around or just above the knees, and vibrant designs representing team identity. These shorts have also gained popularity in fashion beyond basketball, becoming a stylish choice for casual and athleisure wear.

Basting Guns

A basting gun is a hand-held tool used in the fashion design industry to temporarily hold fabric layers together. It is commonly used during the initial stages of the garment construction process, allowing designers to create a mock-up or prototype of the desired design before finalizing the stitches. The basting gun consists of a durable plastic or metal body with a trigger mechanism that drives a small plastic fastener, known as a basting staple, through the fabric layers. These staples are designed to temporarily secure the fabric layers in place, allowing the designer to make any necessary adjustments or alterations before permanently sewing the garment.

Basting Thread

Basting thread is a type of temporary stitching used in fashion design to hold fabric layers together during the construction process. It is often made from a lightweight and strong thread that is easily removable. The purpose of basting thread is to hold fabric pieces in place temporarily while the designer or dressmaker can make adjustments or alterations before permanent stitching. It is especially useful when working with complex or delicate fabrics that may require multiple fittings or adjustments. Basting thread is typically used in various stages of garment construction. It can be used to hold pattern pieces together while cutting out fabric or to temporarily attach seams before final sewing. It is also used for fitting purposes, where it allows the designer or dressmaker to adjust the garment's fit and make any necessary alterations. The thread used for basting is often a contrasting color to the fabric, making it easier to see and remove later. This helps to ensure that the basting stitches are clearly distinguishable from the permanent stitches. Basting thread is typically longer in length compared to regular sewing thread, as it needs to be easily removable without damaging the fabric. It is commonly used with hand stitching techniques, although a machine with a basting stitch setting can also be used for faster and more precise basting. Once the adjustments or alterations have been made, the basting thread is removed by simply pulling it out. This leaves behind the permanent stitching, which may include hand sewing or machine stitching, depending on the preferred technique and the design of the garment. In summary, basting thread is a temporary stitching technique used in fashion design to hold fabric layers together during the garment construction process. It allows for adjustments and alterations before permanent stitching, and is easily removable without damaging the fabric.

Batwing Sweater

A batwing sweater, also known as a batwing top, is a type of loose-fitting sweater that is characterized by its wide and flowing sleeves that resemble the wings of a bat. This style of sweater is popular in the fashion industry due to its unique and stylish design. The batwing sweater typically features a wide neckline that can be either round or V-shaped, although variations with other necklines may also exist. The main highlight of this sweater is its oversized and relaxed fit, which allows for a comfortable and relaxed look. The body of the sweater is usually more fitted compared to the sleeves, creating a contrast in proportions.

Bell-Bottom Pants

Bell-bottom pants, also known as flared pants, are a style of trousers that became popular in the late 1960s and early 1970s. They are characterized by their wide flare at the bottom, starting from the knee or calf and flowing down to the ankle. The name "bell-bottom" refers to the bell-like shape created by the flared cut. Bell-bottom pants gained popularity as a rebellious fashion statement during the counterculture movement of the 1960s. They were associated with the Hippie and Bohemian subcultures, symbolizing a rejection of traditional, mainstream fashion. The style was also influenced by the resurgence of interest in Eastern cultures and the relaxed, free-spirited aesthetics of the era. The design of bell-bottom pants is rooted in practicality. The wide flare at the bottom allows for ease of movement and comfort, especially when paired with boots or platform shoes. The excess fabric sways and flows as the wearer moves, creating a visually striking effect. Bell-bottom pants come in various fabrics, including denim, cotton, and synthetic materials. They can be tailored or loose-fitting, depending on the desired style. The waistband can be high-rise or low-rise, and there may be additional design elements such as pockets or decorative stitching. Over the years, bell-bottom pants have experienced revivals in fashion, often influenced by nostalgia for the 1960s and 1970s. They have been reinterpreted by contemporary designers, incorporating modern elements while retaining the iconic flare. Bell-bottom pants are now considered a classic style with a versatile appeal, suited for both casual and formal occasions. In conclusion, bell-bottom pants are wide-flared trousers that originated in the 1960s and 1970s. They are associated with counterculture fashion and symbolize a rebellious and free-spirited aesthetic. The design provides comfort and ease of movement, and the style continues to be embraced and reinvented in contemporary fashion.

Bell-Sleeve Blouse

A bell-sleeve blouse is a type of women's garment that features sleeves with a distinct bell shape, flaring out at the bottom to create a stylish and fashionable look. The term "bell sleeve" is derived from the shape of the sleeve, which resembles the flared shape of a bell. This type of blouse has gained popularity in the fashion industry and is widely recognized for its unique and eye-catching design. Typically, a bell-sleeve blouse is made from lightweight and flowy fabrics such as chiffon, silk, or cotton. This choice of fabric enhances the loose and flowing nature of the sleeves, allowing them to drape elegantly and create a soft and feminine silhouette. The blouse itself may be fitted or loose, depending on the desired style and the overall design of the garment. Bell-sleeve blouses can come in various lengths, ranging from cropped styles that sit above the waist to longer designs that extend down to the hips or even the knees. The sleeves themselves can also vary in length, with some blouses featuring short bell sleeves that end above the elbow, while others may have long bell sleeves that extend all the way to the wrists. The bell-sleeve blouse is a versatile and trendy piece that can be styled in various ways to suit different occasions and personal preferences. It can be paired with skirts or pants for a sophisticated and feminine look, or worn with jeans for a casual yet fashionable outfit. The blouse can be accessorized with belts, scarves, or statement jewelry to enhance its overall appeal and add a touch of personal style. Due to its unique design and popularity, the bell-sleeve blouse has become a staple in many women's wardrobes. It is often featured in fashion collections and can be found in a wide range of colors, prints, and embellishments. Whether worn for a special occasion, a day at the office, or a casual outing, the bell-sleeve blouse is a fashion-forward choice that adds a touch of elegance and flair to any outfit.

Bell-Sleeve Dress

A bell-sleeve dress is a type of dress characterized by its sleeves that resemble the shape of a bell. The sleeves are flared and typically wide, starting from the shoulder and falling gracefully to the wrist or the forearm. This design feature gives the dress a unique and distinctive look. Bell sleeves can vary in length, with some dresses featuring long sleeves that extend all the way down to the wrist, while others have shorter sleeves that end around the elbow or forearm. The width of the bell sleeve can also vary, with some designs featuring a subtle flare, while others have a more exaggerated and dramatic flare.

Bell-Sleeve Sweater

A bell-sleeve sweater is a fashionable garment that is designed to have sleeves that widen dramatically from the elbow to the wrist, resembling the shape of a bell. This style of sweater has become increasingly popular in the world of fashion due to its unique and eye-catching silhouette. The bell-sleeve sweater is typically made from a variety of materials, including knit fabrics such as wool, cashmere, or acrylic. The choice of fabric can greatly impact the overall look and feel of the sweater, allowing for different levels of warmth, drape, and texture. This versatility makes the bell-sleeve sweater suitable for both casual and dressier occasions. One of the key design elements of a bell-sleeve sweater is the exaggerated width of the sleeves. This detail adds visual interest and creates a sense of movement when the wearer moves their arms. The length of the sleeves can vary, with some sweaters featuring sleeves that end just below the elbow, while others extend all the way to the wrist. Another defining characteristic of the bell-sleeve sweater is the fitted silhouette of the body. While the sleeves flare out dramatically, the body of the sweater is typically more form-fitting, accentuating the natural curves of the wearer's torso. This contrast in volume between the sleeves and the body of the sweater creates a visually striking and balanced look. The bell-sleeve sweater can be styled in various ways to create different fashion statements. It can be paired with high-waisted jeans for a trendy and casual look, or worn with a skirt and heels for a more polished and elegant ensemble. The versatility of this garment allows it to transition seamlessly from day to night, making it a versatile and essential piece in any fashion-savvy individual's wardrobe.

Bermuda Shorts

Bermuda shorts are a type of clothing designed specifically for warm weather and casual occasions. They are typically made of lightweight fabric and feature a length that falls just above the knee. The name "Bermuda shorts" can be traced back to the British Overseas Territory of Bermuda, where this style of shorts is believed to have originated. These shorts are characterized by their tailored fit, often having a flat front and a waistband that sits at or just below the natural waist. They may have a button or hook-and-bar closure, as well as belt loops for added convenience. Bermuda shorts are designed to provide comfort and mobility, making them suitable for activities such as walking, biking, or simply lounging by the beach.

Bias Binding Foot

A bias binding foot is a specialized sewing machine foot that is used in fashion design to attach bias binding to the edges or seams of a garment. Bias binding is a strip of fabric that is cut on the bias, which means it is cut at a 45-degree angle to the straight grain of the fabric. The bias cut gives the binding flexibility, allowing it to be stretched and curved. The bias binding foot is designed to guide the fabric strip smoothly through the sewing machine, ensuring even and accurate stitching. It has a groove or channel that holds the binding in place, as well as a guide that helps to position the fabric correctly. The foot also has a slot or hole that allows the needle to pass through, stitching the binding in place as it moves along the fabric.

Bias Tape Maker Tips

A Bias Tape Maker is a tool commonly used in fashion design to create bias tape. Bias tape is a narrow strip of fabric that is cut at a 45-degree angle to the grainline and is typically used for finishing raw edges, creating decorative accents, and adding stability to seams. The Bias Tape Maker is designed to make the process of creating bias tape quick and efficient. The Bias Tape Maker consists of a metal or plastic device with a slot at one end and a heated plate or iron at the other end. The slot is used to insert a strip of fabric, which is then pulled through the device while applying heat to the fabric. As the fabric is pulled through, the Bias Tape Maker folds the edges of the fabric inward, creating a neat and even fold. The folded fabric is then pressed with the heated plate or iron to set the fold and create the bias tape.

Bias Tape Makers

Bias tape makers are tools used in fashion design to create bias strips, which are narrow strips of fabric cut at a 45-degree angle to the selvage. These strips are used for various purposes in garment construction, such as binding edges, finishing raw edges, or adding decorative details to a garment. The bias tape maker itself is a small tool made of metal or plastic, typically in the shape of a small rectangle or a tube. It has a slot or groove along its length, into which the fabric strip is inserted. The fabric should be cut on the bias, which means it is cut diagonally across the grain of the fabric, allowing it to stretch and curve smoothly around curves and edges.

Bikini Bottom

A bikini bottom is a specific garment designed for women's swimwear. It is a brief-style bottom that is paired with a bikini top to create a complete bikini set. The main purpose of a bikini bottom is to provide coverage and support to the lower body while swimming or engaging in water activities. In terms of fashion design, a bikini bottom plays a crucial role in overall swimwear aesthetics. Designers carefully select fabrics, patterns, and styles to create attractive and comfortable bikini bottoms that complement the entire bikini set. The design of a bikini bottom can vary widely, ranging from classic briefs to hipster, high waist, or string styles. The choice of fabric for a bikini bottom is essential, as it directly impacts both the comfort and durability of the garment. Common materials used in bikini bottom construction include nylon, polyester, spandex, and elastane blend fabrics. These materials offer stretchability, flexibility, and resistance to chlorine and saltwater, ensuring the longevity of the garment. Additionally, the fabric choice also contributes to the overall appearance of the bikini bottom, with options ranging from solid colors to vibrant prints. Designers pay close attention to the fit and construction of a bikini bottom, as it must provide adequate support and coverage while also maintaining a flattering silhouette on the wearer. The bottom's waistband is typically elasticized to ensure a secure yet comfortable fit. Seams are carefully positioned to prevent irritation and enhance the overall fit and structure of the garment. Bikini bottoms are also designed to be versatile, allowing for customization and personalization. Some bottoms have adjustable side ties or drawstrings to provide a customizable fit according to individual preferences. Additionally, designers often incorporate decorative elements such as ruffles, fringes, or embellishments to add visual interest to the garment. In summary, a bikini bottom is a key component of women's swimwear, designed to provide coverage, support, and aesthetic appeal. Fashion designers consider various factors such as fabric choice, fit, construction, and customization options to create a functional and stylish bikini bottom that enhances the overall swimwear ensemble.

Bishop Sleeve Blouse

A bishop sleeve blouse is a type of blouse characterized by its voluminous sleeves that taper at the cuffs. The sleeves are inspired by the wide sleeves commonly seen on religious garments worn by bishops, hence the name. This style of blouse is a popular choice in fashion design, as it adds a touch of elegance and drama to any outfit. The bishop sleeves typically start at the shoulder and gather at the armhole, creating a billowy effect. The sleeves are then fitted at the forearm and end in a tight cuff, often securing with buttons or elastic. This design creates a striking contrast between the voluminous upper sleeve and the more fitted lower sleeve, resulting in a visually interesting silhouette.

Blind Hem Foot

A blind hem foot is a specialized sewing machine foot used in fashion design for creating a nearly invisible hem on garments. It is designed to fold and stitch the fabric in a way that hides the stitches on the right side of the garment, giving it a clean and professional finish. This foot is particularly useful when working with lightweight and delicate fabrics, as it prevents the visibility of bulky stitches that could detract from the overall appearance of the garment. It is commonly used for hemming skirts, dresses, trousers, and other garments where a discreet and seamless hem is desired.

Blocking Mats

Blocking mats in the context of fashion design refers to the process of using foam mats with interlocking squares or grids to stretch and shape fabrics, especially those made from knits or lace. These mats are an essential tool used by designers and garment makers to manipulate and transform fabric into desired shapes and sizes. When working with delicate or stretchy fabrics, blocking mats provide stability and support, preventing the material from warping or stretching out of shape during the construction process. The mats are particularly useful for blocking or stretching patterns, ensuring that the finished garment retains its intended shape and fit.

Board Shorts

Board shorts are a type of swimwear that originate from surf culture. They are typically made from lightweight and quick-drying fabrics such as polyester or nylon, designed to be comfortable and functional in water-based activities. Board shorts are characterized by their knee-length or slightly above-the-knee cut, loose fit, and relaxed style.Board shorts typically feature a drawstring or elastic waistband for easy adjustability and a secure fit. They often have a Velcro or lace-up closure at the front, along with a fly or snap fastening to keep them secure during active movement. Some styles may also have a hook-and-loop fastener or a zipper pocket for storing small essentials, such as keys or a wallet.Board shorts are notable for their bold and vibrant patterns, ranging from tropical prints to geometric designs. They often showcase bright colors, contrasting combinations, or subtle gradients, adding a playful and eye-catching element to beachwear. These patterns often reflect the coastal and nature-inspired themes synonymous with surf culture and the beach lifestyle.The loose fit of board shorts allows for freedom of movement and comfort while engaging in various water activities, such as swimming, surfing, paddleboarding, or beach volleyball. Their length provides adequate coverage and protection against sunburn, sand, or other elements, without hindering mobility or causing discomfort in wet conditions.Board shorts have become a popular choice beyond the beach and are worn as casual summer shorts or sportswear. They are often paired with T-shirts, tank tops, or rash guards, creating a relaxed and effortless look suitable for outdoor activities or leisurely outings. Their versatility and relaxed aesthetic have made board shorts a staple in warm-weather wardrobes and a symbol of the laid-back and carefree beach culture.In conclusion, board shorts are a style of swimwear originating from surf culture, characterized by their knee-length or slightly above-the-knee cut, loose fit, and bold, vibrant patterns. They are designed for comfort, functionality, and freedom of movement in water-based activities, with features such as a drawstring or elastic waistband, Velcro or lace-up closure, and optional pockets. Beyond their water-friendly features, board shorts have become a relaxed and versatile fashion choice suitable for casual and sportswear in warm weather.

Boardshorts

Boardshorts are a type of swimwear that originated in surf culture and have become popular in the fashion industry. They are designed to be lightweight, quick-drying, and comfortable, making them ideal for various water activities such as surfing, swimming, and paddleboarding. These shorts typically feature a loose-fitting, knee-length design with a flat waistband and a single closure system such as a lace-up or Velcro fly. They are often made from a blend of polyester and spandex, allowing for flexibility and ease of movement. Boardshorts may also have a mesh lining on the inside for added support.

Boat Neck Sweater

A boat neck sweater is a type of sweater that is characterized by its wide neckline, which resembles the shape of a boat. It is a popular choice in fashion design, as it adds a stylish and sophisticated touch to any outfit. The boat neck sweater is typically made from soft and comfortable fabrics such as wool, cashmere, or cotton. It is known for its loose and relaxed fit, which makes it a cozy and versatile addition to any wardrobe. The wide neckline of the sweater can be worn off the shoulders, creating an elegant and feminine look.

Bobbin Cases

A bobbin case in the context of fashion design is a small metal or plastic container that holds the bobbin within a sewing machine. It is an essential component of the machine that ensures smooth and precise stitching. The bobbin case is typically located beneath the needle plate, and its main purpose is to hold the bobbin in place while allowing it to rotate freely. The bobbin, which is wound with thread, fits snuggly into the bobbin case, creating a tension that helps regulate the thread's flow during sewing.

Bobbin Winders

A bobbin winder is a crucial tool used in the field of fashion design to wind thread onto bobbins, which are small spools that hold the lower thread in a sewing machine. It is an essential component in the process of creating garments, as well as various types of textile and sewing work. The bobbin winder consists of a simple mechanism that allows for efficient and accurate winding of thread onto bobbins. It typically consists of a spool holder, tensioning device, and a motor or hand-operated mechanism to rotate the spool. The thread is threaded through various guides and tensioning devices before being wound around the bobbin, ensuring that the thread is evenly distributed and tightly wound.

Bobbins

Bobbins are essential tools used in fashion design for the purpose of sewing and thread management. They are small spools that hold thread and are inserted into a sewing machine or handheld sewing tool. The purpose of bobbins is to provide an efficient and organized way to manage the thread during the sewing process. In fashion design, bobbins play a crucial role in ensuring the quality and precision of the stitching. When sewing, the thread from the spool is wound around the bobbin, which is then placed into the bobbin case or shuttle of the sewing machine. As the machine is threaded and operated, the bobbin rotates, releasing the thread and creating the lower thread tension necessary for the formation of stitches.

Bodkin Needles

Bodkin needles are slim and long sewing needles that are commonly used in fashion design and garment construction. They have a sharp point at one end and a small eye at the other end, making them ideal for threading and stitching various types of fabric. These needles are specifically designed for tasks that require precision and control, such as creating intricate designs, sewing delicate fabrics, and making small, precise stitches. They are often used for hand sewing techniques like basting, gathering, and pleating. Bodkin needles are also used for pulling elastic or drawstrings through casings, as their long and slender shape allows them to easily maneuver through tight spaces.

Body Measuring Tools

Body measuring tools in the context of fashion design are devices or instruments used to accurately measure the size and proportions of the human body. These tools are essential for fashion designers to create well-fitted garments that flatter the wearer's body shape and ensure proper fit and comfort. One commonly used body measuring tool is a tape measure. A tape measure consists of a flexible ribbon or tape that can be easily wrapped around the body to measure various body parts such as the chest, waist, hips, and inseam. Tape measures are typically marked with both standard and metric unit measurements, allowing designers to work with different systems of measurement depending on their needs. Another important tool is a dress form or a mannequin. These are three-dimensional models of the human body, often made of foam or padded material and covered in fabric. Dress forms can be adjusted to match specific body measurements, allowing designers to drape and fit garments directly on the form to see how they will look and fit on a real person. Calipers are another type of body measuring tool used in fashion design. These are handheld devices with two arms or jaws that can be opened and closed to measure the thickness or diameter of various body parts. Calipers are particularly useful for measuring body measurements such as the bicep, thigh, and neck circumference. Additionally, a grading ruler is a specialized tool used for scaling patterns in different sizes. It consists of a long, flat ruler with evenly spaced markings that enable designers to increase or decrease the size of patterns accurately and proportionally. In summary, body measuring tools are crucial for fashion designers to ensure the proper fit and proportion of garments. These tools include tape measures, dress forms, calipers, and grading rulers. By accurately measuring and assessing the body, designers can create garments that enhance the wearer's physique and ensure comfort and style.

Bodysuit

A bodysuit is a form-fitting garment that covers the torso and is typically designed to be worn as an undergarment or a part of an outfit. It is commonly made of stretchable fabric, such as cotton, nylon, or spandex, to provide a snug yet comfortable fit. The primary purpose of a bodysuit is to create a seamless and streamlined look when worn underneath clothing, especially tight-fitting or sheer garments. It serves as a foundation piece that helps in shaping and smoothing the silhouette, enhancing body contours, and providing support to the midsection.

Boho Dress

A boho dress, short for bohemian dress, is a fashion design that originated from the bohemian and hippie subcultures of the 1960s and 1970s. It is characterized by its loose and flowy silhouette, vibrant and colorful patterns, and a relaxed and carefree aesthetic. The boho dress is often made from lightweight and breathable materials such as cotton, chiffon, or linen, and typically features an empire waistline, bell sleeves, and a floor-length skirt. However, variations of the boho dress can include midi or mini lengths and different sleeve styles, depending on the current trends and individual interpretations of the bohemian style.

Bolero Jacket

A bolero jacket is a short, waist-length jacket that is open in the front and typically worn by women. It originated in Spain in the 19th century as a traditional garment worn by bullfighters and dancers, but it has since become a popular fashion choice worldwide. The bolero jacket is characterized by its cropped length, usually ending just above the waist or at the waistline. It typically has a fitted silhouette and may feature various sleeve lengths, including long sleeves, three-quarter sleeves, or short sleeves. The design of the bolero jacket can vary widely, with some featuring a collar or lapels, while others are collarless and have a round neckline. One of the key features of a bolero jacket is its versatility. It can be worn as a casual or formal garment, depending on the material and the way it is styled. For a formal look, a bolero jacket made from luxurious fabrics such as silk, satin, or velvet can be paired with an evening gown or a cocktail dress. It adds a touch of elegance and sophistication to the outfit while providing some coverage for the shoulders and arms. On the other hand, a bolero jacket made from more casual fabrics like cotton or denim can be worn with jeans, skirts, or dresses for a more relaxed and casual look. It can be a stylish layering piece that adds some warmth and complements the overall outfit. In colder climates, a bolero jacket can also be paired with a turtleneck or a long-sleeved blouse for added warmth. The bolero jacket has become a popular choice for weddings and other formal occasions. It is often worn by brides who want to cover their shoulders or add a layer of modesty to their bridal attire. Bridesmaids, too, can wear bolero jackets to complement their dresses or add a pop of color to the overall wedding theme. In conclusion, the bolero jacket is a versatile and stylish garment that can be worn for both formal and casual occasions. Its cropped length and open front make it a flattering choice for women of all body types. Whether paired with an evening gown or a casual outfit, the bolero jacket adds a touch of sophistication while providing coverage for the shoulders and arms.

Boning Casings

A boning casing in fashion design refers to a narrow strip of fabric or a specialized channel used to encase boning, which is a rigid or semi-rigid material. The process of boning casings involves sewing a fabric tube or channel to hold the boning material in place within a garment or accessory. Boning casings serve several purposes in fashion design. Firstly, they provide structure and support to a garment or accessory, helping to maintain its shape and prevent it from collapsing or sagging. The boning material, which is typically made of plastic, metal, or synthetic materials, adds rigidity and stiffness to specific areas of the garment where additional support is needed, such as the bodice of a corset or the hemline of a full skirt.

Boning Needles

Boning needles are specialized sewing needles commonly used in fashion design for the purpose of inserting boning into garments. Boning refers to the rigid strips, typically made of steel or plastic, that are used to provide structure and support to certain areas of clothing, such as bodices, corsets, and bustiers. These strips are usually placed along the seams or channels of the garment to help maintain its shape and prevent it from sagging or wrinkling. The boning needle is specifically designed to facilitate the insertion of boning into these garments. It is typically longer and thinner than regular sewing needles, with a sharp point and a slightly curved or hooked end. The curved or hooked end allows for easier maneuvering through the fabric and channels, making it simpler to guide the boning into place. When using boning needles, the fabric is first prepared by creating channels or casings where the boning will be inserted. These channels are usually sewn into the seams or along the edges of the garment, using regular sewing needles and threads. Once the channels are in place, the boning needle is threaded with a strong thread or ribbon, and the boning strip is carefully guided through the channels using the curved or hooked end of the needle. Boning needles are available in various sizes and styles, depending on the specific needs of the garment being constructed. Some may have a larger curve or hook, while others may be straight but extra long to accommodate longer boning strips. The choice of needle will depend on factors such as the thickness of the fabric, the size and type of boning being used, and the desired level of precision and control during the insertion process. In conclusion, boning needles are essential tools for fashion designers and garment makers when working with boning. They are specialized needles designed to facilitate the smooth and precise insertion of boning strips into garments, helping to create structured, well-fitted and aesthetically pleasing designs.

Boning For Corsets

Boning for corsets refers to the supporting materials used in the construction of corsets, a garment commonly worn for aesthetic and shaping purposes. The boning is typically made of rigid strips or spiral steel, and is inserted into channels or casings within the corset fabric. It provides structure, shape, and support to the garment, helping to create the desired silhouette and ensure a proper fit. The boning used in corsets can be categorized into two main types: flat boning and spiral boning. Flat boning is typically made of flat steel strips or rigid plastic, and is used in areas that require a higher level of support and shaping, such as the front busk (the central closure of the corset) and the back lacing panels. Spiral boning, on the other hand, is made of coiled steel and is more flexible, allowing for a greater range of movement and comfort. It is typically used along the sides and curves of the corset to provide support and help maintain the desired shape.

Bootcut Jeans

Bootcut jeans are a style of jeans that are designed to fit snugly through the waist and hips and then gradually flare out starting from the knee, creating a subtle balanced silhouette. This style of jeans was originally popularized in the 1960s and 1970s, and has since become a timeless and versatile choice in the world of fashion design. Bootcut jeans are characterized by their slightly wider hem, which allows enough room for the jeans to be worn over boots. This feature not only adds a touch of practicality but also gives the jeans a relaxed and casual feel. The flare of the jeans is typically subtle, complementing various body types without overwhelming the overall look.

Bouclé Jacket

A bouclé jacket is a type of garment that is characterized by its unique texture and design. It is typically made from bouclé fabric, which is a type of fabric that is created using a special weaving technique. The fabric is known for its looped or curled appearance, which gives the jacket its distinctive look. Bouclé jackets are usually tailored and structured, with a close-fitting silhouette that flatters the wearer's body. They are often waist-length or hip-length, and can be worn as either a casual or formal piece depending on the styling and accessories. The jacket's classic design features a collar, lapels, and buttons down the front, although some modern variations may have different closure methods or no closure at all. One of the key characteristics of a bouclé jacket is its texture. The fabric's looped or curled threads create a three-dimensional quality that adds depth and visual interest to the garment. This texture is not only aesthetically pleasing, but also gives the jacket a warm and cozy feel when worn. Bouclé fabric is typically made from a blend of different fibers, such as wool or synthetic materials, which contributes to its softness and warmth. Bouclé jackets are versatile pieces that can be styled in a variety of ways. They can be paired with a skirt or trousers for a polished and professional look, or worn with jeans for a more casual and laid-back outfit. The jacket can be dressed up with accessories such as statement jewelry or a silk scarf, or dressed down with sneakers or flats for a more relaxed vibe. In conclusion, a bouclé jacket is a fashionable and versatile garment that adds texture and style to any outfit. Its unique fabric and tailored design make it a timeless piece that can be worn for various occasions. Whether dressed up or down, a bouclé jacket is a chic and sophisticated choice for fashion-conscious individuals.

Bouffant Dress

A bouffant dress is a type of formal dress characterized by its voluminous, full-bodied skirt. The term "bouffant" is derived from the French word meaning "puffed out" or "inflated." This style of dress originated in the mid-19th century and has since become synonymous with elegance and femininity. The defining feature of a bouffant dress is its exaggerated skirt, which is typically created by layering multiple underskirts or utilizing stiff materials like tulle or crinoline. The skirt is gathered at the waist to create a flattering, cinched-in silhouette while simultaneously creating a dramatic and eye-catching effect. The overall shape of the dress is often compared to that of a bell or a dome, with a wide and flared skirt that adds a sense of grandeur and sophistication to the design. Bouffant dresses are commonly adorned with intricate detailing, such as embroidery, lace, or beading, which further enhances their luxurious and lavish aesthetic. The bodice of the dress is typically more fitted and structured to contrast with the voluminous skirt, creating a balanced and harmonious silhouette. Necklines can vary, ranging from sweetheart to boat necks, but are often designed to showcase the wearer's décolletage and add a touch of femininity to the overall look. Historically, bouffant dresses were popularized during the Victorian era and were often worn for formal occasions and special events. They were favored by women of high social standing and were seen as a symbol of wealth and status. Today, bouffant dresses continue to be worn for formal events, such as weddings, galas, and red carpet appearances. When styling a bouffant dress, it is important to consider the voluminous nature of the skirt. Pairing it with a fitted top or a tailored jacket can help create a balanced and proportionate look. Accessorizing with delicate jewelry and a pair of high-heeled shoes can add a touch of elegance and sophistication to the overall ensemble.

Boyfriend Jeans

Boyfriend jeans are a type of women's denim pants that are designed to have a loose and relaxed fit, inspired by the idea of borrowing a pair of jeans from a boyfriend. This style of jeans typically features a straight or slightly tapered leg, a mid-rise waist, and a slightly slouchy fit throughout the hips and thighs. Boyfriend jeans first gained popularity in the 1980s and 1990s as a part of the grungy, relaxed aesthetic associated with the rise of hip-hop and indie rock. They were often worn oversized and cuffed at the ankles, paired with oversized flannel shirts and combat boots. The style has since evolved to become a staple in many women's wardrobes.

Bra Extenders

A bra extender is a small accessory that is often used in fashion design to provide extra length and flexibility to a bra band. It is made up of a strip of hook-and-eye closures, similar to those found on the back of a bra, that can be attached to the existing hooks on a bra band to extend its length. These extenders are typically made from a soft and stretchable fabric, such as nylon or spandex, which allows them to easily conform to the shape and size of the wearer's body. They come in various widths to accommodate different bra band sizes and are available in a range of colors to match different bra styles.

Bubble Skirt

A bubble skirt is a type of skirt that is characterized by its voluminous and structured shape, resembling a bubble. It is a popular design in the fashion industry that adds a playful and whimsical touch to any outfit. The defining feature of a bubble skirt is its inflated appearance, which is achieved through the clever use of fabric and construction techniques. Typically, the skirt is gathered at the waistline, creating excess fabric that is then allowed to billow out to create the bubble-like effect. The excess fabric is often cleverly manipulated and shaped through the use of pleats, tucks, or ruching, giving the skirt its unique structure.

Bustier Dress

A bustier dress is a type of formal dress that features a structured bodice resembling a bustier. It is typically designed to fit tightly around the upper body, accentuating the waist and creating a flattering silhouette. The bustier itself is a form-fitting garment that extends from the chest to the waist, providing support and shaping to the bust area. It often features boning or other structural elements, such as underwire or padding, to enhance the shape and provide additional support. The bustier dress takes this design and incorporates it into a dress form.

Bustier Top

A bustier top is a garment that is specifically designed to enhance the shape and support of the bust. It is typically made of structured fabrics such as satin, leather, or lace, and is designed to be tightly fitted and contour the upper body. The main distinguishing feature of a bustier top is its boning, which is sewn into the fabric to provide structure and shape. Boning, typically made of flexible materials such as plastic or metal, helps to create a smooth and streamlined silhouette by cinching in the waist and lifting the bust. This creates an hourglass figure and enhances the curves of the wearer. Due to its fitted design, bustier tops are often worn as standalone garments, rather than as a layering piece. They are commonly used in evening wear and special occasions, such as weddings or formal events. However, lighter and more casual versions of bustier tops also exist, which can be styled with jeans, skirts, or shorts for a more relaxed and trendy look. Bustier tops can vary in styles, with some featuring strapless designs, while others may have thin straps or even sleeves. They can also come in various lengths, from cropped styles that end just above the waist, to longer styles that extend to the hips. The neckline of a bustier top can range from straight across, to sweetheart, to plunging, depending on the desired level of coverage and style. In addition to their aesthetic appeal, bustier tops also serve a functional purpose by providing support to the bust. The boning and structured design help to lift and shape the breasts, providing a flattering and supportive fit. Some bustier tops also have padding or underwire for added support and comfort. Overall, a bustier top is a stylish and versatile garment that accentuates the bust and enhances the curves of the wearer. It is a popular choice for formal occasions and can be paired with a variety of bottoms to create a fashionable and alluring look.

Button Attachments

Button attachments refer to the items or materials used to secure buttons to garments in fashion design. They are essential components in the construction of clothing as they provide a functional and decorative element. The process of attaching buttons to garments involves creating small openings or holes in the fabric, often referred to as buttonholes, to allow the button to pass through and fasten the garment together. The button attachment is then used to secure the button in place, ensuring that it remains securely fastened to the fabric.

Button Sewing Machines

Button sewing machines are specialized sewing machines used in the fashion industry for attaching buttons onto garments. They are designed specifically to streamline the button-sewing process, ensuring accuracy, efficiency, and durability in the finished product. Button sewing machines are equipped with various features that make them suitable for fashion design. They typically have a wide range of buttonhole options and stitch patterns to accommodate different button sizes and styles. This versatility allows fashion designers to experiment with various button placements and designs, enhancing the overall aesthetic appeal of their garments.

Buttonhole Cutter

A buttonhole cutter is a small, sharp tool used in fashion design to create precise and clean buttonholes in fabric. It is an essential tool for garment construction, enabling designers and dressmakers to add functional and decorative buttonholes to their creations. The buttonhole cutter typically consists of a small handle attached to a blade. The blade is thin and sharp, allowing for precise cutting without damaging the surrounding fabric. It is typically made from high-quality stainless steel or carbon steel to ensure durability and sharpness over time. To use a buttonhole cutter, the fabric is first prepared by marking the desired location and size of the buttonhole. This can be done with a ruler and chalk or using specialized marking tools such as a tailor's chalk pencil or fabric marker. Once the buttonhole location is marked, the fabric is securely stabilized using pins or basting stitches to prevent shifting during the cutting process. The buttonhole cutter is then carefully positioned at one end of the marked buttonhole, with the blade parallel to the buttonhole's length. The cutter is gently pressed down and guided along the marked line, cutting through the layers of fabric. The sharp blade easily slices through the material, creating a clean and precise buttonhole in a single pass. After the buttonhole is cut, any loose threads or excess fabric are trimmed away using a pair of sharp scissors. The buttonhole can then be reinforced with stitches or bar tacks to ensure longevity and strength.

Additionally, designers may choose to finish the raw edges of the buttonhole with a zigzag stitch or bound them with bias tape for added durability and aesthetic appeal. Overall, the buttonhole cutter is an indispensable tool for fashion designers and dressmakers, enabling them to create professional-quality buttonholes with ease. Its sharp blade and precise cutting action make it a reliable companion in garment construction, ensuring that buttons can be securely fastened on garments while adding a touch of sophistication and attention to detail.

Camp Shirt

A camp shirt is a type of garment designed for both men and women that originated in the early 20th century. Also known as a Cuban collar shirt or bowling shirt, the camp shirt has become a staple in fashion design due to its unique relaxed and casual style. The defining characteristic of a camp shirt is its open, flat collar that is typically notched and does not fold over. This collar style gives the shirt a more informal and vacation-inspired look. The shirt is typically made from lightweight and breathable fabric such as cotton or linen, making it perfect for warm weather and tropical climates. Camp shirts often feature short sleeves, although long-sleeved variations do exist. The fit of a camp shirt is typically loose and relaxed, allowing for freedom of movement. The shirt is traditionally cut straight across the bottom hem, allowing it to be worn untucked. However, modern variations may include a curved or rounded hem for a more contemporary look. One of the distinguishing features of camp shirts is the use of patterned or printed fabrics. Tropical prints, floral motifs, and retro-inspired designs are commonly seen on camp shirts, adding to their laid-back and vacation vibe. These prints often include vibrant colors and bold graphics, making the camp shirt a standout piece in any outfit. The versatility of the camp shirt allows it to be dressed up or down depending on the occasion. It can be paired with tailored trousers or a pencil skirt for a more polished look, or worn with shorts or jeans for a casual and effortless outfit. The relaxed nature of the camp shirt also makes it a popular choice for resort wear and beach attire. In summary, a camp shirt is a loose-fitting, short-sleeved shirt with an open, notched collar. It is made from lightweight fabric and often features patterned or printed designs. The camp shirt's relaxed style and versatility make it a timeless and popular choice in fashion design.

Cape Blazer

A cape blazer is a unique and stylish garment that combines the elements of a cape and a blazer, creating a modern and sophisticated look. It is a versatile piece that can be worn for both formal and casual occasions, adding a touch of elegance to any outfit. The cape blazer typically features a structured silhouette with a cape-like overlay at the back, which adds drama and movement to the garment. The front of the blazer can vary in design, ranging from a classic blazer lapel to a collarless style.

Cape Sweater

A cape sweater is a type of garment that combines the design elements of a cape and a sweater. It is typically made of knit or woven fabric and is designed to be worn on the upper body. The cape sweater features a loose and flowy silhouette, with a cape-like overlay attached to the back or shoulders of the sweater. The overlay can be of various lengths, ranging from just covering the shoulders to extending all the way down to the waist or even longer. It is often designed to drape elegantly over the body, creating a sophisticated and stylish look. The sweater part of the cape sweater is usually fitted, with long sleeves and a crew or V-neckline. It can be made of a variety of materials, such as wool, cashmere, acrylic, or a blend of fibers. The sweater part provides warmth and comfort, making it suitable for cooler weather or indoor environments where a lightweight layer is desired. Cape sweaters can come in a range of designs and styles. Some may have a single-layer cape overlay, while others may feature multiple layers or cascading ruffles for added dimension and visual interest. The cape overlay can also be embellished with decorative details like buttons, fringes, or embroidery to enhance its aesthetic appeal. When it comes to styling, cape sweaters offer versatility. They can be paired with a variety of bottoms, such as jeans, trousers, or skirts, depending on the desired level of formality. They can be worn for both casual and dressy occasions, depending on the design and fabric choice. The cape overlay adds a touch of drama and uniqueness to the overall outfit, making it a statement piece. Overall, the cape sweater is a fashionable and functional garment that combines the comfort of a sweater with the elegance of a cape. Its loose and flowy silhouette, paired with the warmth of the sweater part, makes it a versatile and stylish option for various fashion-forward individuals.

Cape

A cape is a type of garment that is commonly used in fashion design. It is a sleeveless piece of fabric that is open at the front and drapes over the shoulders and back of the wearer. Capes can be made from a variety of fabrics, including wool, silk, and satin, and they can be decorated with embellishments such as buttons, lace, or embroidery. Capes have a long history in fashion and have been worn by both men and women throughout different time periods. In ancient times, capes were often worn as outerwear to provide warmth and protection against the elements. They were typically made from heavy fabrics and were often lined with fur or other insulating materials. In modern fashion, capes are more commonly worn as a stylish and fashionable accessory. They can be worn over other garments, such as dresses or suits, to add a touch of elegance and sophistication to an outfit. Capes can be long or short in length, with some extending all the way to the floor and others ending around the waist or hips. The versatility of capes makes them a popular choice among fashion designers. They can be designed in a variety of styles, ranging from classic and timeless to modern and avant-garde. Capes can be tailored to fit snugly around the shoulders and back, or they can have a more loose and flowing silhouette. The shape and cut of the cape can also vary, with some designs featuring a pointed hemline, while others have a straight or curved edge. Cap Initially used as a functional garment for protection against the elements, the cape has evolved into a fashionable accessory that can elevate any outfit. Whether used to add a layer of warmth or to make a bold style statement, capes are a versatile and timeless addition to any wardrobe.

Capri Pants

Capri pants are a type of women's clothing that originated in the fashion scene during the mid-20th century. Characterized by their cropped length, Capri pants typically extend to the middle of the wearer's lower leg, between the knee and the ankle. They are often designed to be form-fitting and tailored, accentuating the curves of the leg. Capri pants gained popularity in the 1950s and 1960s and have remained a staple in women's fashion ever since. They were named after the Italian island of Capri, a popular vacation destination for the elite during that time. Capri pants quickly became synonymous with a relaxed and sophisticated Mediterranean style, offering a chic alternative to traditional pants or shorts. In terms of design, Capri pants can vary in their waist height, ranging from low-rise to high-rise. Low-rise Capri pants sit below the waistline, creating a casual and laid-back look. High-rise Capri pants, on the other hand, sit at or above the natural waistline, providing a more polished and retro-inspired aesthetic. Capri pants come in a variety of fabrics, including cotton, linen, denim, and synthetic blends. Lightweight and breathable materials are often preferred, as Capri pants are commonly worn during the warmer months. The style can also feature different closures, such as zippers, buttons, or elastic waistbands, offering versatility in terms of fit and comfort. Capri pants can be styled in numerous ways, making them suitable for various occasions. They can be paired with a tucked-in blouse or a fitted top for a more polished look appropriate for the office or a dinner out. For a more casual ensemble, Capri pants can be paired with a simple t-shirt or a flowy blouse. They can be worn with flats, sandals, or heels, depending on the desired level of formality.

Capsule Collection

A capsule collection, in the context of fashion design, refers to a small and carefully curated selection of essential, timeless and versatile pieces that can be mixed and matched to create a variety of outfits. It is a concise and cohesive collection that typically consists of anywhere between 5 to 15 items, focusing on quality rather than quantity. The purpose of a capsule collection is to provide a minimalist wardrobe solution, offering a range of pieces that can easily be combined to create numerous stylish looks suitable for different occasions. By selecting versatile designs, the collection ensures that each item can complement and enhance the others, maximizing the potential for creating various outfits using a limited number of garments.

Cardigan Vest

A cardigan vest is a type of garment that combines features of both a cardigan and a vest. It is typically made from a lightweight and soft fabric, such as wool or cotton, and is characterized by its sleeveless design and button-front closure. The cardigan vest is designed to be a versatile and functional piece of clothing that can be worn as a layering piece or on its own. It is often worn over a shirt or blouse, providing an extra layer of warmth and style. The sleeveless design allows for ease of movement and added comfort.

Cardigan

A cardigan is a type of knitted garment that is typically worn as a layering piece in fashion design. It is characterized by its open front, which allows for easy wearing and removal, and its long sleeves. Cardigans are typically made from various materials, including wool, cotton, or synthetic fabrics. Cardigans can be found in a variety of styles, lengths, and patterns, making them a versatile option for both casual and formal outings. They can be worn buttoned up for a more polished look or left open for a more relaxed and casual vibe. Some cardigans may also feature additional design elements such as pockets, ribbed trims, or decorative buttons.

Cargo Pants

Cargo Shorts

Cargo shorts are a type of knee-length shorts that are designed with multiple large pockets on the sides and sometimes on the back. They are commonly made from durable and lightweight fabrics such as cotton or nylon, making them ideal for outdoor activities and casual wear during warm weather. The design of cargo shorts is influenced by military uniforms, particularly those worn by soldiers in the field. The large pockets are intended to provide extra storage space for various essentials, such as tools, maps, and other personal items. These pockets are usually secured with flaps and buttons, ensuring the safety and accessibility of the items stored inside.

Cargo Skirt

A cargo skirt is a type of skirt that is inspired by the design of cargo pants. It typically features multiple large pockets, similar to those found on cargo pants, which are often placed on the sides or front of the skirt. These pockets serve both a functional and aesthetic purpose, adding visual interest to the skirt while also providing convenient storage space. The cargo skirt is often made from durable and utilitarian fabrics such as cotton twill or canvas, which further emphasizes its military-inspired origins. The use of these fabrics not only adds to the rugged appeal of the skirt but also ensures that it can withstand wear and tear, making it a practical choice for everyday wear.

Carrot Leg Pants

Carrot leg pants are a style of pants that gained popularity in the world of fashion design. These pants are characterized by their unique silhouette, which tapers towards the ankle, creating a shape reminiscent of a carrot. The design of carrot leg pants is defined by their high waist and relaxed fit around the hips, while gradually narrowing down from the thighs to the ankles. Carrot leg pants are known for their versatility, as they can be worn for both casual and formal occasions. They are often made from lightweight and breathable fabrics such as cotton, linen, or blends that ensure comfort and ease of movement. The high waist of these pants accentuates the waistline, giving the wearer a flattering and feminine silhouette. One of the distinguishing features of carrot leg pants is the pleats that are often found at the front. These pleats add volume to the upper part of the pants, creating a structured look that complements the tapering leg. However, not all carrot leg pants include pleats, as the design can vary depending on the designer's preferences and the overall aesthetic of the pants. The length of carrot leg pants typically falls either just above the ankle or slightly below it. This length allows for various styling options, as the pants can be paired with different types of footwear, from heels to sneakers. The tapered leg creates a slimming effect, making carrot leg pants suitable for a wide range of body types. Carrot leg pants are often worn with tucked-in tops or cropped styles to emphasize the high waist and highlight the unique shape of the pants. They can be styled with blouses, shirts, or even relaxed t-shirts, depending on the desired level of formality. Complete the look with accessories such as belts or statement jewelry to add a personal touch. In conclusion, carrot leg pants are a fashionable and versatile choice in the world of fashion design. Their tapered silhouette, high waist, and unique shape make them a stylish option for both casual and formal occasions. With various styling possibilities, carrot leg pants offer a flattering and fashionable look for individuals wishing to make a statement with their wardrobe.

Carrot Pants

Carrot Pants: Carrot pants, also known as carrot-leg pants, are a style of pants that gained popularity in the 1980s and have remained a staple in fashion since then. The term "carrot" refers to the shape of the pants, which resemble the silhouette of a carrot, with a narrow waist and slightly tapered legs that widen towards the hips. The distinguishing feature of carrot pants is their high waist, which typically sits above the natural waistline, accentuating the waist and creating a flattering hourglass shape. This high-waisted design also allows the pants to be worn with cropped tops or tucked-in blouses, helping to elongate the legs and create a polished, put-together look. Carrot pants often feature pleats or gathers at the waist, which add volume and create a draped effect around the hips. These design details contribute to the pants' relaxed and slightly slouchy fit, making them comfortable for all-day wear. The tapering towards the ankles gives the pants a tailored and sophisticated appearance, making them suitable for both casual and formal occasions. Carrot pants are typically made from lightweight and breathable materials such as cotton or linen, making them perfect for warmer weather. They can come in various lengths, ranging from ankle-length to cropped, allowing for versatility in styling. Carrot pants can be paired with heels for a dressier look or worn with sneakers or flats for a more casual and relaxed outfit. Overall, carrot pants are a stylish and versatile choice for fashion-forward individuals. Their unique shape and high-waisted design make them flattering for different body types, while their comfort and versatility make them a practical option for everyday wear. Whether worn to the office, a social event, or a casual day out, carrot pants can effortlessly elevate any outfit and showcase one's fashion sense and individual style.

Cascade Cardigan

A cascade cardigan, in the context of fashion design, refers to a type of cardigan that features a cascading front, creating a draped effect. It is typically characterized by its loose, open-front silhouette and the way it falls gracefully on the body. The cascade cardigan is known for its versatility and ability to effortlessly enhance any outfit. It can be worn as a lightweight outerwear option or as a layering piece during colder months. The open-front design allows for easy layering over various tops, such as camisoles, t-shirts, or blouses, adding a touch of style and sophistication to any ensemble.

Casting Director

A casting director in the context of fashion design is an individual or a team responsible for selecting models for fashion shows, photo shoots, and other fashion-related events. The casting director plays a vital role in the fashion industry, as they are responsible for finding the right models who will effectively showcase the designer's vision. The primary duty of a casting director is to match the requirements and aesthetic of the fashion designer with the appropriate models. They carefully analyze the designer's clothing line, the theme of the collection, and the desired overall look to ensure that the models chosen complement the brand's identity. When selecting models, casting directors consider various factors, such as height, body proportions, facial features, and individual style. They aim to find models who can bring the designer's creations to life and create a cohesive and visually appealing presentation. Additionally, casting directors also consider diversity and inclusivity, striving to represent a wide range of ethnicities, body types, and ages to reflect the diverse world we live in. Another crucial aspect of a casting director's job is to manage model agencies and scouts. They maintain relationships with these entities and rely on their extensive knowledge of models to find the best potential candidates. Casting directors attend model auditions or go-see events, where they assess models' runway walks, expressions, and poses to determine their suitability for specific fashion projects. Communication is a key skill required for a casting director, as they liaise between the fashion designer and the models. They provide guidance to the models during fittings, ensuring that the garments fit properly and that the models understand the desired style and mood. Casting directors also collaborate with hair stylists, makeup artists, and stylists to create a harmonious overall look for the fashion event. In conclusion, a casting director in fashion design is responsible for selecting models who can effectively showcase a designer's vision. They consider various factors, such as body proportions, facial features, and individual style, while also promoting diversity and inclusivity. A casting director manages relationships with model agencies and scouts, attends auditions, and communicates with both the fashion designer and the models to ensure a successful and visually appealing fashion event.

Catsuit

A catsuit is a one-piece garment that covers the torso, legs, and sometimes arms, typically made of stretchy material such as spandex or latex. It is a popular choice in fashion design for its sleek and form-fitting silhouette. The catsuit is often associated with its iconic design, featuring a high neckline and long sleeves, with the legs extending all the way to the ankles. This full-body coverage accentuates the body's curves, creating a visually appealing and sensual look. The primary purpose of a catsuit in fashion design is to provide a form-fitting and second-skin-like attire that flatters the wearer's figure. The stretchy material used allows for ease of movement and a comfortable fit. The close contact of the fabric against the skin highlights the natural contours of the body, making it a preferred choice for those looking to show off their physique. Catsuits are versatile garments that can be styled in various ways to suit different fashion preferences and occasions. They can be worn as standalone outfits, paired with accessories, or layered with other clothing pieces. The simple yet striking design of the catsuit lends itself well to customization and experimentation, making it a favorite among fashion enthusiasts and designers. In recent years, catsuits have gained popularity beyond the realm of fashion design and have become a staple in performance and entertainment sectors. They are commonly seen in dance performances, stage productions, and even superhero costumes. The sleek and figure-hugging nature of catsuits lends itself well to visually compelling performances, allowing for fluid movements and visually stunning displays on stage or screen. Overall, the catsuit is a versatile and stylish garment in fashion design that offers a form-fitting and flattering silhouette. Its sleek design, comfortable fit, and wide range of styling possibilities make it a popular choice for those looking to make a statement or showcase their physique in a unique and fashionable way.

Chalk Erasers

A chalk eraser is a small, handheld tool used in the field of fashion design to remove marks made by chalk on fabric or other materials. It is typically made of a rectangular or cylindrical block of soft, porous material, such as felt or foam, that is compressed to create a firm yet flexible surface. When fashion designers are working with fabric, they often use chalk to make temporary marks for various purposes. These marks can include guidelines for cutting, sewing, or pleating, as well as notes or symbols to indicate specific instructions or measurements. However, these marks are meant to be temporary and need to be removed before the fabric is used or worn. Chalk erasers are designed specifically for this purpose. The soft and porous material of the eraser allows it to absorb and lift the chalk marks from the fabric without causing any damage or leaving behind any residue. The firm but flexible surface ensures that the eraser can easily glide over the fabric, effectively erasing the marks without smudging or smearing them. The size and shape of chalk erasers can vary depending on the specific needs and preferences of the fashion designer. Some erasers may be larger and more rectangular in shape, allowing for a wider coverage area and easier handling. Others may be smaller and cylindrical, providing more precision and control when erasing delicate or intricate markings. Chalk erasers are an essential tool in the fashion design process as they enable designers to work with precision and accuracy. By using these erasers, designers can easily remove temporary chalk marks without causing any harm to the fabric. This allows them to create garments and accessories with clean, professional finishes.

Chalk Sharpeners

A chalk sharpener, in the context of fashion design, is a small tool used to sharpen tailor's chalk. It is specifically designed to create a fine and precise point on the chalk, allowing fashion designers and garment makers to accurately mark fabric during the garment construction process. The purpose of using tailor's chalk in fashion design is to temporarily mark fabric for various purposes, such as indicating pattern markings, making alterations, or highlighting design details. Tailor's chalk is preferred over other marking tools because it can easily be brushed or washed off without leaving a permanent stain on the fabric.

Chalk Wheels

Chalk wheels, in the context of fashion design, refer to a tool used to mark fabrics during the pattern-making and cutting process. They are primarily used to create temporary markings for precise measurements and cutting lines on various types of fabrics. The chalk wheel consists of a small, cylindrical device made of plastic or metal, which is filled with chalk powder. The wheel itself has a serrated edge that rotates as it is rolled over the fabric, leaving behind a fine line of chalk. This line serves as a guide for the designer or pattern maker when cutting or sewing the fabric. Chalk wheels are an essential tool for ensuring accuracy and precision in garment construction. Chalk wheels are available in different colors, allowing designers to differentiate between different types of markings on a fabric. Some common colors include white, pink, blue, and yellow. The choice of color usually depends on the fabric color and contrast required for visibility. For example, a white chalk wheel is often preferred on dark fabrics, while a pink or blue chalk may be more visible on light-colored fabrics. When using a chalk wheel, it is important to ensure the fabric is properly positioned and taut to prevent any distortion or misalignment of the markings. The wheel should be rolled smoothly and evenly to create a uniform and straight line. If a mistake is made, the chalk marks can be easily removed by brushing or wiping them off with a damp cloth, making it a forgiving and versatile tool. In addition to marking cutting lines, chalk wheels are also useful for indicating other design details such as darts, pleats, notches, and pattern symbols on the fabric. This helps in accurately translating the design from paper to fabric, ensuring all the necessary elements are accurately represented. In conclusion, chalk wheels are an indispensable tool in fashion design for creating temporary markings on fabrics. They enable designers and pattern makers to achieve accuracy, precision, and consistency in the pattern-making and cutting process, resulting in well-fitting and visually appealing garments.

Chemise Dress

A chemise dress is a type of dress that is inspired by the classic chemise undergarment. It typically features a loose and flowing silhouette, often with a straight or A-line shape. The dress is designed to hang loosely on the body, providing a comfortable and relaxed fit. Traditionally, chemise dresses were made from lightweight and breathable fabrics such as cotton or linen, which added to their comfort and ease of wear. However, modern variations of chemise dresses can also be found in a variety of other materials, including silk, chiffon, and polyester. One of the defining features of a chemise dress is its simplicity. Unlike more structured dresses, chemise dresses are typically devoid of intricate details or embellishments. Instead, they rely on the inherent elegance of their minimalist design. This simplicity allows for easy styling and versatility, making chemise dresses suitable for a wide range of occasions. Chemise dresses are known for their relaxed and effortless aesthetic. They are often characterized by loose and billowy sleeves, a low neckline, and a straight or slightly flared silhouette that skims over the body without clinging. Some variations of chemise dresses may also feature smocking or gathering details around the neckline or waist, adding subtle visual interest. The length of a chemise dress can vary, ranging from mini to midi and even maxi lengths. Mini chemise dresses are often popular for more casual settings, while midi or maxi lengths can be appropriate for dressier occasions. The choice of length can also contribute to the overall vibe of the dress, with shorter lengths evoking a more youthful and playful look, and longer lengths exuding elegance and sophistication.

Cigarette Pants

Cigarette pants, also known as slim-fit pants or pencil pants, are a popular style of trousers that are characterized by their narrow and straight cut. These pants are designed to fit closely to the leg, creating a slim and elongated silhouette. Originally popularized in the 1950s by prominent fashion icons such as Audrey Hepburn, cigarette pants have since become a timeless wardrobe staple for both men and women. They are commonly worn in formal and semi-formal settings, as they exude a polished and sophisticated look.

Circle Skirt

A circle skirt is a type of skirt that is characterized by its circular shape and fullness. It is a popular design in fashion due to its feminine and flattering silhouette. The skirt is typically constructed from a single circular piece of fabric, with a hole in the center for the waistband. The length of the circle skirt can vary, ranging from mini to midi to maxi lengths. The waistband is usually fitted and sits at the natural waist, accentuating the waistline and creating an hourglass figure. The skirt then flares out from the waist, creating a flowing and voluminous shape. Circle skirts can be made from a variety of fabrics, including lightweight cotton, flowing chiffon, or even structured denim. The fabric choice will determine the drape and movement of the skirt. A lightweight fabric will create a softer and more fluid look, while a stiffer fabric will add structure and volume to the skirt. The circular shape of the skirt allows for ease of movement and a graceful flow when walking or dancing. The fullness of the skirt gives it a romantic and retro feel, reminiscent of the 1950s fashion era. It is a versatile piece that can be dressed up or down, depending on the occasion. Circle skirts can be styled in many ways, making them a versatile addition to any wardrobe. They can be paired with a fitted blouse for a feminine and polished look, or with a casual t-shirt for a more relaxed and effortless vibe. They can also be layered with a cardigan or jacket for added warmth and style. Overall, a circle skirt is a classic and timeless design in fashion. Its circular shape, fullness, and flattering silhouette make it a popular choice for women of all ages and body types. Whether worn for a special occasion or as an everyday staple, the circle skirt is a versatile and feminine piece that will never go out of style.

Coatdress

A coatdress is a garment that combines the elements of a coat and a dress, creating a unique and versatile piece of clothing. It is typically designed with a tailored and structured silhouette that flatters the figure while providing warmth and modesty. The coatdress incorporates the length and coverage of a coat, often reaching below the knee or even ankle-length, with the design details and style of a dress. The coatdress can be made from a variety of fabrics, including wool, tweed, or even satin, depending on the desired level of formality and occasion. It often features a button or snap closure in the front, extending from the neckline to the hem, allowing for easy wear and removal. The collar of a coatdress can vary, ranging from classic lapels to high necklines, adding a touch of elegance and sophistication. This unique garment is highly versatile and can be styled in various ways to suit different occasions. It can be worn as a standalone piece, paired with heels or boots for a polished and refined look. Alternatively, it can be layered over a blouse or dress, offering warmth and style during colder seasons. The coatdress can also be cinched at the waist with a belt to accentuate the shape and create a more tailored silhouette. Coatdresses are popular choices for formal and semi-formal events, such as weddings, cocktail parties, or business meetings, due to their elegant and sophisticated design. They provide an alternative to traditional coats or jackets, offering a more feminine and glamorous option. The versatility of the coatdress allows it to be dressed up or down, depending on the occasion. In conclusion, a coatdress is a unique garment that combines the elements of a coat and a dress, creating a versatile and stylish option for formal and semi-formal events. Its tailored silhouette, flattering design, and various styling possibilities make it a popular choice among fashion enthusiasts.

Color Matching Tools

The term "color matching tools" refers to a set of resources and techniques used in the field of fashion design to identify and choose an appropriate combination of colors for a particular garment or collection. These tools are essential in creating harmonious and visually appealing designs, as colors have a profound impact on the overall aesthetics and message of a fashion piece. Color matching tools typically consist of various methods and instruments that assist designers in selecting and coordinating colors. One commonly used tool is a color wheel, which is a circular diagram that displays the primary, secondary, and tertiary colors, as well as their relationships and harmonies. Designers can refer to the color wheel to determine which colors work well together and create visually pleasing combinations. For example, complementary colors, which are located opposite each other on the color wheel, often produce a vibrant and striking contrast when used together. In addition to the color wheel, designers may also utilize color swatch books or fabric samples. These books contain small, standardized pieces of fabric in a wide range of colors, allowing designers to physically compare and match different shades. By placing swatches side by side, designers can evaluate how colors interact with one another and ensure that they achieve the desired balance and unity within the design. With the advancement of technology, fashion designers now have access to digital color matching tools. These software programs or applications allow designers to experiment with different color combinations virtually. They provide a wide range of color options and allow designers to easily manipulate and customize hues, saturation, and brightness levels. Digital color matching tools save designers time and effort by providing quick and accurate color matching suggestions. Overall, color matching tools play a crucial role in the fashion design process, enabling designers to create visually appealing and harmonious color palettes. Whether it be through traditional color wheels and swatch books or digital software programs, these tools assist designers in making informed decisions about color, ultimately enhancing the overall aesthetics and impact of fashion designs.

Column Dress

A column dress is a type of formal dress that features a sleek and straight silhouette from the neckline down to the hemline. It is designed to closely follow the natural shape of the body without any added volume or excessive embellishments. With its clean lines and minimalistic design, the column dress exudes an elegant and sophisticated look. It is typically made from luxurious fabrics such as silk, satin, or chiffon, which contributes to its refined and polished appearance.

Corset Top

A corset top is a type of garment that is designed to resemble a corset, which is a fitted undergarment that extends from the bust to the waist. In fashion design, a corset top is typically made from a combination of fabrics, including a strong, boned material like steel or plastic and a softer, more flexible fabric like silk or cotton. The main purpose of a corset top is to accentuate the bust and waist, creating a desired hourglass figure. It is constructed with reinforced boning, which helps to shape and support the upper body. The boning is typically strategically placed along the front, sides, and back of the corset top to provide structure and control. This allows the garment to cinch in the waist and lift the bust, emphasizing the natural curves of the body. Corset tops can vary in style, ranging from traditional Victorian-inspired designs to more contemporary and avant-garde creations. They often feature lace-up closures at the back or front, allowing for adjustable sizing and a personalized fit. The closure is typically secured with a series of eyelets and laces, which can be tightened or loosened to achieve the desired level of compression. Corset tops can be worn as standalone tops or layered with other garments, depending on the desired look. They are commonly paired with high-waisted skirts or pants to highlight the waistline. Additionally, corset tops can be incorporated into various fashion styles, including gothic, steampunk, and vintage-inspired ensembles. While corset tops can be visually striking and fashionable, it is important to note that they can also be restrictive and uncomfortable when worn for extended periods. Therefore, it is essential to consider comfort and mobility when designing and wearing a corset top. Designers often incorporate features like adjustable straps, breathable fabrics, and modern boning materials to enhance both the comfort and aesthetic appeal of corset tops.

Costume Design

Costume design in the context of fashion design refers to the process of creating and visualizing clothing and accessories for theatrical productions, films, television shows, and other performances. It is the art of designing and crafting garments that not only reflect the characters and the time period of the production but also enhance the storytelling and convey the mood and emotions of the narrative. The costume designer, often in collaboration with the director and other members of the production team, begins by immersing themselves in the script or the story. They analyze the characters, their backgrounds, personality traits, and relationships to ensure that the costumes accurately represent their individuality and contribute to the overall narrative arc. Research plays a crucial role in the costume design process. The designer studies historical periods, cultural references, and trends relevant to the production to create authentic and believable costumes. They may also draw inspiration from various sources such as art, literature, and fashion history to bring a unique and creative perspective to the costumes. Once the conceptualization phase is complete, the designer moves on to the practical aspects of costume design, which include sketching the initial ideas, selecting fabrics, and creating patterns. They consider factors like color, texture, and silhouette to ensure that the costumes enhance the actors' performances and allow for easy movement on stage or on camera. Costume fittings and alterations are another essential part of the process. The designer works closely with the performers to ensure the costumes fit properly, are comfortable to wear, and allow for necessary adjustments during the performances. Accessories like hats, shoes, and jewelry are also carefully chosen to complement the overall look and add finishing touches to the costumes. Throughout the production stage, the costume designer collaborates with other members of the production team, such as set designers, lighting designers, and makeup artists, to ensure a cohesive visual aesthetic. They coordinate with the wardrobe department to manage the costumes' construction, maintenance, and changes throughout the performances. In conclusion, costume design is a crucial aspect of fashion design that involves creating and visualizing garments and accessories for performances. It requires a combination of artistic creativity, research, and practical skills to bring characters and narratives to life through clothing.

Costume Jewelry

Costume jewelry, also known as fashion jewelry or imitation jewelry, refers to decorative accessories that are made from inexpensive, non-precious materials. Unlike fine jewelry, which is typically crafted from precious metals and gemstones, costume jewelry is designed to be affordable and accessible to a wider range of consumers. Costume jewelry can include a wide variety of items, such as necklaces, bracelets, earrings, rings, brooches, and hair accessories. These pieces are often made from materials like base metals, plastic, glass, wood, or even fabric. While they may not be made from precious metals like gold or silver, costume jewelry can still be creatively designed and stylish, allowing individuals to express their personal style without breaking the bank.

Couture Techniques

Couture Techniques refer to the specialized skills and methods used in high-end fashion design to create garments of exceptional quality and craftsmanship. These techniques involve meticulous attention to detail, precision sewing, and the use of luxurious and often rare materials. Couture garments are typically created by highly skilled artisans, such as couturiers and seamstresses, who possess advanced knowledge and expertise in garment construction. One of the key aspects of couture techniques is the emphasis on handwork. Unlike mass-produced garments, couture pieces are predominantly hand-sewn, allowing for a level of precision and customization that is not achievable through machine sewing alone. This hand-stitching ensures that each seam, dart, and pleat is perfectly executed, resulting in a garment with impeccable fit and structure. Another hallmark of couture techniques is the use of intricate embellishments and embroidery. Couturiers skillfully incorporate techniques such as beading, featherwork, and lace appliqué to add a unique, ornamental touch to their creations. These embellishments are often painstakingly applied by hand, further showcasing the artisan's skill and attention to detail. In addition to handwork and embellishments, couture techniques also involve advanced pattern making and draping skills. Couturiers are trained in creating custom patterns that accurately capture the client's measurements and desired fit. They are also adept at draping fabric directly on the dress form, allowing for precise and sculptural garment construction. Overall, couture techniques represent the pinnacle of craftsmanship in fashion design. They require exceptional skill, patience, and attention to detail to create garments that are not only visually stunning but also of the highest quality. Through the use of handwork, embellishments, and advanced pattern making, couturiers are able to transform fabrics into works of art that are unique, luxurious, and truly one-of-a-kind.

Couturier

A couturier is a highly skilled fashion designer who creates custom-made garments for individual clients. The term "couturier" is derived from the French word "couture," which means "dressmaking" or "sewing." In the world of fashion design, a couturier is recognized for their expertise in creating exquisite and unique clothing pieces that are tailored to fit the client's specific measurements and preferences. A couturier is known for their attention to detail, precision, and ability to bring a client's vision to life through their designs. They possess an extensive knowledge of textiles, garment construction techniques, and fashion trends, which allows them to create high-quality and luxurious pieces. Couturiers often work closely with clients to understand their personal style, body shape, and occasion for which the garment is intended. They use this information to design and craft one-of-a-kind garments that not only complement the client's individuality but also enhance their confidence and self-expression. Unlike ready-to-wear fashion designers who produce clothing in standard sizes for mass production, couturiers prioritize the art of bespoke tailoring. Every garment created by a couturier is meticulously handcrafted, using premium materials and techniques that are time-consuming and require exceptional skills. Couturiers may also incorporate elements of hand embroidery, lacework, or beadwork into their creations, elevating the garments to wearable works of art. Due to the exclusive nature of their craft, couturiers primarily serve a niche clientele who appreciate the exceptional craftsmanship and exclusivity offered by custom-made clothing. The garments created by couturiers are known for their superior fit, ultimate comfort, and impeccable finish. They are worn for special occasions such as weddings, red carpet events, or any event where the wearer desires a unique and exceptional ensemble that reflects their style and personality. In the fashion industry, the title of "couturier" is highly esteemed and reserved for designers who have established themselves as masters of their craft. The couturier's signature style and meticulous attention to detail set them apart from other designers, contributing to their legacy and recognition in the world of fashion.

Cowl-Neck Top

A cowl-neck top is a type of clothing item in fashion design characterized by its unique neckline. The cowl-neck top features a loose and draped neckline that creates a soft, elegant, and feminine look. The neckline is typically created by folding over a generous amount of fabric, creating a draped effect that falls gracefully from the shoulders to the chest area. This draped fabric forms a gentle cowl shape, hence the name of the garment. Due to its distinct neckline, the cowl-neck top offers a unique and stylish alternative to traditional necklines such as crew necks, V-necks, or boat necks. The draped fabric adds volume and texture to the garment, enhancing its visual appeal and giving it a sophisticated touch. Cowl-neck tops are versatile and can be found in a variety of styles, fabrics, and lengths. They can be sleeveless, short-sleeved, or long-sleeved, allowing for different options depending on the season or occasion. The length of the top can range from cropped styles to longer tunic-length options, catering to various preferences and body types. This type of top can be worn in both casual and formal settings, depending on the fabric and design details. Lighter fabrics such as chiffon or cotton are more suitable for casual occasions, while silk or satin materials can lend an air of sophistication, making them suitable for more formal events. The cowl-neck top can be easily paired with skirts, pants, or jeans, making it a versatile and fashion-forward choice.

Crewneck Sweater

A crewneck sweater is a type of knitwear that is characterized by its round neckline and long sleeves. It is a popular and versatile garment in the fashion industry, particularly in the autumn and winter seasons. The crewneck sweater was originally inspired by the traditional uniform worn by rowers in the early 20th century. Its round neckline was designed to provide comfort and ease of movement, while its long sleeves offered warmth during cold weather. Over time, the crewneck sweater has evolved and become a staple in both men's and women's wardrobes.

Crochet Hooks

Crochet hooks are essential tools in fashion design that are used to create intricate and delicate designs using the crochet technique. These hooks are specifically designed with a long shaft and a hook at one end to facilitate the process of interlocking loops of yarn or thread to create decorative and textural patterns. The crochet technique is widely used in fashion design to add intricate details, patterns, and embellishments to garments, accessories, and even footwear. It involves creating a series of interconnected loops using the crochet hook to form fabrics or designs that can range from simple to complex, depending on the desired effect.

Crop Top

A crop top is a type of garment that is designed to expose the midriff, typically ending just above or below the navel. It is often made from lightweight fabrics such as cotton or jersey and is popularly worn by women as a stylish and fashionable option. The crop top first gained popularity in the 1940s as a practical garment for women participating in sports activities. It provided freedom of movement and allowed for better ventilation during physical activities. However, it wasn't until the 1960s and 1970s that the crop top began to be embraced as a fashion statement.

Cropped Blazer

A cropped blazer is a type of jacket that is characterized by its shorter length, typically ending above the waistline. It is a versatile and stylish garment that is often worn as a fashionable outerwear piece or as part of a tailored suit ensemble. The cropped blazer is designed to be more fitted and tailored in comparison to traditional blazers, which typically have a longer length that falls at or below the hips. This shorter length gives the cropped blazer a more modern and youthful appearance. One of the key features of a cropped blazer is its silhouette. It is typically more structured and streamlined, with a slightly tapered waist and a defined shoulder line. This creates a flattering and polished look that can enhance the overall shape of the wearer. Cropped blazers come in a variety of styles, fabrics, and colors to suit different fashion preferences and occasions. They can be made from materials such as wool, tweed, linen, or even leather, which can give the blazer a more edgy and contemporary vibe. One of the most popular ways to wear a cropped blazer is to pair it with high-waisted bottoms, such as skirts, trousers, or jeans. This combination creates a balanced and proportionate look, as the shorter length of the blazer highlights the waist and elongates the legs. In addition to its fashion-forward style, the cropped blazer also offers practicality and versatility. It can be worn in both formal and casual settings, making it a go-to choice for various occasions. Whether it's for a business meeting, a social event, or a night out, the cropped blazer adds a touch of sophistication and chicness to any outfit. Overall, the cropped blazer is a fashion staple that combines style and functionality. Its shorter length, structured silhouette, and diverse range of fabrics make it a versatile piece that can elevate any look.

Cropped Flare Pants

Cropped flare pants are a type of trousers that are characterized by their wide and flared silhouette, which starts to flare out below the knee and continues to widen towards the hem. These pants are designed to have a cropped length, typically hitting above the ankle but below the calf, hence the term "cropped" flare pants. The flare in cropped flare pants refers to the exaggerated width of the pant legs, which creates a bell-like or trumpet-like shape. This flared shape adds volume and movement to the pants, giving them a distinct and eye-catching aesthetic. The flared silhouette also creates a balancing effect, as it visually offsets the width of the hips and thighs, creating a more proportionate and elongated silhouette. Cropped flare pants can be made from a wide range of fabrics, including denim, cotton, linen, or even more luxurious materials like silk or velvet. They can be designed to have a high-rise, mid-rise, or low-rise waist, depending on the desired style and fit. The waistband of these pants can feature various closure options, such as buttons, zippers, or hooks. These pants are versatile and can be styled in different ways to suit various occasions and personal preferences. They can be dressed up or down, depending on the choice of accompanying garments and accessories. For a casual daytime look, cropped flare pants can be paired with a simple t-shirt or blouse and sandals or sneakers. For a more formal or evening look, they can be paired with a stylish blouse or blazer and heels. The popularity of cropped flare pants has surged in recent years, as they offer an alternative to the traditional straight or skinny trousers. They have become a staple in many women's wardrobes, offering a fashionable and flattering option for those who want to add some flair to their outfits while maintaining comfort and style.

Cropped Jeans

Cropped jeans refers to a style of jeans that are tailored to end above the ankle, often with a raw or frayed hem. This design creates a shorter length compared to traditional full-length jeans. Cropped jeans are crafted to fit snugly around the waist and hips, while tapering down the leg and ending just at or slightly above the ankle. They are typically made from denim fabric, but can also be found in other materials such as cotton or twill. The cropped length of these jeans allows for a more contemporary and relaxed look. It is a versatile style that can be dressed up or down, depending on the occasion. Cropped jeans are a popular choice for warmer seasons, as they provide a breezy and lightweight feel, making them suitable for casual and outdoor activities. They are also a go-to option for those who want to show off their footwear, as the shorter length allows shoes to be more prominently displayed.

Cropped Sweater

A cropped sweater is a type of garment designed for the upper body that has a shortened length, typically ending above the waistline or hips. The main purpose of a cropped sweater is to provide a stylish and trendy option for layering or wearing on its own, particularly in the context of fashion design. This type of sweater typically features a fitted or slightly relaxed silhouette and is often made from a variety of fabric materials such as cotton, wool, or synthetic blends. The cropped length allows for versatile styling options, as it can be paired with high-waisted bottoms like jeans, skirts, or trousers to create a fashionable and balanced look.

Culotte Jumpsuit

A culotte jumpsuit is a fashionable garment that combines the style of culottes with the convenience and versatility of a jumpsuit. Culottes are wide-legged pants that resemble a skirt or a divided skirt, while jumpsuits are one-piece garments that combine a top and pants in one. The fusion of these two styles creates a unique and contemporary fashion piece that is both stylish and practical. The culotte jumpsuit is known for its wide and flowing legs, which allow for ease of movement and a relaxed, comfortable fit. The legs typically end at or below the knee, creating a wide and airy silhouette. This design element adds a touch of femininity and elegance to the overall look of the jumpsuit.

Culottes

Culottes, in the context of fashion design, refer to a specific type of women's trousers that are cut to resemble a skirt. This garment typically falls below the knee or mid-calf length, and is characterized by its wide-legged silhouette. Culottes are known for their unique combination of comfort and style, making them a popular choice among fashion enthusiasts. Originally developed in the late 19th century as a practical alternative to the restrictive clothing worn by women at the time, culottes have since evolved into a versatile fashion statement. They are often crafted from lightweight, flowing fabrics such as linen, cotton, or silk, allowing for ease of movement and breathability. One of the defining features of culottes is their wide leg openings, which create the illusion of a skirt when the wearer is in motion. This design element adds a touch of femininity and elegance to the overall look. Culottes also typically feature a high waist, which helps to elongate the legs and accentuate the waistline. When it comes to styling culottes, there are countless possibilities. They can be dressed up or down, depending on the occasion. For a polished and sophisticated look, culottes can be paired with a tailored blazer and a fitted blouse. This combination is perfect for professional settings or formal events. For a more casual and relaxed ensemble, culottes can be teamed with a loose-fitting t-shirt or a cropped top. Adding a pair of sneakers or sandals can further enhance the laid-back vibe. Culottes can also be worn with heels or wedges for a chic and elevated look. Overall, culottes play a significant role in contemporary fashion design. They offer a practical and stylish alternative to skirts and trousers, effortlessly combining comfort and elegance. Whether worn to the office, a social gathering, or a casual outing, culottes are a versatile wardrobe staple that allow individuals to express their personal style while staying comfortable and chic.

Cultural Exchange In Fashion

Cultural Exchange in Fashion refers to the process of sharing and incorporating elements of different cultures into the design and production of clothing and accessories. It involves the dissemination and adoption of traditional clothing, textiles, symbols, techniques, and aesthetics from one culture to another. The concept of Cultural Exchange in Fashion is rooted in the recognition that fashion is not limited to a single culture or geographic location. It acknowledges that fashion is a dynamic and ever-evolving expression of identity and creativity, influenced by various cultural, historical, social, and economic factors. Cultural Exchange in Fashion promotes the cross-pollination of ideas, styles, and techniques, resulting in the creation of unique and diverse fashion designs.

Cutoff Shorts

Cutoff shorts, also known as denim shorts or jean shorts, are a type of garment that is characterized by its shortened length. These shorts are typically made from denim fabric, which is known for its durability and versatility. Cutoff shorts feature a straight or slightly tapered leg, with the hemline cut off above the knee. The edges of the cutoff shorts are often left frayed or distressed for a more casual and worn-in look. The cutoff style is achieved by cutting off the legs of a pair of jeans or shorts, either by the wearer or by the manufacturer.

Cutout Bodysuit

A cutout bodysuit is a form-fitting garment designed to cover the torso and legs, similar to a one-piece swimsuit. What sets it apart is the presence of strategically placed cutouts or openings on the fabric. These cutouts can vary in shape, size, and location, adding a touch of uniqueness and edginess to the overall design. Cutout bodysuits are popular in the fashion industry as they combine the comfort and versatility of a bodysuit with the daring and sensual appeal of exposed skin. The cutouts are strategically placed to reveal specific parts of the body, such as the midriff, sides, back, or neckline, while still maintaining a certain level of coverage. Designers often use various techniques to create the cutouts, including laser cutting, slashing, or creating intricate patterns. This allows for a wide range of design possibilities, whether it's a single, large cutout or multiple smaller ones. The placement of the cutouts can also be customized to flatter specific body shapes or draw attention to certain areas. Cutout bodysuits can be made from different materials, such as stretchy spandex, lycra, or other synthetic fabrics that provide a snug and comfortable fit. The choice of fabric can greatly influence the overall look and feel of the garment, from a more athletic and sporty appearance to a sultry and elegant vibe. These bodysuits are often worn as standalone pieces, paired with high-waisted bottoms, skirts, or pants. They can be styled for both casual occasions or dressed up for more formal events, depending on the design and accompanying accessories. The versatility of cutout bodysuits makes them a popular choice among fashion enthusiasts, allowing for endless possibilities in creating unique and personalized outfits. In conclusion, a cutout bodysuit is a fashion garment that combines the figure-hugging fit of a bodysuit with strategically placed cutouts to expose specific areas of the body. They come in various shapes, sizes, and designs, offering a stylish and daring option for both casual and formal wear.

Cutting Mats

A cutting mat, in the context of fashion design, refers to a specialized tool or surface used for cutting fabric, patterns, and other materials during the garment construction process. Made from a durable, self-healing material such as PVC or high-density polyethylene, cutting mats provide a smooth, non-slip surface that protects the underlying work surface while ensuring clean and accurate cuts. Cutting mats are an essential element in the fashion designer's toolkit as they offer various benefits. Firstly, they provide a protective layer for the work surface, be it a table or a cutting table. The self-healing nature of the mat ensures that any cuts or incisions made on its surface close up, preventing permanent damage. This not only prolongs the lifespan of the mat but also protects the underlying work surface from scratches, nicks, and marks caused by cutting tools such as rotary cutters or scissors. Additionally, cutting mats are designed with measurements and grid lines that aid in precise and consistent cutting. These grids are typically marked in both inches and centimeters, allowing fashion designers to accurately measure and cut fabrics according to their designs. The grids not only provide a guide for cutting straight lines but also assist in measuring and aligning patterns, ensuring symmetry and accuracy in the final garment construction. The non-slip nature of cutting mats is another valuable feature, particularly when working with slippery or delicate fabrics. By preventing shifting or sliding, cutting mats provide stability and control during the cutting process, enabling fashion designers to achieve clean and precise cuts. This is especially important when working with intricate designs or complex patterns that require careful attention to detail. In conclusion, a cutting mat is an indispensable tool for fashion designers as it offers protection, precision, and stability during the fabric cutting process. By providing a durable and self-healing surface with measurements and grids, cutting mats streamline garment construction, resulting in high-quality and professional-looking designs.

Denim Playsuit

The denim playsuit is a one-piece garment that is designed for women and is typically made from denim fabric. It is a popular and fashionable clothing item that is widely worn during the warmer months or in casual settings. The playsuit combines the convenience and ease of a jumpsuit with the versatility and casual vibe of denim, making it a versatile and trendy choice for many fashion-conscious individuals. The design of the denim playsuit typically features a fitted bodice with a button or zipper closure at the front or back. The bodice can be sleeveless, short-sleeved, or long-sleeved, depending on the style and personal preference. The bottom half of the playsuit consists of shorts that can be in various lengths, ranging from mid-thigh to knee-length. One of the key features of the denim playsuit is its use of denim fabric, which is a sturdy and durable cotton twill textile that is known for its rugged and casual appearance. Denim is typically blue in color, although it can also come in other shades such as black, white, or even pastel colors. The fabric is often washed or distressed to give it a worn-in look, adding to the overall casual aesthetic of the playsuit. The denim playsuit can be styled in numerous ways to create different looks. It can be paired with sneakers and a denim jacket for a relaxed and casual outfit, or dressed up with heels and statement accessories for a more chic and polished ensemble. The playsuit is also a versatile piece that can be worn during various occasions, such as picnics, brunches, beach trips, or even nights out on the town. In conclusion, the denim playsuit is a fashionable and versatile garment that combines the convenience of a jumpsuit with the casual and rugged vibe of denim. Its popularity lies in its ability to be dressed up or down, depending on the occasion and personal style. With its fitted bodice, shorts bottom, and use of denim fabric, the playsuit offers a fashionable and contemporary option for women seeking a trendy and effortless outfit choice.

Digital Drawing Pens

A digital drawing pen, also known as a stylus, is a tool specifically designed for fashion designers to create digital sketches and illustrations on digital drawing tablets or screens. It provides a more precise and natural drawing experience compared to using a mouse or touchpad. These pens are equipped with pressure-sensitive tips that can detect different levels of pressure applied by the designer. This feature allows for varying line thickness and opacity, mimicking the effects of traditional drawing techniques such as shading and cross-hatching.

Digital Fabric Printing Machine

A digital fabric printing machine, in the context of fashion design, refers to a technologically advanced device used to print intricate and vivid patterns or designs onto various types of fabrics. This machine revolutionizes the traditional method of fabric printing by providing a faster, more efficient, and more versatile alternative. With the advent of digital fabric printing machines, fashion designers can bring their ideas to life with greater ease and creativity. These machines utilize digital technology to reproduce complex designs, vibrant colors, and even photographic images onto fabrics, allowing for limitless design possibilities.

Digital Fashion Design

Digital fashion design is the process of creating and visualizing clothing and accessories using computer software and technology. It combines elements of traditional fashion design with digital tools to enhance creativity, streamline the design process, and enable virtual prototyping. With digital fashion design, designers can create and modify garments and accessories digitally, without the need for physical materials. This allows for faster iterations and experimentation, as well as reducing waste and costs associated with traditional production methods. The use of computer-aided design (CAD) software is a central aspect of digital fashion design. Designers can use CAD tools to create virtual prototypes of their ideas, manipulating patterns, colors, and textures to explore different design possibilities. This enables them to visualize and refine their concepts before committing to physical production. Another important aspect of digital fashion design is the ability to simulate and preview how garments will look and behave on the human body. Virtual fitting tools allow designers to virtually dress 3D avatars with their creations, adjusting fit and proportions to ensure the best possible result. This not only saves time and resources but also improves the accuracy and realism of the design process. Furthermore, digital fashion design facilitates collaboration between different stakeholders in the industry. Designers can easily share their digital files with manufacturers, pattern makers, and other team members, ensuring efficient communication and reducing errors in the production process. Additionally, digital fashion design opens up new possibilities for customization and personalization. With digital technologies, designers can create dynamic and interactive clothing, integrating sensors, lights, and other elements to enhance functionality and user experience. In conclusion, digital fashion design revolutionizes the traditional fashion design process by leveraging computer software and technology. It allows for faster iterations, virtual prototyping, precise fit adjustments, and improved collaboration. Digital fashion design not only enhances creativity and efficiency but also opens up new possibilities for customization and innovation in the fashion industry.

Digitizing Tablets

A digitizing tablet, in the context of fashion design, refers to a specialized device that allows fashion designers to create digital sketches and illustrations of their designs. It comprises a flat surface with a pressure-sensitive pad that captures and translates hand-drawn sketches into digital format. Unlike traditional paper and pencil drawings, digitizing tablets offer numerous advantages for fashion designers in terms of efficiency, accuracy, and versatility. By using a digitizing tablet, fashion designers can quickly and easily create and modify their designs digitally. The pressure sensitivity of the tablet allows designers to vary the thickness and opacity of their lines, replicating the natural feel and texture of traditional drawing techniques. This flexibility enables designers to experiment, refine, and iterate their ideas more efficiently than through traditional manual methods. Additionally, digitizing tablets provide designers with the ability to work directly within design software applications, such as Adobe Illustrator or CorelDRAW, enhancing their digital drawing capabilities. This integration allows designers to easily transfer their hand-drawn sketches onto the computer screen and manipulate them further by adding colors, patterns, and other design elements. This versatility fosters creativity as designers can explore different concepts and visualizations, saving time and effort in the design process. Moreover, digitizing tablets enable fashion designers to maintain a digital archive of their sketches and illustrations. This digital repository offers convenience and accessibility, allowing designers to easily retrieve and reuse their previous designs, eliminating the need for physical storage of paper-based drawings. It also facilitates collaboration among designers, as digital files can be easily shared, reviewed, and edited by multiple individuals simultaneously. In summary, digitizing tablets, particularly in the realm of fashion design, revolutionize the way designers conceptualize and create their designs. They offer a digital alternative to traditional sketching techniques, enabling designers to work more efficiently, accurately, and creatively. With their integration into design software applications, digitizing tablets enhance and streamline the design process, ultimately contributing to the advancement and innovation of the fashion industry.

Distressed Jeans

p { margin-bottom: 10px; text-align: justify; text-justify: inter-word; } Distressed jeans, also known as ripped jeans or grunge jeans, are a type of denim pants that have intentionally been treated to have a worn-out or aged appearance. This popular fashion trend emerged in the mid-1980s and has continued to evolve ever since. Distressing techniques involve fabric manipulation, which may include cuts, abrasions, bleach splatters, or chemical washes. These techniques create a fashionable and edgy look by giving the fabric a distressed, vintage, or grunge aesthetic. Distressing techniques aim to mimic the natural wear and tear that occurs over time on denim fabric. By strategically distressing certain areas such as knees, thighs, or pockets, the jeans give the impression of being well-loved and broken in. This deliberate damage contrasts with the clean and pristine appearance of non-distressed jeans, offering a rebellious and non-conventional style statement. Distressed jeans can vary in the degree of distressing, ranging from mild rips or frays to heavily torn or shredded designs. Designers often experiment with distressing techniques to create unique and innovative looks. Some popular techniques include sanding, tearing, scraping, or using chemicals to create faded or discolored patches. These techniques can be applied to jeans of different styles, such as skinny jeans, boyfriend jeans, or bootcut jeans, allowing for versatility in design and interpretation. The distressed jeans trend has gained popularity across various fashion subcultures, including punk, grunge, and streetwear. It has become an iconic symbol of youth rebellion, effortlessly blending style and attitude. Distressed jeans are often paired with casual or street-style outfits, complemented by graphic tees, oversized sweaters, leather jackets, or sneakers. This style has also transitioned to high fashion, with luxury brands incorporating distressed jeans into their collections. While distressed jeans were initially seen as a sign of rebellion against traditional fashion norms, they have since become widely accepted and embraced as a mainstream fashion staple. They offer individuals the ability to express their personal style and attitude through clothing, creating a lived-in and effortlessly cool look. Distressed jeans have become a timeless and versatile piece in fashion design, showcasing the evolution of denim as a fabric and its continued influence on contemporary trends.

Draping Tools

Draping tools are essential instruments used in the field of fashion design. They are used to shape and manipulate fabric directly on a dress form or mannequin, allowing designers to create unique and three-dimensional garments. These tools enable designers to experiment with different draping techniques, explore various silhouettes, and bring their design ideas to life. The primary draping tool used in fashion design is the dress form or mannequin. This tool acts as a three-dimensional representation of the human body, allowing designers to drape fabric on it to achieve the desired fit and shape. Dress forms come in various sizes and proportions, ensuring that designers can design for different body types and sizes.

Drawstring Pants

A drawstring pant is a type of trousers that features an adjustable waistband with a drawstring closure. These pants are designed to be comfortable, casual, and easy to wear. The drawstring waistband is a defining characteristic of these pants and is typically made of a flexible material, such as elastic or cotton. The drawstring itself is usually made of a matching or contrasting fabric and can be adjusted to fit the wearer's waist securely. Drawstring pants are popular in various fashion contexts due to their versatility and functional design. They are commonly seen in casual and leisurewear, as they provide a relaxed fit and allow for easy movement. Many athletic brands also incorporate drawstring pants into their activewear collections to offer comfort during workouts or other physical activities. These pants can be found in a variety of fabrics, including cotton, linen, jersey, and blended materials. The relaxed fit of drawstring pants makes them suitable for warm weather, as the loose cut allows for breathability and airflow. They are often associated with summer fashion and beachwear due to their easygoing aesthetic. Drawstring pants come in a range of styles, including wide-leg, tapered, and jogger. Wide-leg drawstring pants are loose fitting throughout the legs, creating a flowing silhouette. Tapered drawstring pants are more fitted around the hips and thighs and gradually narrow towards the ankles. Jogger-style drawstring pants have a relaxed fit and are gathered at the ankles, often featuring ribbed cuffs. These pants can be styled in various ways depending on the desired look. They can be paired with a simple T-shirt or tank top for a casual ensemble or dressed up with a blouse or button-down shirt for a more polished appearance. Drawstring pants also lend themselves well to layering, as they can be worn with sweaters, jackets, or cardigans.

Dress Forms

A dress form, also known as a dressmaker's dummy or a mannequin, is a three-dimensional representation of the human body used in fashion design. It serves as a tool for fashion designers to create and alter clothing designs before they are produced for consumers. The dress form is typically made of a solid material, such as fiberglass or foam, and is shaped to mimic the proportions and contours of the human body. It has various adjustable features, such as height, chest circumference, waist measurement, hip size, and shoulder width, to accommodate different body sizes and shapes. These adjustable features allow fashion designers to accurately visualize how their designs will fit on a real person.

Dressmaker's Tracing Paper

Dressmaker's tracing paper is a specialized tool used in the field of fashion design. It is a thin, translucent paper that allows designers to transfer and trace patterns onto fabric or other materials without the need for direct cutting or marking. This paper is commonly used in the process of creating garments, especially when precision and accuracy are crucial. The use of dressmaker's tracing paper simplifies the pattern transfer process by providing a temporary outline on fabric. Designers can place the paper between the pattern and the fabric, then use a tracing wheel or stylus to apply pressure and create a transferred line. This method allows for easy replication of a pattern onto multiple pieces of fabric, ensuring consistency in the final garment. The tracing paper is available in a variety of sizes to accommodate different pattern dimensions and can be easily trimmed to fit specific requirements. It is often used alongside a cutting mat or surface to protect the underlying table or work area from damage caused by the tracing wheel. Additionally, the paper's translucent nature allows designers to align patterns accurately and adjust placements as necessary before committing to any permanent marks on the fabric. Once the pattern is transferred, designers can proceed with cutting and sewing the fabric pieces together, confidently knowing that the alignment and proportions of the garment will remain intact. Dressmaker's tracing paper offers an efficient and reliable way to preserve patterns while minimizing the risk of mistakes or inaccuracies. In conclusion, dressmaker's tracing paper is an essential tool in fashion design that enables precise pattern transfer onto fabric. Its thin and translucent nature allows for easy alignment and adjustments, ensuring accuracy in garment construction. By simplifying the pattern replication process, it contributes to the overall efficiency and quality of the designer's work.

Duffel Coat

A duffel coat is a type of outerwear that originated in Belgium and is typically made of heavy wool material. It is known for its distinctive design featuring a toggle-fastening front, hood, and large patch pockets. The coat is named after the town of Duffel in Belgium, where the fabric used to make these coats was originally produced. The duffel coat has become a timeless classic in the world of fashion, offering both style and functionality. Its popularity can be attributed to its practical features, including its warmth and durability. The thick wool material provides excellent insulation, making it ideal for cold weather conditions. The coat's hood provides additional protection against rain and wind, making it a practical choice for outdoor activities. One of the main distinguishing features of the duffel coat is its toggle-fastening front. Instead of buttons or zippers, the coat is secured with a series of toggles made from wood or horn. This design element adds a unique touch to the coat, setting it apart from other outerwear options. The toggles are not only aesthetically pleasing but also easy to use, allowing for quick and effortless fastening and unfastening of the coat. The large patch pockets on the front of the duffel coat add both style and functionality. These pockets provide convenient storage space for small items like keys, phones, or gloves. They also add visual interest to the coat, enhancing its overall design aesthetic. Due to its versatility and timeless appeal, the duffel coat has remained a popular choice in fashion for many decades. It can be dressed up or down, making it suitable for various occasions and outfit combinations. Whether paired with jeans and boots for a casual look or worn over a dress for a more polished ensemble, the duffel coat adds a touch of sophistication to any outfit. In conclusion, a duffel coat is a type of outerwear made of heavy wool material, featuring a toggle-fastening front, hood, and large patch pockets. It offers both style and functionality, making it a popular choice in fashion design. The coat's distinctive design elements, including its toggle fastenings and patch pockets, set it apart from other outerwear options. Its versatility and timeless appeal make it a wardrobe staple for both men and women.

Duffle Bag Coat

A duffle bag coat is a type of outerwear that is designed to resemble a duffle bag in both appearance and functionality. It is typically made of a sturdy, waterproof material such as nylon or cotton twill and is often lined with a warm and insulating fabric, such as fleece or faux fur. The defining characteristic of a duffle bag coat is its unique construction, which features a large, oversized silhouette with a loose, boxy fit. This creates a relaxed and casual look that is both stylish and practical. The coat is typically cut to fall just above the knee or mid-thigh, providing ample coverage and protection from the elements. One of the key design elements of a duffle bag coat is its front closure, which typically consists of toggles or looped fastenings. These closures are reminiscent of the traditional fastenings found on duffle bags, adding to the coat's overall aesthetic. Some duffle bag coats may also feature a concealed zipper or button placket underneath the toggles for added convenience and security. Additionally, many duffle bag coats are equipped with a generous hood, which provides additional protection against wind, rain, and snow. The hood is often adjustable, allowing the wearer to customize the fit and coverage. Some duffle bag coats may also feature a removable or detachable hood, providing versatility for different weather conditions or personal preferences. The overall design of a duffle bag coat prioritizes practicality and functionality. Its oversized silhouette allows for layering underneath, making it suitable for colder temperatures. The sturdy outer material and insulating lining ensure durability and warmth, making it a popular choice for outdoor activities or winter excursions. In terms of styling, duffle bag coats are versatile and can be paired with a variety of outfits. They can be worn casually with jeans and sneakers for a relaxed and effortless look or dressed up with tailored trousers and boots for a more polished ensemble. The neutral colors and minimalist design of duffle bag coats make them a timeless and versatile addition to any wardrobe.

Duster Cardigan

A duster cardigan is a versatile fashion garment that combines the characteristics of a duster coat and a cardigan. It is usually made from lightweight, soft, and flowing materials such as cotton, linen, or knit fabric. The duster cardigan typically features an open front, long sleeves, and a length that extends below the waist, often reaching the mid-thigh or knee. Designed as a layering piece, the duster cardigan provides comfort, style, and functionality. Its loose and unstructured silhouette allows for easy movement and a relaxed fit, making it suitable for a variety of body types and occasions. The open front design of the duster cardigan provides a flattering and elongating effect, creating a vertical line that visually lengthens the body. This makes it an ideal garment for both casual and more formal dress codes. With its versatile nature, the duster cardigan can be worn throughout all seasons. In warmer weather, it can serve as a lightweight outerwear option, offering a sense of coverage and added style to an outfit. During the cooler months, it can be layered over t-shirts, blouses, or sweaters, providing an extra layer of warmth and texture. The duster cardigan can be paired with a wide range of clothing items, including jeans, trousers, skirts, and dresses. It can effortlessly elevate a simple jeans-and-t-shirt combination, adding a touch of sophistication and trendy flair. For a more elegant look, it can be worn over a dress or paired with a skirt and blouse ensemble, creating a cohesive and polished appearance. In terms of styling, the duster cardigan offers endless possibilities. It can be styled with a belt to define the waist and create a more tailored look. Additionally, it can be accessorized with statement jewelry, scarves, or hats to enhance its overall aesthetic. The duster cardigan also lends itself well to layering with other clothing items, such as blazers, vests, or even other cardigans, allowing for creative and personalized styling options.

Duster Coat

A duster coat is a long, loose-fitting outer garment typically made from lightweight fabric. It is a versatile piece of clothing that can be worn by both men and women, and is often used as a protective layer during mild weather conditions or as a fashionable statement in various settings. The duster coat is characterized by its length, which typically falls below the knee and can even extend to the ankles. This elongated silhouette provides ample coverage and protection, making it suitable for different occasions and climates. The coat is usually constructed with a relaxed fit, allowing for ease of movement and layering over other clothing items. Originally, duster coats were designed for practical purposes, particularly for horseback riders and drivers. The coat's length helped prevent dust and dirt from settling on the wearer's clothes, hence the name "duster." Its lightweight fabric, such as cotton or linen, allowed for breathability and comfort during long rides. In the context of modern fashion design, the duster coat has transcended its utilitarian origins and has become a stylish addition to any wardrobe. It can be found in a variety of fabrics, including but not limited to wool, silk, polyester, and suede, catering to different style preferences and weather conditions. The duster coat's versatility lies in its ability to effortlessly elevate any outfit. It can be dressed up or down, depending on the occasion. For a more casual look, it can be paired with jeans or leggings and a simple top. Alternatively, it can add a touch of elegance when worn over a dress or tailored pants. Its loose fit allows for layering underneath, making it suitable for transitional seasons or unpredictable weather. The style of the duster coat can vary, with some featuring buttons or a belt to cinch the waist, while others maintain a more open-front design. This allows for different ways of styling and individual expression. Additionally, the coat may include pockets, which add functionality to the garment. Overall, the duster coat is a versatile and fashionable outerwear option. Its length, lightweight fabric, and loose fit make it suitable for various weather conditions and styles. Whether used for its practical purposes or as a statement piece, the duster coat remains a timeless and essential addition to any fashion-conscious individual's wardrobe.

Eco-Friendly Materials

An eco-friendly material in the context of fashion design refers to a substance or fabric that is produced using processes and materials that have a minimal negative impact on the environment. Sustainable fashion has gained significant attention in recent years due to the growing awareness of the fashion industry's contribution to pollution, waste generation, and resource depletion. As a result, designers and brands are increasingly seeking alternatives to conventional materials that are harmful to the environment.

Elastic Threaders

Elastic threaders are tools used in fashion design to insert elastic through casings or channels in garments. They consist of a thin, flexible wire with a loop at one end and a handle at the other. The looped end is used to grasp the elastic, and the wire is then threaded through the casing, guiding the elastic through as it goes. Elastic threaders are commonly used in the construction of garments that require adjustable waistbands, such as skirts, pants, and shorts. They make it easier to insert elastic into casings, ensuring a smooth and even distribution of the elastic throughout the garment.

Embroidery Floss Organizers

An embroidery floss organizer is a tool used in fashion design to efficiently store and categorize embroidery floss, which is a type of thread commonly used in embroidery and needlework. It consists of a compact container or holder with individual compartments or slots to accommodate various colors and types of floss. The purpose of an embroidery floss organizer is to provide fashion designers with a convenient and organized way to manage their embroidery floss collection. By keeping the floss neatly arranged and separated, designers can easily access the specific colors they need for their projects, saving time and effort in the process.

Embroidery Hoops

Embroidery hoops are essential tools in the world of fashion design. These circular frames are made of wood or plastic and are used to hold fabric taut and in place while hand embroidery is being done. The purpose of using an embroidery hoop is to ensure that the fabric remains stable and doesn't pucker or warp during the embroidery process. The hoop provides tension to the fabric, keeping it taut and preventing any wrinkles or folds that could interfere with the accuracy and precision of the embroidery stitches. Fashion designers often use embroidery hoops to create intricate and detailed designs on garments and accessories. By securing the fabric in the hoop, they can easily maneuver the needle and thread to create precise stitches and patterns. The hoop acts as a guide, helping the designer maintain even tension and control over the embroidery process. Embroidery hoops come in various sizes to accommodate different projects. Smaller hoops are used for delicate and intricate designs, while larger hoops are ideal for larger areas of embroidery. Some hoops even have adjustable mechanisms that allow the designer to increase or decrease the tension on the fabric as needed. In addition to their practical function, embroidery hoops can also be used as decorative elements in fashion design. Hoops with decorative designs or embellishments can be incorporated into garments or used as accessories on their own. They add a unique and artistic touch to the overall aesthetic of the design. To use an embroidery hoop, the fabric is placed between the inner and outer rings of the hoop. The fabric is then pulled taut and secured in place by tightening the screw or adjusting the mechanism of the hoop. The hoop is held in one hand while the other hand is used for the embroidery stitches. As the stitching progresses, the hoop can be easily rotated or repositioned to access different areas of the fabric. Overall, embroidery hoops are essential tools for fashion designers, providing stability and precision during the embroidery process. They ensure that the fabric remains taut and wrinkle-free, allowing for accurate and intricate embroidery designs. Whether used purely for function or incorporated into the design itself, embroidery hoops play a vital role in the world of fashion design.

Embroidery Machines

An embroidery machine is a specialized device used in fashion design to create intricate designs and patterns on fabric. It automates the process of embroidery, which involves stitching thread or yarn onto a fabric surface to create decorative designs or patterns. Embroidery machines come in various types, including single-head machines, multi-head machines, and computerized machines. Single-head machines are designed for small-scale production or personal use, while multi-head machines are used for larger-scale production. Computerized machines are the most advanced type of embroidery machines and offer a wide range of features and capabilities.

Embroidery Thread Holders

Embroidery thread holders are essential tools used in the field of fashion design to organize and manage different types of threads used in embroidery work. These holders are specifically designed to keep embroidery threads neatly arranged and tangle-free, allowing fashion designers to easily access and use the required threads for their creations. The main purpose of embroidery thread holders is to provide a convenient storage solution that keeps threads in optimal condition. This helps fashion designers in saving time and avoiding frustration that may arise when dealing with tangled or misplaced threads. By keeping the threads in an organized manner, these holders ensure that designers have easy access to the specific colors and types of threads they require for their designs.

Embroidery Thread Organizers

An embroidery thread organizer is a tool used in fashion design to keep embroidery threads organized and easily accessible. It is a storage system specifically designed to hold and display various types and colors of embroidery threads. The purpose of an embroidery thread organizer is to help fashion designers efficiently manage their embroidery threads during the design process. It allows designers to easily see and access different colors and types of threads, reducing the time and effort required to select the right thread for a particular project. Additionally, an organized thread storage system ensures that threads remain untangled and free from knots or other damage, ensuring their quality and usability.

Embroidery Threads

Embroidery threads, in the context of fashion design, are fine strands of colored yarn or thread used to create intricate and decorative embroidery designs on fabric. These threads are specially designed to be strong, durable, and resistant to fading, ensuring longevity and quality in the finished embroidery piece. Embroidery threads come in a wide variety of colors, textures, and finishes, allowing fashion designers to bring their creative visions to life through intricate stitches and patterns. The choice of thread color and type can significantly impact the overall aesthetic of the embroidery, creating depth, dimension, and visual interest.

Embroidery

Embroidery is a technique used in fashion design where decorative designs, patterns, or motifs are created on fabric using various types of stitches. It is a traditional form of embellishment that adds texture, depth, and intricacy to garments, accessories, and home furnishings.The process of embroidery involves the use of a needle and thread, or in some cases, a specialized embroidery machine, to stitch designs onto a piece of fabric. The designs can range from simple and geometric to complex and highly detailed, depending on the desired effect.In fashion design, embroidery is often used to enhance the aesthetic appeal of garments. It can be applied to a variety of fabrics, including cotton, silk, wool, and synthetic materials, and can be used on both woven and knit fabrics. Embroidery can be found on a wide range of apparel items, such as dresses, blouses, jackets, and skirts, as well as accessories like handbags, shoes, and hats.Embroidery can be done using a variety of techniques, each resulting in a different effect. Some commonly used embroidery techniques include satin stitch, cross-stitch, chain stitch, and appliqué. These techniques can be combined or used individually to create unique and visually appealing designs.Traditionally, embroidery was done by hand, with skilled artisans meticulously stitching each design. However, with advancements in technology, embroidery can now also be done using computerized embroidery machines. These machines are capable of creating intricate and precise designs in a fraction of the time it would take to do them by hand.Embroidery can be used to convey a variety of messages and meanings in fashion design. It can be used to represent cultural or ethnic identity, showcase craftsmanship and artistry, or simply add a touch of luxury and sophistication to a garment. The choice of embroidery design, thread color, and placement on the garment can all contribute to the overall aesthetic and message of the piece.In conclusion, embroidery is a technique used in fashion design to create decorative designs on fabric using various types of stitches. It adds texture, depth, and intricacy to garments and accessories, enhancing their aesthetic appeal. Embroidery can be done by hand or using computerized machines, and it can convey different messages and meanings depending on the design and placement.

Empire Waist Dress

An empire waist dress is a style of dress that is characterized by a high waistline that sits just below the bust, creating a fitted bodice and a flowing skirt that falls loosely over the hips and waist. This design creates a flattering silhouette that accentuates the bust and elongates the overall appearance of the body. The empire waist dress originated in ancient Greece and became popular during the Regency era in the early 19th century. It was revived again in the 1960s with the rise of bohemian and hippie fashion, and has remained a classic and timeless style ever since.

Empowerment Through Fashion

Empowerment Through Fashion refers to the concept of using fashion as a means to inspire and uplift individuals, allowing them to gain a sense of confidence, control, and self-expression. It involves the design and creation of clothing and accessories that not only enhance one's appearance but also promote a positive mindset and overall well-being. This approach to fashion design recognizes the transformative power that clothing can have on a person's mindset and self-perception. It goes beyond mere aesthetics and explores the potential of fashion to shape and empower individuals by aligning their outward appearance with their inner values and aspirations.

Environmental Sustainability

Environmental sustainability in the context of fashion design refers to the practice of designing, producing, and consuming fashion items in a way that minimizes negative impacts on the environment, both in the short and long term.This involves considering the entire lifecycle of a fashion product, from the sourcing of raw materials to its disposal, in order to reduce its ecological footprint. Fashion designers who prioritize environmental sustainability aim to minimize waste, pollution, and resource depletion throughout every stage of the design process.

Ethical And Socially Responsible Fashion

Ethical and socially responsible fashion can be defined as a design approach that takes into consideration the environmental, social, and ethical aspects of the fashion industry. It involves the production and consumption of clothing that is mindful of its impact on both the planet and the people involved in its creation. From an environmental perspective, ethical and socially responsible fashion aims to minimize the negative effects of the industry on the planet. This includes using sustainable materials, implementing eco-friendly production processes, and reducing waste and pollution. Designers may choose to use organic fabrics, recycled materials, or innovative eco-friendly technologies to create their garments. They may also adopt practices such as zero-waste production, where all fabric remnants are utilized, or implement recycling programs to ensure the circularity of their products. When it comes to social responsibility, ethical fashion considers the well-being of the workers involved in the production process. This means ensuring fair wages, safe working conditions, and the absence of child or forced labor. Designers who prioritize social responsibility may choose to work with suppliers and manufacturers that adhere to international labor standards and certifications, such as Fair Trade or SA8000. They may also engage in partnerships with organizations or cooperatives that support marginalized communities and provide them with employment opportunities. Ethical and socially responsible fashion also embraces transparency and consumer education. Designers who value ethical practices are transparent about their production processes, supply chains, and the origins of their materials. They strive to educate consumers about the impact of their fashion choices, encouraging them to make more conscious decisions and supporting a shift towards a more sustainable and ethical fashion industry.

Eyelet Tools

Eyelet tools are essential equipment used in fashion design for creating eyelets, which are small round openings made in fabric or leather to serve both functional and decorative purposes. These tools consist of various components, including a punch, an anvil, and a setter, that work together to form a complete eyelet setting system. The punch is a pointed tool with a cylindrical shape, often made of metal or plastic. It is used to create a hole in the fabric or leather, where the eyelet will be inserted. The punch is typically held in one hand and struck with a mallet or hammer to pierce the material. It is crucial to align the punch perpendicular to the fabric's surface to ensure precise and clean holes. The anvil, also known as a base or die, is a flat surface made of metal or hard plastic. It provides support to the fabric during the eyelet-setting process. The anvil usually has a concave cavity that fits the shape of the eyelet to hold it securely in place. The fabric or leather is placed on top of the anvil, with the hole aligned directly above the cavity. The setter is a specialized tool used to fix the eyelet into the hole created by the punch. It consists of a cylindrical stem with a flat or convex head. The stem is inserted through the eyelet from the front side of the fabric or leather. Then, the setter's head is placed on top of the eyelet from the backside of the material. The setter is struck with a mallet or hammer, compressing the eyelet's rim against the anvil. This action secures the eyelet in place and creates a neat finish on both sides of the material. Eyelet tools are commonly used in a variety of fashion design applications, such as creating laces, ribbons, or decorative trims. They are particularly popular for garments like corsets, bodices, and shoes, where eyelets are essential for tightening or lacing up. Additionally, eyelets can add an aesthetic touch to clothing and accessories, allowing designers to incorporate unique patterns and designs into their creations. In conclusion, eyelet tools are indispensable instruments in fashion design that facilitate the creation of eyelets by punching holes in fabric or leather and securing the eyelets in place. They enable designers to add both functionality and decorative elements to their garments and accessories, enhancing the overall appeal of their creations.

Fabric Bias Binding

Fabric bias binding refers to a narrow strip of fabric that is cut on the bias, a 45-degree angle from the straight grain of the fabric, and is used to finish raw edges or add decorative accents in fashion design. Bias binding is created by cutting across the bias grain of the fabric, which allows for optimal stretch and flexibility. This results in bias binding being able to smoothly curve around rounded edges without puckering or pulling. It is often used on garments where the fabric requires extra ease and movement, such as armholes, necklines, and hems.

Fabric Chalk

Fabric chalk is a useful tool in the field of fashion design, commonly used to temporarily mark fabric during the pattern making and garment construction process. It is a type of tailor's chalk specifically designed for use on textiles.Fabric chalk comes in various forms, including sticks, pencils, and markers, and is typically made from a soft, crumbly substance that easily adheres to fabric without leaving a permanent mark. The chalk is specifically formulated to be easily transferable onto fabric, allowing designers and garment makers to easily mark their fabric with precise lines and patterns.One of the main advantages of fabric chalk over other marking tools is its temporary nature. The marks made with fabric chalk are easily erasable and can be removed by simply brushing or washing the fabric. This makes it an excellent choice for marking fabric during the construction process, as it allows designers to make adjustments or changes as needed without leaving permanent traces on the fabric.Fabric chalk is particularly useful in pattern making, where precise markings are essential for accurate cutting and sewing. Fashion designers often use fabric chalk to transfer the shape and placement of pattern pieces onto fabric, ensuring that the final garment is cut and sewn accurately. The chalk lines can also be used to indicate seam allowances, darts, pleats, and other important construction details.In addition to pattern making, fabric chalk is also commonly used in garment alterations and modifications. Tailors and seamstresses rely on fabric chalk to mark areas that need to be taken in, let out, or adjusted in any way. The temporary nature of the chalk marks allows for easy changes and adjustments throughout the fitting process.Overall, fabric chalk is an indispensable tool in the fashion industry. Its ease of use, temporary nature, and versatility make it a preferred choice for pattern making, garment construction, and alterations. Whether used by professional designers or DIY enthusiasts, fabric chalk is an essential tool for accurately marking fabric and bringing fashion designs to life.

Fabric Dye Kits

Fabric dye kits are a set of materials used by fashion designers to add color to fabrics in a controlled and precise manner. These kits typically include various components such as the dye itself, fixing agents, applicators, and instructions. In the world of fashion design, fabric dye kits are an essential tool for creating unique and customized garments, costumes, and accessories. The primary purpose of fabric dye kits is to alter the color of textiles, allowing designers to achieve specific visual effects and express their creativity. The dyes included in these kits are typically formulated to work on a wide range of fabrics, including natural fibers like cotton, silk, and linen, as well as synthetic materials such as polyester and nylon. This versatility makes fabric dye kits suitable for use in various fashion design projects. With fabric dye kits, designers have the freedom to experiment with different color combinations, gradients, and patterns. By immersing or applying the dye onto fabrics, they can create vibrant and eye-catching designs that are unique to their vision. The inclusion of fixing agents in these kits ensures that the dye adheres to the fabric and maintains its color even after washing or exposure to sunlight. Applicators, such as brushes, sponges, or spray bottles, are often included in fabric dye kits to provide designers with different techniques for applying the dye onto fabrics. This allows for greater precision and control, enabling them to achieve intricate details or large-scale color transformations. The instructions provided with the kits guide designers on the proper use of the dye, ensuring optimal results. Overall, fabric dye kits are indispensable tools for fashion designers looking to add a personal touch to their creations. By offering a wide range of colors, applicators, and fixing agents, these kits empower designers to explore the possibilities of color and express their artistic vision through textiles. Whether it's for a runway collection, costumes for a film or theater production, or simply for personal projects, fabric dye kits are a reliable and versatile resource in the world of fashion design.

Fabric Dye Removers

Fabric dye removers are chemical products used in fashion design to remove or lighten unwanted color from fabric. They are specifically formulated to break down and remove synthetic or natural dyes from various types of fabric without damaging the fabric's integrity. When working with fabric, designers often encounter situations where they need to change the color of a garment or undo a dyeing mistake. This is where fabric dye removers come into play. These products are designed to effectively remove dye particles from the fabric, allowing designers to correct coloring errors, create unique color patterns, or prepare the fabric for re-dyeing. Fabric dye removers typically contain active ingredients such as reducing agents or bleach, which chemically react with the dye molecules. The chemical reaction breaks the bonds between the fabric and dye, making it easier to remove the color. Depending on the type and strength of the fabric dye remover, the original color can be partially or completely eliminated. It is important to note that fabric dye removers may not work on all types of fabric or dyes. Some fabric dye removers are formulated specifically for certain types of fabric, such as cotton or synthetics, while others are more versatile and can be used on a variety of fabrics. Additionally, certain dyes may be more resistant to removal, requiring stronger or repeated applications of the fabric dye remover. When using fabric dye removers, it is essential to follow the instructions provided by the manufacturer. This includes properly diluting the product, applying it to the fabric evenly, and allowing sufficient time for the dye remover to work. It is also important to consider the fabric's colorfastness and stability before using a fabric dye remover, as some fabrics may be more prone to damage or discoloration.

Fabric Glue

Fabric glue is a type of adhesive specifically designed for use in fashion design. It is a liquid mixture that is used to bond fabrics together, eliminating the need for sewing. The glue is applied directly to the fabric, creating a strong and permanent bond when it dries. Fabric glue is commonly used in various aspects of fashion design, including the creation of garments, accessories, and costume design. It offers several advantages over traditional sewing methods, such as speed, ease of use, and the ability to bond different types of fabrics together.

Fabric Manipulation

Fabric manipulation in the context of fashion design refers to the techniques and processes used to alter the shape, texture, and structure of fabric to create unique and innovative designs. It involves the manipulation and transformation of fabric through various methods, such as folding, pleating, twisting, tucking, gathering, and draping. These techniques offer fashion designers the opportunity to add depth, dimension, and visual interest to their creations, allowing them to push the boundaries of traditional fabric usage. Fabric manipulation can be seen as a form of sculpture, as designers sculpt and mold the fabric to create three-dimensional shapes and forms.

Fabric Marking Tools

Fabric marking tools are essential instruments used in the field of fashion design to create precise and accurate markings on fabric. These tools are specifically designed to aid fashion designers in various stages of the design process, including pattern drafting, cutting, and sewing. One of the most commonly used fabric marking tools is the tailor's chalk, which is a soft, colored chalk that can be easily applied and removed from fabric. Tailor's chalk is used to transfer pattern markings onto fabric, allowing designers to accurately cut and sew their garments. Another popular fabric marking tool is the water-soluble fabric marker, a pen-like tool that creates temporary markings on fabric. These markers come in a variety of colors and are especially useful for creating detailed markings on dark or patterned fabrics.

Fabric Paints

Fabric paints are specialized paints that are designed to be applied directly onto fabric surfaces. They are commonly used in fashion design to add color, patterns, and unique designs to garments and accessories. Fabric paints are available in various formulations and colors, allowing designers to create customized and long-lasting designs on fabric. These paints are specifically formulated to adhere to fabric fibers, resulting in a durable and flexible finish. They are made with pigments that are finely ground and suspended in a medium that allows for easy application and blending. Fabric paints are available in different types, such as acrylic, oil-based, water-based, and fabric markers, each with its own characteristics and applications. Acrylic fabric paints are commonly used as they provide vibrant colors and have good adhesion to most fabric types.

Fabric Pattern Cardstock

Fabric pattern cardstock refers to a type of sturdy paper or cardboard material that is used by fashion designers for creating and documenting various fabric patterns. It is an essential tool in the fashion design process as it allows designers to visualize and organize their ideas before executing them in the actual fabric. This cardstock is typically available in standard sizes, such as 8.5 x 11 inches, which makes it convenient for designers to work with. It is often blank or features grid lines or dots, which aid in accurate pattern drafting. Some cardstock may also have a matte or glossy finish, depending on the designer's preference.

Fabric Pattern Drafting Paper

Fabric Pattern Drafting Paper is a specialized type of paper used in the field of fashion design. It is an essential tool for creating, designing, and visualizing the patterns that will be used to construct garments. This paper serves as a blueprint for fashion designers, allowing them to develop and refine their designs before cutting into the actual fabric. It provides a structured and precise representation of the garment's shape, measurements, and construction details. Pattern drafting is the process of creating a template from which the fabric pieces will be cut and sewn together. This involves taking measurements, interpreting design sketches, and translating them into a pattern that will result in a well-fitting and aesthetically pleasing garment. Fabric Pattern Drafting Paper typically features a grid or dot matrix, which helps designers maintain the correct proportions and scale of the pattern. The grid lines or dots assist in drawing and aligning the various components of the pattern, such as the neckline, sleeve, waistline, and hemline. Designers can use different tools, such as rulers, curves, and tracing paper, in conjunction with the fabric pattern drafting paper to create precise and accurate patterns. They can make adjustments, modifications, and variations to the pattern, ensuring the desired fit and design elements are achieved. This specialized paper also allows designers to explore and experiment with different design options, such as collars, pleats, gathers, and darts. It provides a platform for designers to bring their creative ideas to life, visualize how the garment will look when sewn, and make any necessary revisions or improvements. Overall, fabric pattern drafting paper plays a crucial role in the fashion design process. It enables designers to translate their visions into tangible patterns, guiding them in the creation of garments that are both fashionable and functional. It offers a precise and structured approach to pattern development, ensuring accurate measurements and proportions, and facilitating the construction of well-crafted garments.

Fabric Pattern Drafting Pencils

Fabric pattern drafting pencils are essential tools used in the field of fashion design. These pencils are specifically designed for creating patterns on fabric, which are used as templates for cutting and sewing garments. Pattern drafting is the process of creating a 2-dimensional blueprint for a garment, allowing designers to visualize the shape, size, and proportions before cutting and sewing the fabric. Fabric pattern drafting pencils play a critical role in this process by allowing designers to accurately mark the fabric with precise measurements and guidelines. These pencils are typically made with a fine, sharp lead that enables designers to make precise markings on a variety of fabrics. The lead is usually firm enough to create clear lines, but also gentle enough to avoid damaging the fabric. This allows designers to create patterns with accuracy and ease. Fabric pattern drafting pencils come in a range of hardness levels, allowing designers to choose the appropriate pencil for their specific needs. Harder pencils with a higher lead hardness are ideal for creating small, detailed markings, while softer pencils with a lower lead hardness are better suited for larger, bolder lines. In addition to their hardness levels, fabric pattern drafting pencils also come in various colors. This allows designers to differentiate between different parts of the pattern or make specific markings for sewing instructions. The color options also enable designers to create patterns on a wide range of fabric colors, ensuring visibility and clarity. Overall, fabric pattern drafting pencils are indispensable tools for fashion designers, enabling them to accurately create patterns on fabric. These pencils provide designers with the precision and control they need to bring their designs to life, ensuring that the final garments are well-fitting and visually appealing.

Fabric Pattern Weights

Fabric pattern weights are essential tools used in the field of fashion design. They are small, weighted objects that are used to hold down patterns and fabric pieces during the cutting and sewing process. The main purpose of fabric pattern weights is to keep patterns and fabrics in place, preventing them from shifting or moving while being cut or sewn. This ensures accurate and precise cutting of the fabric, resulting in a well-finished garment.

Fabric Rolling Machines

A fabric rolling machine is a mechanical device used in the field of fashion design to roll and store large rolls of fabric. It is an essential tool in the industry as it allows for efficient and organized fabric handling. The main purpose of a fabric rolling machine is to neatly roll and store fabric rolls, ensuring that they are free from wrinkles, creases, and other forms of damage. This is particularly important in the fashion design process as the quality and appearance of the fabric can greatly impact the final garment.

Fabric Scissors

Fabric scissors, also known as dressmaker shears, are specialized cutting tools used in the field of fashion design. These scissors are designed specifically for cutting fabric, ensuring clean and precise cuts without causing fraying or damage to the material. One of the key features of fabric scissors is their long and sharp blades. The length of the blades allows for longer, smoother cuts, while the sharpness ensures that the fabric is cleanly cut without leaving any jagged edges. This is particularly important when working with delicate or intricate fabrics, as any fraying or uneven edges can affect the overall appearance and quality of the garment. In addition to their long and sharp blades, fabric scissors also have a serrated or zigzag edge. This edge helps to prevent the fabric from slipping or shifting while cutting, providing better control and accuracy. It also helps in reducing fatigue, as the serrated edge acts as a grip that holds the fabric in place during the cutting process. Fabric scissors usually have larger handles compared to regular scissors. These larger handles provide a comfortable grip and allow for better control and maneuverability. This is especially important when cutting through multiple layers of fabric or when performing intricate cuts and details. When using fabric scissors, it is important to use them exclusively for cutting fabric and avoid using them for other materials, such as paper or plastic. This is because cutting other materials can dull the blades or cause them to become misaligned, which can affect the cutting performance and result in less precise cuts. Regular maintenance and care of fabric scissors is crucial to ensure their longevity and cutting performance. It is recommended to keep the blades clean and dry, and to periodically sharpen them to maintain their sharpness. Some fabric scissors also come with a protective case or sheath, which should be used when storing the scissors to prevent accidental damage or dulling of the blades.

Fabric Seam Rollers

A fabric seam roller is a tool used in fashion design to flatten and smooth fabric seams during the garment construction process. It is a cylindrical tool typically made of wood or plastic, with a rounded surface that allows for even pressure distribution when working with fabric. The primary purpose of a fabric seam roller is to help create neat and professional-looking seams. When two pieces of fabric are sewn together, there is often a resulting ridge or bump where the seam is located. This can be especially prominent when working with heavier fabrics or fabrics with a nap or texture. By using a fabric seam roller, designers can press the seam to one side or open it up, ensuring the fabric lies flat and smooth.

Fabric Selvage Cutters

Fabric selvage cutters are specialized tools used in the fashion design industry to remove the selvage edges from fabric. The selvage is the tightly woven edge of a fabric that runs parallel to the fabric's lengthwise grain. It is usually a different texture or color than the rest of the fabric and may contain important information such as the manufacturer's name or fabric content. When creating garments or other textile products, fashion designers often need to remove the selvage edges to achieve a clean finish and ensure the fabric hangs properly. Fabric selvage cutters are designed to delicately and precisely trim these edges without damaging the rest of the fabric.

Fabric Serrated Tracing Wheel

A fabric serrated tracing wheel is a tool used in the field of fashion design to transfer patterns onto fabric. It consists of a handle and a serrated wheel made of metal or plastic. The wheel has sharp edges that are designed to puncture the pattern paper, allowing the user to trace the pattern onto the fabric with precision. The serrated edges of the wheel create small perforations along the pattern lines, which can then be used as a guide for cutting the fabric or marking important points such as darts or pleats. This allows the designer or seamstress to accurately replicate the pattern on different pieces of fabric, ensuring consistency and accuracy in the final garment.

Fabric Sourcing

Fabric sourcing in the context of fashion design refers to the process of researching, selecting, and acquiring suitable fabrics and materials for the creation of garments and accessories. It involves finding reliable suppliers or manufacturers who can provide the desired type, quality, and quantity of fabrics needed for a particular fashion collection or project. During fabric sourcing, fashion designers consider various factors including the desired aesthetics, functionality, and cost of the fabric. They typically start by conducting thorough research to identify potential fabric options that align with their design vision and meet the requirements of the intended garments. This research may involve visiting fabric trade shows, browsing fabric catalogues, trend forecasting, and consulting industry resources. Once potential fabrics are identified, designers reach out to suppliers or manufacturers to request fabric samples and gather information on factors such as composition, weight, texture, color-fastness, durability, and care instructions. These details are crucial for ensuring that the selected fabrics are suitable for the planned garments and will meet the expectations of the end consumers. Designers also consider the sourcing location and production practices of fabrics. Ethical and sustainable sourcing is increasingly important in the fashion industry, with designers opting for fabrics that are produced using environmentally friendly methods and fair labor practices. This involves researching the supply chain and certifications of the fabric suppliers to ensure that the materials align with their ethical values. The fabric sourcing process also includes negotiating prices, lead times, and minimum order quantities with the fabric suppliers. Designers aim to strike a balance between the desired quality and cost-effectiveness to ensure profitability and competitiveness in the market. Once the negotiations are finalized, purchase orders are placed, and fabrics are acquired for further development and production.

Fabric Stencils

Fabric stencils are tools used in fashion design to create patterns or designs on fabric using a cutout template. A fabric stencil is typically made of a durable material such as plastic or cardboard, with the design cut out of it. The stencil is placed on top of the fabric, and paint or dye is applied over the cutout area to transfer the design onto the fabric. The use of fabric stencils allows fashion designers to easily and accurately replicate intricate patterns or designs onto fabric. They are commonly used in various stages of the design process, from creating initial sketches and prototypes to producing finished garments. Fabric stencils offer a versatile and cost-effective way to add unique and detailed embellishments to garments, accessories, and home textiles. When using fabric stencils, designers have the freedom to choose from a wide range of designs, including geometric patterns, floral motifs, abstract shapes, or even custom designs created by the designer. Stencils can be purchased pre-made from art supply stores, or they can be handcrafted by the designer to suit their specific design needs. To use a fabric stencil, the designer first secures the fabric in place to ensure it does not move during the stenciling process. The stencil is then carefully positioned on top of the fabric, with the desired design area aligned with the fabric's surface. The designer can use tape or weights to hold the stencil in place securely. Once the stencil is in position, the designer can apply the paint or dye onto the fabric using various methods, such as brushstrokes, sponging, or spraying. It is important to apply the paint evenly and avoid excessive saturation that may cause bleeding or smudging of the design. After the paint has been applied, the stencil is carefully lifted off, revealing the transferred design on the fabric. To create more intricate designs or layered effects, designers can use multiple stencils in succession. This allows for the creation of depth and dimension in the final design. The choice of paint or dye colors also plays a significant role in the overall outcome, as different colors can create contrasting or harmonious effects. Overall, fabric stencils are valuable tools in fashion design, allowing designers to add detailed and intricate patterns to their creations. They provide a versatile and cost-effective way to enhance the aesthetics of garments and textiles, making them an essential component of the design process for many fashion designers.

Fabric Stretch Gauge

A fabric stretch gauge is a tool used in the fashion design industry to measure the amount of stretch in a fabric. It is designed to determine the elasticity of various types of textiles, which is an important factor in garment construction and design. The fabric stretch gauge consists of a small device with a calibrated scale or numerical markings. It typically has a straight edge and curved edge, which are used to measure the stretch by pulling the fabric in different directions. The stretch is measured by securing one end of the fabric to the straight edge of the gauge and pulling the fabric across the curved edge. The amount of stretch is then read off the scale or numerical markings.

Fabric Stretchers

A fabric stretcher is a device used in fashion design to stretch and manipulate fabrics. It is typically made of a sturdy frame, often constructed from wood or metal, and consists of two adjustable bars that can be moved closer together or further apart. These bars are equipped with clamps or pins to securely hold the fabric in place. The purpose of a fabric stretcher is to create tension in the fabric, allowing the designer to accurately measure and cut patterns, or to reshape and reposition garments during the fitting process. Fabric stretchers come in different sizes and designs to accommodate various types of fabrics and garments. They are especially useful for fabrics that are prone to stretching, such as knits or loosely woven materials. By applying controlled tension to the fabric, the stretcher helps prevent distortion and maintains the desired shape and dimensions.

Fabric Stretching Frames

Fabric stretching frames, also known as stretchers, are specialized tools used in the field of fashion design. These frames consist of a rigid structure made of wood or metal, with adjustable clamps or pins that secure the fabric in place. The purpose of fabric stretching frames is to provide a smooth and taut surface for pattern making, draping, and garment construction. In the world of fashion design, accuracy and precision are crucial. Fabric stretching frames help designers achieve these qualities by creating a stable platform to work on. The fabric is stretched and secured tightly across the frame, allowing designers to manipulate and shape it with ease. This is particularly useful when working with delicate fabrics that tend to shift or wrinkle during the design process. Fabric stretching frames offer several benefits to fashion designers. Firstly, they provide a consistent and even surface, ensuring that the fabric remains flat and smooth. This is essential for pattern making, as any distortions or irregularities in the fabric can affect the fit and drape of the final garment. Additionally, the stretched fabric allows designers to accurately align and match patterns or motifs, resulting in a cohesive and visually appealing finished product. Furthermore, fabric stretching frames facilitate the process of draping. Draping involves using fabric to create three-dimensional shapes directly on a dress form or mannequin. By stretching the fabric over the frame, designers can drape it in a controlled manner, experimenting with different folds, pleats, and gathers. This technique helps them visualize how the fabric will behave when worn, enabling them to make adjustments and achieve the desired silhouette. Another application of fabric stretching frames is in garment construction. Once the fabric has been draped and the pattern has been finalized, the stretched fabric can be used as a reference for cutting and sewing. The taut surface helps maintain the shape and grain of the fabric, allowing for precise cutting and sewing techniques. This ensures that the final garment matches the intended design and fits the wearer accurately.

Fabric Swatch Books

Fabric Swatch Ring Sets

Fabric Swatch Ring Sets are a collection of small fabric samples that are attached to a sturdy ring. They are commonly used in the field of fashion design as a convenient and practical tool for designers to gather and organize different fabric options for a specific project. These sets typically include a variety of fabric swatches that showcase different colors, patterns, textures, and materials. The swatches are carefully selected to provide a comprehensive range of options for the designer to consider when creating or planning a garment or collection.

Fabric Testing Kits

Fabric testing kits are essential tools used by fashion designers to assess the quality and performance of fabrics before incorporating them into their designs. These kits consist of a collection of instruments, materials, and instructions that allow designers to conduct various tests on fabrics to ensure they meet the desired standards. The main purpose of fabric testing kits is to evaluate the durability, strength, and suitability of fabrics for specific fashion applications. These tests help designers make informed decisions about which fabrics to use for different types of garments or accessories.

Fabric Transfers

Fabric transfers in the context of fashion design refer to the process of applying pre-designed or printed designs or patterns onto fabric surfaces. This technique allows fashion designers to add intricate details, graphics, or logos to garments, accessories, or other textile items. Fabric transfers can be achieved through various methods, including heat transfers, screen printing, and digital printing techniques. Heat transfers, also known as iron-on transfers, involve applying a design or pattern by using heat and pressure to transfer the image from a transfer paper or film onto the fabric. This method is commonly used for single-color or limited-color designs. The transfer paper is placed on the fabric, and then heat is applied using an iron or heat press machine, causing the design to adhere to the fabric. Heat transfers are often used to create personalized t-shirts, bags, or other fabric items.

Fair Isle Cardigan

A Fair Isle cardigan is a type of garment that is commonly used in the field of fashion design. It is characterized by the use of a particular knitting technique known as Fair Isle knitting, which originated in the Fair Isle, a small island in Scotland. This technique involves knitting with two or more colors of yarn in a single row, using different colors to create intricate patterns and designs. The patterns typically feature geometric shapes, repeating motifs, and contrasting colors, creating a visually striking and unique appearance.

Fair Isle Sweater

A Fair Isle sweater is a type of knitted garment that originated in the Fair Isle, a small island in

Scotland. It is characterized by its intricate and colorful pattern, which typically consists of multiple stranded motifs. The sweater is knitted using the Fair Isle technique, also known as stranded knitting, where two or more colors are carried along the row, creating a fabric with distinct colorwork. The Fair Isle sweater is traditionally made from wool, which provides warmth and durability. It is typically knitted in a tight gauge to ensure a close fit and to enhance its insulation properties. The sweater often features a crew neck, long sleeves, and ribbed cuffs and hem for a snug and comfortable fit. The Fair Isle pattern is what sets this sweater apart from other knitted garments. It is characterized by its geometric motifs, such as diamonds, zigzags, and stars, as well as nature-inspired elements like trees, flowers, and animals. The pattern is created by alternating the colors of the yarn in a specific sequence, often repeating the motifs across the sweater. Traditionally, the Fair Isle sweater uses a limited color palette, with natural shades like gray, cream, and brown combined with bright hues like red, blue, and green. However, modern interpretations may incorporate a wider range of colors to create bolder and more contemporary designs. The Fair Isle sweater has become a timeless classic in fashion, known for its cozy and stylish appeal. It is a versatile garment that can be dressed up or down, making it suitable for various occasions. Whether paired with jeans for a casual look or worn over a shirt for a more sophisticated ensemble, the Fair Isle sweater adds a touch of elegance and charm to any outfit.

Fashion Accessory

A fashion accessory refers to an item that complements and enhances an individual's outfit or overall appearance. It is a non-essential item that adds an extra touch of style, personality, and uniqueness to a person's ensemble. Fashion accessories can be worn or carried, and they include a wide range of items such as jewelry, handbags, hats, scarves, belts, sunglasses, watches, and shoes. Unlike essential clothing pieces like shirts, pants, and shoes, fashion accessories are not required for basic functionality or protection. Instead, they serve as decorative embellishments that contribute to the overall aesthetic appeal of an outfit. These accessories often reflect the current fashion trends and can be used to convey personal style, cultural heritage, social status, or simply enhance an individual's confidence and self-expression.

Fashion Activism

Fashion Activism refers to the use of fashion as a means of expressing and advocating for social, political, and environmental change. It involves the conscious decision to design, produce, and consume fashion in a way that promotes ethical and sustainable practices, challenges societal norms, and raises awareness about various issues. As a form of activism, fashion becomes a tool for self-expression, enabling individuals to visually communicate their beliefs, values, and concerns. Through clothing, accessories, and other fashion items, people can convey powerful messages, spark conversations, and provoke thought. Fashion activists use their designs to challenge traditional notions of beauty, disrupt oppressive systems, and promote inclusivity, diversity, and individuality. One aspect of fashion activism is its focus on ethical and sustainable practices. This involves considering the entire lifecycle of a fashion product, from the sourcing of materials to its disposal. Fashion activists prioritize using materials that are socially and environmentally responsible, such as organic or recycled fabrics, and employ manufacturing processes that minimize waste, pollution, and exploitation of workers. They also aim to create fashion items that are durable, timeless, and can be repurposed or recycled, reducing the reliance on fast fashion and its negative impact on the environment. Fashion activism also extends to addressing social and political issues. Fashion designers who engage in this form of activism often tackle subjects such as gender equality, racial justice, LGBTQ+ rights, and body positivity. By creating designs that challenge stereotypes, break gender norms, or celebrate diversity, they strive to promote inclusivity and empower marginalized communities. They also use fashion as a platform to address other social issues, such as labor rights, fair trade, and consumerism, shedding light on the interconnectedness of the fashion industry and global inequalities. Fashion activism is a form of creative resistance, allowing individuals to express their values and concerns through their personal style. It encourages consumers to make conscious choices and supports the development of a more transparent, equitable, and sustainable fashion industry. By using fashion as a means of activism, designers and consumers alike can contribute to positive social change and the creation of a more compassionate and responsible world.

Fashion Alterations

Fashion alterations refer to the process of modifying or adjusting garments to fit a specific individual's body shape or to achieve a desired style. It is an essential aspect of fashion design as it allows for customization and ensures that clothing fits well and flatters the wearer. Alterations can involve various techniques such as taking in or letting out seams, shortening or lengthening hems, adjusting waistlines, or reshaping sleeves. These adjustments are typically made by hand or with the use of a sewing machine, depending on the complexity of the alteration. Fashion designers or tailors may perform these alterations themselves, or individuals may seek the services of a professional seamstress or tailor.

Fashion Alumni Network

The Fashion Alumni Network is a platform designed to connect individuals who have graduated from fashion design programs or have a background in the fashion industry. It serves as a means of networking, collaboration, and resource sharing for fashion professionals. By joining the Fashion Alumni Network, members gain access to a community of like-minded individuals who share a passion for fashion and a common educational background. This network allows members to connect with alumni from their own fashion school or program, as well as those from other institutions, creating a vast and diverse professional network. Networking is a crucial component of career development in the fashion industry, as it opens doors to new opportunities, collaborations, and mentorship. The Fashion Alumni Network provides a platform for members to build and expand their professional connections, fostering relationships that can lead to job opportunities, partnerships, and industry insights. In addition to networking, the Fashion Alumni Network also offers resources and support for members. This includes access to job boards, internships, and career development resources specific to the fashion industry. Members can also share knowledge, experiences, and industry news through forums, discussions, and articles. Furthermore, the Fashion Alumni Network organizes events, such as workshops, panel discussions, and fashion shows, to facilitate learning, inspiration, and collaboration among members. These events provide a platform for showcasing talent, exchanging ideas, and staying updated with the latest trends and developments in the fashion industry. In summary, the Fashion Alumni Network serves as a valuable platform for fashion professionals to connect, network, and collaborate with fellow fashion design alumni. It provides resources, support, and opportunities for career development and offers a sense of community and belonging within the fashion industry.

Fashion Analytics

Fashion analytics is a field of expertise that applies data analysis techniques to the fashion industry, with the aim of gaining insights and making data-driven decisions in the design and production of fashion products. It involves the collection, processing, and analysis of various types of data related to fashion, such as customer preferences, market trends, sales figures, social media buzz, and production costs. By analyzing this data, fashion designers and industry professionals can better understand the ever-changing dynamics of the fashion market and make informed decisions regarding product design, pricing, marketing strategies, and inventory management.

Fashion Appliqué

Fashion Appliqué refers to the decorative technique used in fashion design where a piece of fabric is placed on top of another fabric and attached using various stitching or adhesive methods. The appliqué fabric can be of a different color, pattern, or texture to create contrast and add visual interest to the garment or accessory. Appliqué is a versatile technique that can be used on different types of fabrics, such as cotton, silk, denim, or leather, and can be applied to various fashion items, including clothing, bags, shoes, and accessories. It allows designers to personalize and customize their creations by adding unique and eye-catching elements.

Fashion Archive

Fashion Association

Fashion Association refers to a group or organization that brings together industry professionals, designers, retailers, models, manufacturers, and other individuals or businesses involved in the world of fashion. It serves as a platform for collaboration, communication, education, and promotion within the fashion industry. These associations play a crucial role in advancing the fashion industry by fostering relationships between various stakeholders and providing a collective voice for the industry. They aim to promote and support the growth, development, and sustainability of fashion design and related businesses. Fashion associations may engage in a wide range of activities, including organizing fashion shows, exhibitions, and networking events. These events serve as opportunities for designers to showcase their work, connect with buyers and potential clients, and establish themselves in the industry. Fashion associations also often provide resources and support for emerging designers, mentoring programs, and scholarships to nurture new talent. In addition to hosting events, fashion associations may also conduct research and analysis on industry trends, market demands, and consumer behavior. This information helps designers and fashion businesses stay relevant and make informed decisions regarding product development, pricing, marketing strategies, and overall business operations. By staying updated on industry trends and consumer preferences, fashion associations offer valuable insights and guidance to their members. Furthermore, these associations frequently collaborate with educational institutions, supporting fashion design programs and providing students with internship opportunities, scholarships, and access to industry connections. This collaboration between fashion associations and educational institutions helps bridge the gap between classroom learning and real-world industry experiences. Overall, fashion associations play an integral role in the fashion industry by bringing together professionals, facilitating collaboration and communication, providing resources and support, and promoting industry growth and development. Through their efforts, they strive to strengthen the fashion ecosystem, foster innovation, and contribute to the cultural and economic significance of fashion design.

Fashion Athleisure

Fashion athleisure refers to a clothing trend that combines elements of both athletic and leisure wear, resulting in a fashionable and comfortable style. It is a modern approach to fashion design that caters to the growing demand for versatile clothing that can be worn in various settings, including casual outings, workout sessions, and even social events. The concept of athleisure emerged as a response to the increasing focus on health and fitness in contemporary society. With more people incorporating exercise into their daily routines, there was a need for clothing that could seamlessly transition from the gym to everyday activities, without sacrificing style or comfort. A key characteristic of fashion athleisure is the use of technical fabrics and construction techniques typically associated with sportswear. These fabrics, such as moisture-wicking materials and four-way stretch fabrics, offer functional benefits like breathability, flexibility, and durability. This allows individuals to engage in physical activities while maintaining a fashionable appearance. The design aesthetic of fashion athleisure often includes elements such as slim silhouettes, minimalistic details, and neutral color palettes. This understated approach creates a versatile wardrobe that can easily be mixed and matched, providing endless styling options. Fashion athleisure also embraces the concept of layering, allowing individuals to adapt their outfits to different weather conditions or occasions. Furthermore, fashion athleisure blurs the lines between traditional gendered clothing. It challenges traditional notions of femininity and masculinity by offering gender-neutral silhouettes and designs. This inclusive approach allows individuals of all genders to express their personal style in a way that aligns with their preferences and comfort level. In conclusion, fashion athleisure is a clothing trend that combines athletic and leisure elements to create fashionable and comfortable outfits. It caters to the demand for versatile clothing that can be worn in various settings and embraces functional fabrics and minimalistic design aesthetics. By challenging traditional gender norms, fashion athleisure promotes inclusivity and self-expression.

Fashion Avant-Garde

Fashion Avant-garde is a term used in the realm of fashion design to describe innovative and unconventional approaches to clothing and accessories creation that challenge traditional norms and conventions. It is a movement that pushes the boundaries of fashion, introducing new and daring concepts that often go beyond the realm of practicality and functionality. Avant-garde fashion designers are known for their experimental and visionary designs, taking inspiration from various sources such as art, architecture, culture, and technology. They strive to break away from established norms, rejecting mainstream fashion trends and embracing unconventional materials, shapes, and techniques.

Fashion Award

Fashion Award is a prestigious recognition given in the field of fashion design. It acknowledges exceptional talent, innovation, and creativity exhibited by fashion designers. This accolade celebrates the high level of skill and vision demonstrated in the creation and presentation of fashion collections, garments, and accessories. A Fashion Award is typically granted by renowned fashion organizations, industry experts, or institutions involved in promoting and supporting the fashion industry. The purpose of this award is to honor individuals or fashion houses that have made significant contributions to the fashion world and have had a profound impact on fashion trends, aesthetics, and cultural influences. The criteria for receiving a Fashion Award vary depending on the specific organization or institution that presents it. Generally, the recipient is selected based on their artistic vision, originality, craftsmanship, and the impact of their work on the industry or society as a whole. The award may also consider factors such as innovation, sustainability, and social responsibility. The Fashion Award is often accompanied by a ceremony or event, where industry professionals, designers, celebrities, and media converge to acknowledge and celebrate the achievements of the awardee. This event not only showcases the work of the winner but also serves as a platform for emerging designers to gain exposure and recognition. Receiving a Fashion Award can significantly boost a designer's reputation and career. It enhances their visibility within the fashion industry and opens doors to new collaborations, partnerships, and opportunities. The award serves as a validation of their talent and expertise, making them more sought after by clients, fashion houses, and retailers. Ultimately, a Fashion Award distinguishes individuals or fashion houses as influential leaders in the fashion design sphere. It showcases their ability to shape and redefine the ever-evolving landscape of fashion, leaving a lasting impact on the industry's aesthetics, trends, and cultural significance. In conclusion, a Fashion Award is a highly esteemed recognition given to outstanding fashion designers, honoring their exceptional creativity, innovation, and influence within the fashion industry. It serves as a platform to celebrate their artistic achievements and to inspire and empower future generations of fashion designers.

Fashion Awards

Fashion Awards are prestigious events held to recognize and celebrate the achievements and contributions of individuals in the field of fashion design. These annual ceremonies bring together industry professionals, designers, models, celebrities, and fashion enthusiasts to honor outstanding talent, innovation, and creativity in the fashion world. The purpose of Fashion Awards is to acknowledge and celebrate the exceptional work and success of designers, both established and emerging, who have made a significant impact on the fashion industry. These awards serve as a platform for showcasing the diversity, artistry, and craftsmanship of fashion designers and their collections. They provide recognition and encouragement to those who have demonstrated exceptional talent, vision, and skill in the fashion design field.

Fashion Bag

A fashion bag, also known as a handbag or purse, is a stylish accessory designed to carry personal belongings. It is an essential accessory for both men and women, complementing their outfit and adding a finishing touch to their overall look. Fashion bags come in a variety of shapes, sizes, and materials, allowing individuals to express their personal style and meet the demands of their daily activities. They are made from various materials such as leather, fabric, and synthetic materials, each offering its own unique look and feel.

Fashion Beading

Fashion Beading is a technique used in the field of fashion design that involves the application of beads to clothing, accessories, or other fashion items. It is a decorative method that adds texture, sparkle, and visual interest to garments, making them more unique and visually appealing. The process of fashion beading typically starts with choosing the appropriate beads, which can vary in size, shape, color, and material. Commonly used beads include glass, crystal, plastic, metal, and pearl. Once the beads are selected, they are secured to the fabric or material using various techniques such as sewing, embroidery, or gluing. Fashion beading can be applied to a wide range of clothing and accessories, including dresses, tops, skirts, jackets, handbags, shoes, and jewelry. The placement of beads on the garment can vary depending on the desired design and effect, ranging from scattered or clustered patterns to intricate motifs and embellishments. The use of fashion beading allows designers to create stunning and intricate designs that elevate the aesthetic value of the garments. Beads can be used to create various effects, such as adding shine and shimmer, creating three-dimensional texture, or enhancing specific areas of the garment. They can be arranged in patterns, shapes, or motifs to complement the overall design or convey a specific theme or concept. Overall, fashion beading is a versatile and creative technique that adds a touch of glamour and luxury to fashion items. It requires a keen eye for design, attention to detail, and skillful craftsmanship. Fashion designers and artisans use this technique to transform ordinary garments into unique works of art, showcasing their creativity and expertise in the field of fashion design.

Fashion Belt

A fashion belt is a type of accessory that is worn around the waist to enhance the overall look and style of an outfit. It is typically made of a variety of materials such as leather, fabric, or metal and is often embellished with different embellishments, patterns, and designs to add visual interest. The main purpose of a fashion belt is to cinch in the waist and create definition, which can help to create a more flattering silhouette. It can be worn with a wide range of garments, including dresses, skirts, pants, and jumpsuits, and can be used to either highlight or accentuate certain areas of the body.

Fashion Bespoke Suit

A bespoke suit in the context of fashion design is a custom-made suit that is meticulously tailored to fit an individual's specific measurements and preferences. It is a sartorial masterpiece that is created with utmost precision and attention to detail, resulting in a suit that is unmatched in quality and fit. The process of creating a bespoke suit involves several steps, beginning with a thorough consultation with the client to understand their style, body shape, and personal preferences. Measurements are then taken in order to create a pattern that is unique to the individual. This pattern is then used to cut the fabric, ensuring that every piece is perfectly aligned and symmetrical. After the fabric is cut, it is meticulously hand-stitched by skilled craftsmen, who take great care to ensure that every seam, stitch, and buttonhole is flawlessly executed. The suit is then fitted on the client multiple times throughout the construction process, allowing for any necessary adjustments to be made to ensure a perfect fit. A bespoke suit is characterized by its attention to detail, with features such as hand-sewn buttonholes, pick stitching, and functional cuffs. The fabric used is of the highest quality, often sourced from renowned fabric mills and made from luxurious materials such as wool, silk, or cashmere. What sets a bespoke suit apart from off-the-rack or made-to-measure suits is the level of personalization and customization it offers. The client has the freedom to choose every aspect of the suit, from the fabric and color to the style of lapels, pockets, and buttons. This ensures that the suit truly reflects the client's personal style and preferences. A bespoke suit is a timeless investment that exudes elegance and sophistication. It is an embodiment of craftsmanship and artistry, created to enhance the wearer's confidence and make a lasting impression. Whether for a special occasion, business attire, or simply to elevate one's personal style, a bespoke suit is the epitome of refinement in the world of fashion.

Fashion Black Tie

A black tie attire in fashion design is a formal dress code typically worn at evening events or special occasions. It is characterized by a specific set of garments that create an elegant and sophisticated look. The term "black tie" refers to the black silk bow tie that is an essential part of this dress code. The key elements of a black tie outfit for men include a black tuxedo or dinner jacket, a white dress shirt, a black formal waistcoat or cummerbund, formal trousers with a satin stripe on the outer leg, black patent leather shoes, and of course, the black silk bow tie. Men may also choose to wear a black or white formal dinner jacket instead of a traditional tuxedo. Accessories such as cufflinks, studs, and a pocket square can be added to enhance the formal look. For women, a black tie attire typically consists of a long formal gown, preferably in dark colors such as black, navy, or deep burgundy. The dress should be made from luxurious fabrics such as silk, satin, or velvet and may feature elegant embellishments like sequins or lace. Styles can vary from A-line to mermaid silhouettes, with options for strapless, long sleeves, or off-the-shoulder designs. It is important to opt for a tasteful and modest neckline and a floor-length hemline. Women can complement their gown with accessories like statement jewelry, a clutch purse, and high heels. The black tie dress code represents a higher level of formality compared to semi-formal attire. It is often requested for events such as black-tie galas, formal weddings, or prestigious award ceremonies. By adhering to the black tie guidelines, individuals can exude elegance and refinement, demonstrating their appreciation for timeless fashion. In conclusion, black tie attire in fashion design refers to a formal dress code that includes a black tuxedo or dinner jacket for men and a long formal gown for women. By following the specific guidelines of this dress code, individuals can create a polished, sophisticated look, perfect for special evening events.

Fashion Blog

A fashion blog is a type of online platform that focuses on sharing information, opinions, and ideas related to fashion design. It serves as a virtual space where fashion enthusiasts, professionals, and designers can express and discuss their thoughts, experiences, and trends. Through a fashion blog, designers can showcase their collections, provide insights into their creative process, and share their inspirations. They can use images, videos, and written content to communicate their vision to their audience. Furthermore, fashion blogs often feature interviews with designers, giving readers a deeper understanding of their work and the industry as a whole.

Fashion Blogger

A fashion blogger is a person who creates and manages a website or social media platform dedicated to sharing their personal experiences, thoughts, and opinions on fashion design and the latest trends in the industry. Through written content, photographs, and sometimes videos, fashion bloggers provide insights into their own fashion choices, styling tips, product reviews, and advice on how to incorporate various fashion pieces into everyday outfits. They often collaborate with brands and designers, showcasing their collections and promoting new product launches.

Fashion Blogging

Fashion blogging is a form of online writing where individuals share their perspective, insights, and opinions on various aspects of fashion design. It functions as a platform for fashion enthusiasts to express their creativity, knowledge, and personal style preferences. In the world of fashion design, blogging plays a crucial role in connecting fashion lovers, designers, and brands. It serves as a digital space where individuals can share their thoughts on fashion trends, styling tips, fashion events, and product reviews. Fashion bloggers often share their own personal experiences related to fashion, such as shopping hauls, outfit inspirations, and fashion-related stories. Fashion blogging serves as a source of inspiration for both fashion designers and enthusiasts. These blogs showcase the latest trends, innovative designs, and unique styles. They provide valuable insights into the evolving fashion industry, helping readers stay updated with the latest happenings. Additionally, fashion bloggers often partner with brands to promote their products or collaborate on fashion-related projects. Through their blogs, they provide an avenue for designers and brands to reach a wider audience and create brand awareness. They often feature sponsored content, such as product reviews or outfit styling incorporating the brand's items. By doing so, they contribute to the promotion and marketing strategies of fashion companies. Fashion bloggers also play a role in shaping the industry's trends. Their influence can be seen in the rise of influencer marketing, where brands collaborate with popular bloggers or social media personalities to endorse their products. These collaborations have the potential to greatly impact consumer behavior and fashion choices. In summary, fashion blogging is an online platform for individuals passionate about fashion design to express their creativity, share their perspectives on fashion, and influence the industry. It connects fashion lovers, designers, and brands, providing inspiration and insight into the world of fashion. Through collaborations and endorsements, fashion bloggers contribute to brand awareness and shape consumer trends.

Fashion Bohemian Style

The fashion Bohemian style, also known as boho style, is a distinctive aesthetic that emerged in the 1960s and 1970s and is characterized by a relaxed and nonconformist approach to fashion. It draws inspiration from the Bohemian lifestyle, which emphasizes individuality, creativity, and free-spiritedness. The Bohemian style is often associated with nature, art, and the unconventional. It incorporates various elements such as flowing and loose-fitting clothing, vibrant colors and patterns, and a mix of vintage and ethnic pieces. Fabrics commonly used in this style include cotton, linen, and silk, which contribute to the comfort and free movement of the garments.

Fashion Book

A fashion book, in the context of fashion design, refers to a comprehensive publication that showcases, explores, and documents various aspects of the fashion industry. It serves as a reference tool and source of inspiration for fashion designers, stylists, and fashion enthusiasts. The fashion book typically features a wide range of content, including but not limited to fashion photography, runway images, designer profiles, trend analysis, historical references, and interviews with industry professionals. It offers a visual representation of fashion trends, designs, and styling techniques, along with informative text to provide context and insights.

Fashion Boutique

A fashion boutique is a specialized retail store that sells clothing, accessories, and other fashion-related products. It offers a curated selection of merchandise catered to a specific target market or style aesthetic. Boutique stores are characterized by their distinct and unique offerings, as well as their personalized customer service. Unlike large department stores, fashion boutiques typically have a smaller physical footprint and a more intimate shopping experience. They often carry limited quantities of each product, creating a sense of exclusivity and rarity. This limited stock allows boutique owners to carefully curate their inventory, ensuring that each item embodies their vision and brand identity. One of the key aspects of a fashion boutique is its focus on individuality and personal style. Boutique owners and employees are trained to provide personalized styling advice and assistance to customers. They have a deep understanding of current fashion trends and can help customers find items that best suit their body type, preferences, and occasion. In addition to clothing, fashion boutiques may also carry accessories such as jewelry, handbags, belts, and shoes. Some boutiques may even stock home decor items that align with their brand's aesthetic. By offering a range of complementary products, boutiques provide customers with a one-stop shopping experience where they can find complete outfits and accessories all in one place. In recent years, many fashion boutiques have expanded their presence online, allowing customers to shop from the comfort of their own homes. Online boutiques often offer a wider selection of products and sizes, further expanding their reach and customer base. Overall, fashion boutiques play a significant role in the fashion industry by providing a platform for emerging designers, unique brands, and distinctive styles. Through their carefully curated selections and personalized customer service, they offer a shopping experience that is both unique and memorable.

Fashion Brand Collaboration

Fashion Brand Collaboration refers to the strategic alliance or partnership between two or more fashion brands or designers, with the aim of creating a joint collection, product line, or marketing campaign. This collaborative effort combines the unique strengths and resources of each brand, leading to the development of innovative and exclusive products that cater to a wider audience and elevate the overall brand image. In the highly competitive fashion industry, brand collaborations have become increasingly popular as a means to gain a competitive edge, increase brand exposure, and tap into new consumer markets. These collaborations allow fashion brands to leverage each other's expertise, creativity, and brand equity to create products that are more desirable and have a higher perceived value. By joining forces, brands can share the costs of production, marketing, and distribution, making collaborations a cost-effective way to reach new customers and drive sales. Brand collaborations are often driven by shared values, aesthetic sensibilities, or target markets. They can be temporary, limited-edition partnerships or long-term strategic alliances. The collaboration may involve joint design and production, where designers from both brands work together to create a cohesive collection that represents the essence of both brands. Alternatively, it can take the form of co-branding, where the brands create a product by blending their distinctive design elements or logos. The benefits of fashion brand collaborations extend beyond financial gains and market expansion. Collaborations allow brands to tap into each other's loyal customer base, gaining exposure to new potential customers who may not have been previously aware of or interested in their brand. Collaborations can also create a buzz and generate excitement around the brands, driving social media engagement and increasing brand visibility. Additionally, collaborations offer an opportunity for brands to experiment with new ideas and push creative boundaries, resulting in fresh and innovative designs that captivate consumers. Overall, fashion brand collaborations are a powerful tool in the fashion industry, allowing brands to leverage each other's strengths, reach new audiences, and create unique and captivating products that stand out in a highly competitive market.

Fashion Brand

A fashion brand is a label or name assigned to a collection of clothing and accessories created by a fashion designer or design house. It represents the overall aesthetic, style, and image that the designer or design house wants to convey to its target audience. A fashion brand is not just about the physical products it produces, but also encompasses the values, ideals, and personality associated with the brand. It is a combination of the visual elements such as the logo, typography, and color palette, as well as the messaging and storytelling that accompanies the brand.

Fashion Branding Workshop

A fashion branding workshop is a formal educational event that focuses on the development and promotion of a fashion brand. It is specifically designed for individuals and professionals in the fashion industry who want to enhance their understanding of branding and apply it to their own fashion designs. During a fashion branding workshop, participants are introduced to the fundamental concepts of branding and its importance in the context of fashion. They learn how to create a unique brand identity that aligns with their design aesthetic and target market. The workshop covers various branding strategies, including brand positioning, brand personality, and brand differentiation. Participants gain insights into how successful fashion brands have effectively built and communicated their brand messages to connect with their customers. The workshop also highlights the significance of market research and competitor analysis in shaping a fashion brand. Participants learn how to identify their target audience and understand their needs and preferences. They explore techniques for conducting competitor analysis to gain a competitive edge in the market and position their brand effectively. In addition to theoretical knowledge, a fashion branding workshop provides practical insights and tools for brand development. Participants are guided through the process of creating a brand identity, including designing a brand logo, selecting brand colors, and establishing brand guidelines. They learn about the importance of consistent branding across all touchpoints, such as packaging, promotional materials, and online presence. A fashion branding workshop also explores the role of storytelling in brand communication. Participants discover how to craft compelling brand narratives that resonate with their target audience and create an emotional connection. They learn how to effectively communicate their brand story through various channels, such as social media, websites, and fashion shows. Overall, a fashion branding workshop equips fashion designers with the knowledge and skills to strategically develop and promote their fashion brand. It enables them to establish a strong brand identity that sets them apart from competitors and resonates with their target market. By understanding the fundamentals of branding and applying them to their designs and marketing efforts, participants are able to create a brand that is recognized, desired, and trusted in the fashion industry.

Fashion Branding

Fashion Branding is the process of creating a unique and recognizable brand identity for a fashion label or company. It involves establishing an overall brand strategy, which includes defining the brand's values, positioning, target audience, and visual identity. In the context of fashion design, branding plays a crucial role in differentiating a fashion brand from its competitors and building a strong relationship with consumers. A well-executed fashion branding strategy helps to create a brand image that resonates with the target audience and fosters brand loyalty and recognition. First and foremost, fashion branding involves defining the brand's values and unique selling propositions. This step requires understanding the target audience and their preferences, as well as identifying the brand's key strengths and competitive advantages. By clearly defining the brand's values and unique selling propositions, fashion designers can establish a strong brand positioning that sets them apart from other brands in the market. Once the brand values and positioning are established, the next step in fashion branding is to develop a visual identity for the brand. This includes designing a logo, selecting brand colors, and creating a distinctive typography style. The visual identity should align with the brand's values and target audience, as it will be used across various brand touchpoints, such as packaging, advertising, and website design. By consistently applying the visual identity across all brand materials, fashion designers can strengthen brand recognition and create a cohesive brand experience. In addition to visual identity, fashion branding also extends to other brand touchpoints, such as brand messaging and communication. This involves crafting a unique brand voice and tone that reflects the brand's personality and resonates with the target audience. Fashion designers should carefully consider the language they use in brand communications, including advertising campaigns, social media posts, and product descriptions. Overall, in the context of fashion design, fashion branding is the process of creating a distinct brand identity that resonates with the target audience. Through defining the brand's values, establishing a visual identity, and developing a unique brand voice, fashion designers can differentiate their brands and build strong connections with consumers.

Fashion Brocade

Fashion Brocade refers to a type of fabric that is commonly used in the field of fashion design. It is characterized by its intricate and often raised patterns, which are typically woven into a richly colored background. Brocade fabric is known for its opulent and luxurious appearance, making it a popular choice for formal attire and special occasion garments. The patterns found in brocade are often inspired by historical or cultural references, such as floral motifs, paisley designs, or geometric shapes.

Fashion Business Casual

Fashion Business Casual is a dress code that combines elements of professional attire with more relaxed and informal clothing. It is commonly adopted in professional environments that allow for greater flexibility and creativity in personal style, such as creative industries, start-ups, and certain modern office settings. The concept of Fashion Business Casual emerged as a response to the changing dynamics of the workplace and the desire for more comfortable and expressive clothing options. It acknowledges the need for individuals to feel comfortable and at ease while still maintaining a level of professionalism and presenting a polished appearance. The key elements of Fashion Business Casual include a blend of formal and informal clothing. It typically includes tailored separates, such as blazers, dress pants, or skirts, paired with more casual and relaxed pieces like shirts, blouses, or sweaters. This combination creates a balance between formality and comfort, allowing individuals to express their personal style while still adhering to professional norms. While Fashion Business Casual allows for a wider range of clothing options compared to traditional business attire, it is important to maintain a sense of appropriateness and professionalism. Certain clothing items, such as jeans, t-shirts, shorts, and sneakers, are generally not considered appropriate for Fashion Business Casual. It is advisable to opt for clothing that is well-fitted, clean, and wrinkle-free to achieve a polished look. Accessories also play a role in Fashion Business Casual. They can be used to add personality and flair to an outfit, but one should exercise moderation and avoid excessive or distracting accessories. Simple and classic accessories, such as a watch, belt, or small pieces of jewelry, are ideal choices to enhance the overall appearance without overpowering the outfit. Overall, Fashion Business Casual allows individuals to express their personal style and creativity while maintaining professionalism in the workplace. It provides a comfortable and versatile alternative to the more strict and formal business dress code, fostering a more relaxed and inclusive work environment.

Fashion Business Models

Fashion business models refer to the various strategies and approaches that fashion designers and companies adopt to create, market, and sell their products in the fashion industry. These models encompass the entire process of designing, manufacturing, and retailing fashion items, as well as the business structures and strategies employed to ensure their success. The fashion industry is highly dynamic and competitive, requiring designers and companies to constantly innovate and adapt to changing market trends. Fashion business models serve as frameworks that guide these entities in making strategic decisions and organizing their operations to meet consumer demands while achieving profitable outcomes. There are several key fashion business models that designers and companies can choose from based on their goals, resources, and target market. One common model is the traditional wholesale model, where designers create collections which are then sold to retailers who, in turn, sell the products to consumers. This model allows designers to focus primarily on the creative aspects of fashion design while relying on retailers to handle marketing and sales. Another popular fashion business model is the direct-to-consumer (D2C) model, in which designers bypass traditional retailers and sell their products directly to consumers through their own channels, such as e-commerce websites or flagship stores. This model allows for greater control over pricing, branding, and customer relationships, but requires designers to invest in marketing and distribution infrastructures. Some fashion brands adopt a hybrid business model, combining elements of both wholesale and D2C approaches. They may sell their products through select retailers while also maintaining their own online and offline stores. This allows for greater market reach and diversification of revenue streams. Additionally, there are fashion business models that focus on sustainability and ethical practices. These models prioritize environmentally friendly materials, fair trade practices, and transparent supply chains to meet the increasing demand for socially conscious fashion. By aligning their business practices with sustainability principles, designers and companies can cater to consumers who value ethical fashion. In conclusion, fashion business models encompass the strategies and approaches employed by fashion designers and companies to create, market, and sell their products. These models can range from traditional wholesale models to direct-to-consumer approaches, as well as hybrid models and sustainable business practices. By choosing the right business model, fashion entities can navigate the complexities of the industry and achieve long-term success.

Fashion Business Seminar

A fashion business seminar is a specialized event that focuses on providing valuable knowledge and skills relevant to the fashion industry. It is designed for individuals interested in pursuing a career in fashion design, brand management, retail, or any other aspect of the fashion business. During a fashion business seminar, industry experts and experienced professionals share their insights, experiences, and expertise in various areas of the fashion industry. The seminar typically includes presentations, panel discussions, workshops, and interactive sessions that cover a wide range of topics related to fashion design, marketing, production, distribution, and retailing.

Fashion Buyer

A fashion buyer is a professional who works in the fashion industry and is responsible for selecting and purchasing the merchandise that will be sold in retail stores. They are the link between the fashion designers and the consumers, as they have a keen eye for trends and an understanding of the target market's preferences. The role of a fashion buyer involves several key tasks. Firstly, they research the latest fashion trends by attending fashion shows, browsing online platforms, and reading fashion magazines. By staying updated on the current styles and designs, they can make informed decisions about which items to purchase and stock in their stores. Once the research is complete, the fashion buyer must establish relationships with suppliers and negotiate the best prices for the merchandise. They need to have strong communication and analytical skills to analyze suppliers' offerings and compare them with market demands and competitors' prices. This allows them to ensure that they are making cost-effective decisions while still providing high-quality fashion items to their customers. Another crucial aspect of a fashion buyer's job is forecasting and planning. They need to anticipate consumer demands and market trends to determine the quantities of each item that should be purchased. This involves analyzing sales reports, monitoring inventory levels, and evaluating the performance of previous purchases. By carefully planning their inventory, fashion buyers can avoid overstocking or understocking and optimize sales and profits. In addition to selecting and purchasing merchandise, fashion buyers also have a role in promoting and marketing the products. They collaborate with the marketing and visual merchandising teams to plan effective promotional campaigns and create visually appealing displays to attract customers. This requires creativity and an understanding of the brand's image and target audience. In summary, a fashion buyer is responsible for selecting and purchasing the fashion merchandise for retail stores. They research fashion trends, establish relationships with suppliers, negotiate prices, forecast demand, and collaborate with marketing teams. Through their expertise and understanding of the fashion industry, they contribute to the success of retailers by ensuring that the right products are available to consumers at the right time.

Fashion Buyer's Guide

A fashion buyer's guide is a comprehensive resource that provides information and guidance on the various aspects of buying fashion merchandise for retail purposes. It serves as a reference tool for fashion buyers, offering insights on the latest trends, brands, designers, and market strategies. Within the context of fashion design, a fashion buyer's guide plays a crucial role in the decision-making process. It assists designers and retailers in selecting the right products to stock their stores or online platforms. The guide typically covers a wide range of topics, including fashion forecasting, product sourcing, merchandising, and inventory management.

Fashion Buying

Fashion buying is a process within the fashion industry where individuals or teams are responsible for selecting and purchasing clothing and accessories to be sold in retail stores, online platforms, or through other distribution channels. This role involves a combination of trend analysis, market research, negotiation, budgeting, and merchandising skills to ensure the products chosen align with the target market and meet the company's financial goals. The fashion buying process typically starts with trend forecasting and analysis. Buyers need to stay on top of current and emerging fashion trends by attending fashion shows, browsing fashion magazines, and monitoring social media platforms. They need to understand the preferences and tastes of their target audience and anticipate future purchasing behaviors. Once the trends are identified, fashion buyers collaborate with designers, suppliers, and manufacturers to select the merchandise for their stores. They evaluate various collections, considering factors such as quality, price, style, and brand reputation. Buyers negotiate with suppliers to secure the best terms, including price, delivery schedule, and exclusivity agreements. After the merchandise is selected, fashion buyers work closely with visual merchandisers and marketing teams to develop strategic merchandising plans that maximize sales and profitability. This may involve creating product assortments, determining pricing strategies, and planning promotional activities. Buyers also need to analyze and understand sales data and consumer feedback to make informed decisions for future product selections and adjustments to the inventory. In addition to the creative aspects, fashion buying also requires strong analytical and financial skills. Buyers need to develop budgets, track expenses, and monitor inventory levels to ensure profitability and avoid overstocking or understocking situations. They need to analyze sales performance, identify trends, and adapt their purchasing strategies accordingly. In summary, fashion buying is a vital function within the fashion industry that involves selecting and purchasing clothing and accessories to meet the demands and preferences of the target market. It requires a combination of fashion knowledge, trend forecasting, negotiation skills, and business acumen to maximize sales and drive profitability.

Fashion Calendar

A fashion calendar is a tool used in the fashion design industry to organize and plan events, such as fashion shows, presentations, launches, and other important dates and deadlines. It serves as a guide for designers, brands, retailers, journalists, and other industry professionals to stay informed about upcoming fashion-related happenings. The purpose of a fashion calendar is to streamline the process of scheduling and coordinating various events within the fashion industry. It helps designers and brands to plan their collections, determine the timing for runway shows or presentations, and ensure that their products are ready for market at the right time. It also allows retailers to plan their buying seasons and promotions accordingly. A fashion calendar typically includes key dates such as fashion weeks, trade shows, and industry events held in different cities around the world. Fashion weeks are the most significant events in the calendar, where designers showcase their collections on the runway. These events attract international attention and set the trends for the upcoming seasons. In addition to fashion weeks, the calendar also includes other events like trunk shows, showroom presentations, and product launches. Trunk shows and showroom presentations provide an opportunity for designers to showcase their collections directly to buyers and potential customers. Product launches, on the other hand, are used to introduce new trends, collaborations, or collections to the market. Moreover, the fashion calendar helps journalists and fashion reporters to keep track of important events and plan their coverage. They use the calendar as a reference to attend runway shows, schedule interviews with designers, and report on emerging trends in the industry. Overall, a fashion calendar serves as a centralized source of information for the fashion industry, ensuring that everyone involved in the design, production, promotion, and reporting of fashion is on the same page. It helps to maximize efficiency, minimize conflicts, and foster collaboration among designers, brands, retailers, journalists, and other industry stakeholders.

Fashion Campaign

A fashion campaign is a coordinated marketing strategy that aims to promote a specific fashion brand, collection, or product. It typically involves a series of visual, digital, and/or print advertisements that showcase the brand's designs and convey its aesthetic, values, and message to the target audience. The purpose of a fashion campaign is to create awareness, generate interest, and ultimately drive sales by creating a strong and memorable brand presence. It serves as a powerful tool to establish or reinforce the brand's identity, create desire among consumers, and position the brand as a leader in the industry.

Fashion Capital

The term "Fashion Capital" refers to a city or location that is recognized as a global hub for the fashion industry. It generally denotes a place that is influential in terms of fashion design, production, and trends, serving as a significant center for the creation, marketing, and consumption of fashion products. A fashion capital often possesses several key characteristics that distinguish it from other cities. Firstly, it is home to a concentration of renowned fashion designers, fashion houses, and influential industry figures. These individuals and establishments play a crucial role in shaping the overall aesthetic, innovation, and style direction within the fashion community. Secondly, a fashion capital attracts and cultivates a diverse and vibrant fashion scene. This includes hosting major fashion weeks and events where designers from around the world showcase their latest collections. These events offer a platform for designers to gain exposure, establish connections, and gain recognition within the industry. Furthermore, a fashion capital typically boasts a rich cultural heritage and history in relation to fashion and textile production. It may have a long tradition of craftsmanship, artisanal skills, and specialized manufacturing techniques that contribute to the city's reputation as a premier fashion destination. In addition, a fashion capital is often characterized by a strong retail sector, with a multitude of high-end boutiques, luxury department stores, and concept stores. These establishments attract both local and international shoppers, contributing significantly to the overall economy of the city. Moreover, a fashion capital serves as a center for education and research in fashion design and related fields. It may be home to renowned fashion schools and institutions that offer comprehensive programs and resources for aspiring designers, further enhancing the city's influence and fostering the development of talent. In conclusion, a fashion capital is a city or location that holds prominence and recognition within the global fashion industry. It combines elements such as influential designers, fashion events, cultural heritage, retail infrastructure, and educational institutions to create a dynamic and thriving fashion ecosystem.

Fashion Capitals

A fashion capital refers to a city or a region that serves as a prominent hub for the fashion industry, playing a significant role in the production, design, and distribution of clothing and accessories. These fashion capitals are widely recognized for their influence and innovation in setting trends, shaping styles, and fostering creativity within the fashion world. These cities are characterized by a concentration of fashion businesses, including designer studios, fashion houses, ateliers, textile mills, showrooms, and retail stores, attracting talented individuals and industry professionals from around the globe. They often host fashion weeks, trade shows, and industry events that bring together designers, buyers, media, and fashion enthusiasts to showcase and promote upcoming collections, establish business connections, and provide a platform for networking and collaboration.

Fashion Career Fair

A fashion career fair is an event specifically organized for individuals interested in pursuing a career in fashion design. It provides a platform for various fashion companies, brands, and industry professionals to showcase their work, recruit new talent, and connect with aspiring fashion designers. During a fashion career fair, attendees have the opportunity to interact with representatives from different fashion companies and learn about the career opportunities available in the fashion industry. These representatives may include designers, stylists, merchandisers, brand managers, and other professionals who play a key role in the fashion design process.

Fashion Casting

A fashion casting is a crucial step in the fashion design process where designers select models who will showcase their clothing collections on the runway or in print campaigns. It involves a rigorous selection process to find the most suitable models who embody the aesthetic and vision of the designer. In a fashion casting, designers and their casting directors review portfolios and attend casting calls to view potential models. They assess various factors like physical attributes, personality, and ability to effectively portray the desired image and style. Models are evaluated based on their height, body proportions, flexibility, and overall appearance.

Fashion Casual Style

Fashion Casual Style refers to a clothing style that strikes a balance between comfort and sophistication. It is a popular fashion trend that incorporates relaxed and laid-back elements into one's outfit while still maintaining a level of fashion-forwardness. Characterized by its effortless and approachable nature, Fashion Casual Style allows individuals to express their personal style in a more relaxed and comfortable way. It offers a departure from formal, dressier attire and provides a more relaxed alternative without sacrificing style or fashionability.

Fashion Charity

A fashion charity refers to a nonprofit organization that focuses on using fashion as a means to raise funds, awareness, and support for various charitable causes. These organizations utilize the power and influence of the fashion industry to make a positive impact on society by addressing social, environmental, and humanitarian issues. Fashion charities often collaborate with fashion designers, brands, and industry professionals to create unique fundraising events, campaigns, and initiatives. These efforts aim to engage and involve the fashion community and general public in supporting important causes and making a difference through their love for fashion.

Fashion Chic Style

The fashion chic style is a design aesthetic that embraces a sophisticated and elegant look, characterized by understated confidence, timeless pieces, and attention to detail. It is a style that exudes glamour and sophistication while maintaining a sense of effortless grace. When it comes to fashion chic style, simplicity and minimalism are key. Clean lines, tailored cuts, and classic silhouettes are at the forefront, creating a refined and polished look. The focus is on quality over quantity, with a few well-chosen pieces that can be mixed and matched to create a variety of stylish outfits.

Fashion Chiffon

Fashion Chiffon is a lightweight and sheer fabric commonly used in the fashion industry. It is made from synthetic fibers, such as polyester, nylon, and rayon, or natural fibers, such as silk or cotton. The word "chiffon" originates from the French language, which means "rag" or "cloth." The characteristic feature of fashion chiffon is its soft and flowing texture, which gives garments an elegant and romantic appearance. It is a popular choice for designing evening wear, bridal gowns, and high-end couture due to its luxurious look and feel.

Fashion Cocktail Attire

Cocktail attire is a formal dress code that is typically worn to social events or parties held in the evening. It is a semi-formal style that falls between casual wear and formal evening wear, and is often referred to as the "little black dress" or the "cocktail dress." The essence of cocktail attire lies in its versatility and elegance. It allows individuals to showcase their personal style while adhering to the expected level of sophistication for the occasion. The dress code is characterized by refined yet modern silhouettes, flattering cuts, and attention to detail.

Fashion Collection Presentation

A fashion collection presentation is an important event in the field of fashion design. It is a formal showcase of a designer's collection, where garments and accessories are displayed to potential buyers, industry professionals, and the media. The purpose of a fashion collection presentation is to introduce and promote the designer's new collection to the target audience. It serves as an opportunity for the designer to present their creative vision, craftsmanship, and aesthetic choices. The presentation allows the audience to understand the inspiration behind the collection, the materials used, and the overall design concept. Typically, a fashion collection presentation takes place in a designated venue, such as a runway, showroom, or presentation space. The designer carefully curates the presentation, ensuring that the garments and accessories are arranged in a visually appealing and cohesive manner. Each look is styled and displayed to showcase its unique attributes and to convey the desired mood and message of the collection. The presentation itself may take various forms, depending on the designer's preferences and the nature of the collection. It can involve models walking down a runway, posing or standing in designated areas, or even interactive installations where the audience can experience the collection in a more immersive way. The designer may also incorporate music, lighting, and other elements to enhance the overall atmosphere and create a memorable experience for the audience. Fashion collection presentations are crucial for establishing the designer's brand image and reputation. They provide an opportunity for industry professionals, such as buyers and editors, to view the collection up close and make informed decisions regarding potential collaborations, purchases, or press coverage. Media coverage of the presentation can generate buzz, increase brand visibility, and attract potential customers. In conclusion, a fashion collection presentation is a formal event where a designer presents their new collection to a targeted audience. It showcases the designer's creative vision, craftsmanship, and aesthetic choices, aiming to promote the collection and establish the designer's brand image. The presentation is carefully curated and can take various forms, providing an opportunity for industry professionals to make informed decisions and generating media coverage for the designer.

Fashion Color Palette

A fashion color palette refers to a carefully curated set of colors that are specifically chosen and used within the context of fashion design. It serves as a guide for designers, enabling them to create cohesive and harmonious color schemes for their clothing or accessory collections. The color palette is crucial in fashion design as it plays a major role in determining the overall aesthetic and mood of a collection. It helps convey the designer's intended message, whether it is a bold and vibrant look, or a soft and delicate feel.

Fashion Columnist

A fashion columnist is a professional writer or journalist who specializes in writing about fashion design. They typically work for newspapers, magazines, or online publications, and their primary role is to provide insightful and informative commentary on the latest trends, styles, and fashion events. The fashion columnist plays a crucial role in the fashion industry by offering expertise, analysis, and opinions about various aspects of fashion design. They are knowledgeable about different designers, brands, collections, and fashion shows, and they use their expertise to provide readers with a deeper understanding of the fashion world.

Fashion Competition

A fashion competition is an event in the fashion industry where fashion designers compete against each other to showcase their talent, creativity, and skills in designing clothing and accessories. It serves as a platform for designers to exhibit their unique styles and interpretations of fashion trends. Participants in a fashion competition are typically required to create and present a collection of outfits that adhere to a specific theme or concept. They are given the opportunity to unleash their artistic vision and demonstrate their ability to create cohesive and innovative designs. Fashion competitions may focus on various aspects of fashion design, such as haute couture, streetwear, sustainable fashion, or bridal wear. Judges, who are usually eminent figures in the fashion industry, evaluate the designs based on factors like originality, craftsmanship, construction techniques, use of materials, and overall presentation. They consider how well the participants have interpreted and executed the given theme, as well as the level of skill and creativity demonstrated in their designs. The winner or winners of a fashion competition often receive recognition, prestige, and valuable opportunities to further their career in the fashion industry. They may be offered internships or collaborations with established fashion brands, exposure in renowned fashion publications, or invitations to showcase their designs on prestigious runways or at other fashion-related events. Fashion competitions serve as an important platform for emerging designers to gain exposure and make a name for themselves in the highly competitive fashion industry. They provide a valuable opportunity for designers to network with industry professionals, gain feedback on their work, and receive recognition for their talent and hard work.

Fashion Concept Development

Fashion Concept Development is the process of transforming an initial idea or inspiration into a fully developed and cohesive fashion collection. It involves the exploration, research, and refinement of various elements such as theme, color palette, fabric selection, silhouette, and detailing to create a unique and compelling fashion design. At the heart of Fashion Concept Development lies creativity and innovation. It is a critical stage in the design process where fashion designers translate their creative vision into wearable and marketable garments. The concept development phase serves as the foundation for the entire design process, guiding designers in making informed decisions regarding the overall direction and aesthetic of their collection. During Fashion Concept Development, designers typically start by researching and gathering inspiration from various sources such as art, culture, history, nature, or current trends. This research helps them to develop a strong concept or theme that will act as the narrative or story behind their collection. Once a concept is established, designers begin to explore and develop other crucial elements of the collection, such as the color palette. Colors play a fundamental role in fashion design as they evoke emotions and set the tone for the overall aesthetic. Designers carefully select colors that complement their concept and convey the desired mood and message of the collection. Fabric selection is also a crucial aspect of Fashion Concept Development. Designers consider the weight, texture, drape, and durability of fabrics to ensure they align with the desired silhouette and overall aesthetic of the collection. Different fabric choices can greatly impact the final outcome of the design, as they can enhance or detract from the intended concept. Silhouette and detailing are further explored during the concept development phase. Designers experiment with various shapes, proportions, and construction techniques to create unique and innovative garments. They consider how these elements interact with the concept, ensuring that each design reflects the overall theme and narrative. Fashion Concept Development is a dynamic and iterative process. Designers constantly refine and reassess their ideas, making adjustments based on feedback, market research, or their own intuition. It requires a balance of creativity and practicality, as designers aim to create designs that are not only aesthetically pleasing but also commercially viable. In conclusion, Fashion Concept Development is the creative and strategic process that takes an initial fashion idea and transforms it into a cohesive and marketable fashion collection. It encompasses the exploration and refinement of various elements such as theme, color palette, fabric selection, silhouette, and detailing to bring the designer's vision to life.

Fashion Concept Sketches

Fashion Concept Sketches are visual representations or drawings created by fashion designers to communicate their design ideas for a collection or specific garments. These sketches are an essential part of the design process as they allow designers to visualize and conceptualize their ideas before translating them into actual garments. The main purpose of fashion concept sketches is to convey the designer's creative vision and provide a clear representation of the proposed designs. They typically include details such as the silhouette, color scheme, fabric choice, and other design elements that define the aesthetic of the collection.

Fashion Conference

A fashion conference is an industry event that brings together professionals from the fashion design field to discuss and showcase the latest trends, innovations, and challenges in the fashion industry. It serves as a platform for designers, retailers, manufacturers, stylists, journalists, and other fashion enthusiasts to connect, learn, and exchange ideas. The primary goal of a fashion conference is to provide a collaborative environment where attendees can gain insights into the current state of the industry and explore future possibilities. Through keynote speeches, panel discussions, workshops, and exhibitions, participants can expand their knowledge, refine their skills, and stay up-to-date with emerging fashion trends.

Fashion Consultant

A fashion consultant is a professional who offers expert advice and guidance to individuals or organizations in the field of fashion design. They possess a deep knowledge and understanding of current fashion trends, styles, fabrics, and accessories. A fashion consultant works closely with clients to help them discover and develop their personal style, while also taking into consideration their body shape, skin tone, and lifestyle. They provide recommendations on clothing, footwear, accessories, and even hairstyles that will best suit the client's preferences and needs. The role of a fashion consultant extends beyond simply suggesting what to wear. They also assist clients in creating a cohesive wardrobe by helping them choose versatile pieces that can be mixed and matched, ensuring maximum use of existing clothing items. They may also advise on the appropriate colors, patterns, and textures that flatter the client's unique features. In addition to working with individual clients, fashion consultants often collaborate with designers, retailers, and fashion companies. They contribute their expertise by providing insights into market trends, evaluating product lines, and offering suggestions for improvement. To excel in their role, fashion consultants need to stay updated with the latest fashion shows, industry news, and emerging designers. They must possess a keen eye for detail, a sense of creativity, and strong communication skills to effectively convey their ideas and recommendations to clients. Overall, a fashion consultant plays a significant role in helping individuals and organizations navigate the ever-changing world of fashion. Through their knowledge and expertise, they guide their clients towards making informed fashion choices that align with their personal style, body type, and lifestyle.

Fashion Cotton

Fashion Cotton is a type of fabric commonly used in the fashion industry for various applications. It is a versatile and widely favored material due to its natural qualities and aesthetic appeal. Cotton is a soft, natural fiber that comes from the cotton plant, which is primarily grown in warm climates. It has been cultivated for thousands of years and has become one of the most popular fibers in the fashion industry. Fashion Cotton is known for its breathability, moisture-absorbing properties, and comfort. It allows air to circulate freely, making it an ideal choice for clothing in warm weather. The fabric also has excellent moisture-wicking capabilities, keeping the wearer dry and comfortable. These properties make it suitable for both casual and formal wear, as well as sportswear and loungewear. In addition to its functional qualities, Fashion Cotton is highly versatile and can be easily dyed, printed, and manipulated. It can be woven into various textures and patterns, such as twill, satin, and plain weaves, making it suitable for a wide range of fashion designs. The fabric takes colors well, resulting in vibrant and long-lasting hues. Fashion Cotton is also known for its durability and strength. It can withstand regular wear and tear, making it a practical choice for everyday clothing. However, it is important to note that the quality and thickness of the fabric can vary, affecting its longevity. When designing with Fashion Cotton, fashion designers often consider its natural properties and characteristics. They utilize its breathability and comfort to create garments that promote ease of movement and wellbeing. The fabric's ability to hold vibrant colors and patterns allows designers to experiment with bold and expressive designs. In summary, Fashion Cotton is a versatile fabric widely used in the fashion industry. It offers breathability, moisture-absorbing properties, and comfort, making it suitable for various clothing applications. Its versatility, durability, and aesthetic appeal make it a favored choice among fashion designers.

Fashion Council

A Fashion Council is an organization comprised of industry professionals, designers, fashion experts, and key stakeholders within the fashion industry. It is responsible for promoting, supporting, and shaping the direction of the fashion design sector. The main objective of a Fashion Council is to foster collaboration, innovation, and growth within the fashion industry. It serves as a platform for designers to showcase their collections, exchange ideas, and receive guidance and mentorship from experienced professionals. The council also plays a crucial role in promoting local and emerging designers, providing them with exposure and opportunities to establish their brands nationally and internationally. Additionally, a Fashion Council serves as a bridge between the fashion industry and the government, advocating for policies and initiatives that facilitate the growth and development of the sector. It actively engages with policymakers to address issues such as intellectual property rights, copyright protection, and trade regulations, ensuring a conducive environment for fashion designers to thrive. Furthermore, a Fashion Council organizes industry events, fashion weeks, and shows to showcase the talent and creativity of designers. These events not only provide a platform for designers to present their collections to buyers, retailers, and the media but also serve as a source of inspiration for future fashion trends. The council sets the standards for fashion shows and helps designers navigate the complex world of runway presentations, styling, and production. In conclusion, a Fashion Council plays a pivotal role in the fashion design industry by supporting and promoting designers, fostering collaboration, advocating for industry-friendly policies, and organizing fashion events. It serves as a beacon of creativity, excellence, and innovation, shaping the future of fashion design.

Fashion Critic

A fashion critic is a professional who assesses and evaluates clothing designs, styles, trends, and overall fashion sense. They provide their opinion and analysis on various aspects of fashion, including garments, accessories, hair, makeup, and overall visual presentation. A fashion critic closely observes fashion shows, collections, and fashion events to gain a deep understanding of the latest trends and styles. They analyze the craftsmanship, materials, and construction techniques used in garments and accessories. They also pay attention to the colors, patterns, and textures employed by designers in their collections. When evaluating fashion designs, a critic considers the level of creativity, originality, and innovation exhibited by the designer. They assess whether the collection aligns with current trends or offers a unique perspective. A fashion critic also evaluates how well the designer has executed their vision and the cohesiveness of the overall collection. In addition to assessing the garments themselves, a fashion critic pays attention to how they are styled and accessorized. They evaluate the hair, makeup, and overall styling choices made by fashion designers and stylists. They analyze how well these elements enhance and complement the clothing designs. A fashion critic often writes reviews and articles for fashion magazines, blogs, newspapers, and other media outlets. They provide detailed critiques of fashion shows, collections, and individual designs. Their goal is to provide readers with valuable insights and opinions that can help them navigate the ever-changing world of fashion. Overall, a fashion critic serves as an authority and guide for individuals seeking to stay informed and make informed fashion choices. They play a crucial role in shaping public opinions and perceptions about fashion trends, designers, and the industry as a whole.

Fashion Curator

A Fashion Curator is a professional who is responsible for selecting and showcasing fashion pieces in a curated and meaningful way. They have a deep knowledge and understanding of fashion trends, styles, and history, and they use this expertise to curate collections for various purposes like exhibitions, fashion shows, magazines, and online platforms. The primary role of a Fashion Curator is to curate fashion collections that tell a story or convey a specific theme. They carefully select garments, accessories, and other fashion artifacts that align with the desired narrative or concept. This involves researching, exploring different fashion eras, and analyzing the contemporary fashion landscape to find the most relevant pieces that fit the desired aesthetic and message. A Fashion Curator also collaborates with designers, brands, and institutions to create exhibitions or displays that showcase fashion as a form of art. They work closely with designers to understand their creative vision and curate collections that highlight their unique style and craftsmanship. They also collaborate with museums, galleries, and fashion institutions to bring their curated collections to the public and educate them about fashion history and cultural impact. In addition to curating fashion collections, a Fashion Curator is responsible for organizing fashion shows and events. They liaise with designers, models, hairstylists, makeup artists, and other professionals to ensure that the event runs smoothly and represents the curated collection in the best possible way. They have a keen eye for detail and aesthetics, and they oversee the entire production process, from conceptualization to execution. Overall, a Fashion Curator plays a crucial role in the fashion industry by presenting fashion as a form of art and storytelling. They bridge the gap between creativity and commerce by curating collections that are visually appealing, intellectually stimulating, and commercially viable. Their expertise in fashion history and trends allows them to create unique and captivating exhibitions, displays, and events that engage and inspire fashion enthusiasts worldwide.

Fashion Customization

Fashion customization refers to the process of personalizing or modifying fashion designs to suit individual preferences and tastes. It involves taking a pre-existing clothing item or accessory and making alterations to its design, style, or fit in order to create a unique and personalized fashion statement. This customization can be done through various means, such as tailoring, embellishments, additions or subtractions of components, or changes to colors and patterns. By customizing their fashion pieces, individuals can express their individuality, creativity, and personal style, and establish a distinctive image or brand.

Fashion Denim

Fashion denim is a term used in fashion design to refer to a specific type of fabric that is commonly used in the creation of jeans and other denim clothing items. Denim is a sturdy cotton fabric that is woven in a way that creates a distinctive diagonal pattern known as a twill weave. This fabric is then typically dyed with indigo, resulting in its characteristic deep blue color. In fashion design, denim has become an iconic material that is associated with casual and versatile clothing styles. Fashion designers often incorporate denim into their collections to create a range of different looks, from rugged and edgy to classic and timeless. Denim can be used to create a variety of garment types, including jeans, jackets, shirts, skirts, and dresses.

Fashion Design Competition

A fashion design competition is a prestigious event that allows aspiring fashion designers to showcase their creativity, talent, and skills. It serves as a platform for designers to present their unique and innovative designs to a panel of industry experts, including renowned designers, fashion professionals, and stakeholders. The primary objective of a fashion design competition is to identify and recognize emerging talents in the field of fashion design. Participants are given an opportunity to demonstrate their ability to conceptualize and create original fashion pieces that are aesthetically pleasing, marketable, and reflective of current fashion trends. The competition often focuses on specific themes, trends, or concepts that designers need to incorporate into their designs. During the competition, participants are required to present a collection of garments or outfits that embody their interpretation of the given theme. They are expected to showcase their proficiency in various aspects of the design process, including research, sketching, fabric selection, color coordination, pattern making, and garment construction. Attention to detail, creativity, originality, and craftsmanship are key factors that judges consider when evaluating the designs. The competition is typically divided into multiple rounds, allowing designers to progress through each stage based on their performance and the judges' assessments. In addition to presenting their designs, participants may also be required to articulate their design concepts, inspirations, and target market to the judges. This allows the designers to demonstrate their understanding of the fashion industry and their ability to communicate their ideas effectively. Winners of a fashion design competition are often rewarded with valuable prizes, scholarships, mentorship programs, internships, or opportunities to showcase their collections at renowned fashion events or runways. These accolades serve as a catalyst for their career growth and provide them with valuable exposure and recognition within the fashion industry. In summary, a fashion design competition is a highly esteemed event that provides aspiring fashion designers with a platform to showcase their creativity, gain industry recognition, and propel their careers forward. It challenges designers to push their boundaries, think outside the box, and create outstanding fashion pieces that resonate with the judges, industry professionals, and consumers.

Fashion Design Portfolio

A fashion design portfolio is a collection of original and curated work that showcases a fashion designer's creativity, skills, and ideas. It is a valuable tool used by fashion designers to communicate their design aesthetic, technical abilities, and potential to prospective employers, collaborators, or clients. Within a fashion design portfolio, designers typically include a variety of materials such as sketches, illustrations, technical drawings, fabric swatches, photographs of finished garments, and sometimes even runway or editorial images. These materials aim to demonstrate the designer's ability to conceptualize and develop unique and visually compelling fashion designs. Each piece included in a fashion design portfolio is carefully selected to highlight a designer's strongest work and illustrate their artistic vision. The portfolio may be organized by theme, collection, or specific design projects, allowing viewers to understand the designer's creative process and aesthetic direction. This organization provides a cohesive narrative that helps potential employers or clients envision how the designer's style and skills align with their own brand or project needs. Additionally, a fashion design portfolio often includes supporting documentation such as design concept statements, fabric sourcing information, and technical specifications. These details offer further insight into the designer's thought process and demonstrate their attention to detail and professional approach to the design process. A well-executed fashion design portfolio not only showcases a designer's technical skills but also reflects their ability to develop cohesive and marketable collections. It should convey their understanding of current fashion trends, cultural influences, and industry standards. Moreover, it should demonstrate their ability to interpret and reinterpret these trends into innovative and unique designs that have the potential to resonate with a target audience. In the highly competitive world of fashion design, a strong portfolio can be the key to opening doors and securing professional opportunities. Therefore, fashion designers invest significant time and effort in curating their portfolios, ensuring they are visually striking, effectively communicative, and demonstrate their potential to contribute to the ever-evolving world of fashion.

Fashion Design Software

A fashion design software refers to a computer program that allows fashion designers to create, design, and visualize their clothing collections digitally. It serves as a tool to streamline and enhance the design process, enabling designers to bring their ideas to life in a digital format before proceeding to the physical production phase. By utilizing a fashion design software, designers can create detailed sketches, renderings, and technical drawings using a variety of tools such as digital pencils, brushes, and color palettes. These software applications often include pre-loaded templates and libraries of garment patterns, textiles, and accessories that can be used as a starting point or customized according to the designer's vision. The main purpose of fashion design software is to provide designers with a virtual platform where they can experiment with different styles, shapes, colors, and fabrics in a cost-effective and time-efficient manner. It allows them to visualize how their designs would look on a 3D model or a flat pattern, enabling them to make modifications and adjustments before sending their designs to production. Moreover, fashion design software also facilitates communication and collaboration between designers, patternmakers, and manufacturers. It allows for the easy sharing of digital files and designs, as well as the ability to annotate and provide feedback directly on the software. This fosters a more efficient workflow and reduces errors and misinterpretations during the production process. Overall, a fashion design software is an essential tool for modern-day fashion designers, providing them with a platform to explore their creativity, improve productivity, and bring innovative designs to life. It combines artistry and technology, enabling designers to create stunning collections with precision and speed, ultimately revolutionizing the fashion industry.

Fashion Designer Showcase

A fashion designer showcase refers to an event or platform where fashion designers present their latest collections or designs to a target audience, which usually includes buyers, press, and industry professionals. It serves as a way for designers to showcase their creativity, innovation, and craftsmanship, while also gaining exposure and potential business opportunities. During a fashion designer showcase, designers typically organize a runway show, where models walk down a catwalk or runway wearing the designer's garments or accessories. The show is carefully curated and choreographed to highlight the designer's vision and aesthetic. This includes the selection of music, lighting, and overall ambiance, all of which contribute to creating a captivating and memorable experience for the audience. Designers may also choose to showcase their work through presentations, exhibitions, or installations. These alternative formats allow for a more intimate and interactive experience, where attendees can examine the details and construction of the garments up close, or engage in conversations with the designer themselves. Alongside the presentation of their collections, fashion designer showcases often include opportunities for networking and business development. Buyers from retail stores or boutiques attend the event to preview the collections and potentially place orders for their stores. This direct interaction between designers and buyers is an essential part of the fashion industry's supply chain, enabling designers to establish relationships and secure distribution channels for their products. Furthermore, the press coverage generated from a fashion designer showcase is instrumental in promoting the designer and their brand. Fashion journalists and editors attend these events to report on the latest trends and emerging talents, which can significantly impact a designer's visibility and reputation. This media exposure contributes to the overall success and longevity of a designer's career. In conclusion, a fashion designer showcase is a platform for designers to present their collections to a targeted audience, including buyers and press. It plays a pivotal role in promoting designers' creativity, facilitating business opportunities, and enhancing their brand's reputation within the fashion industry.

Fashion Director

A Fashion Director is a key role in the fashion industry, responsible for overseeing and directing the overall creative vision and styling of a fashion brand or publication. They play a crucial role in the artistic and commercial success of a fashion brand by curating and guiding the design team, ensuring that the collections align with the brand's aesthetic and target audience. In the context of fashion design, the Fashion Director is responsible for developing and defining the brand's visual identity, setting the tone for the collections, and establishing the brand's distinctive style. They work closely with designers, merchandisers, and buyers to determine the direction and themes for each season's collection. Their creative eye and artistic sensibility enable them to conceptualize and translate trends into innovative and appealing designs that resonate with the brand's target market. Moreover, the Fashion Director is involved in the creative process from start to finish. They are responsible for selecting fabrics, colors, and materials, ensuring that they align with the brand's aesthetic and quality standards. They also oversee fittings and ensure that the garments fit and drape perfectly, making necessary adjustments to achieve an impeccable fit. Additionally, the Fashion Director collaborates with photographers, models, and stylists to create captivating and impactful visual campaigns and editorial shoots. Furthermore, the Fashion Director is responsible for staying abreast of industry trends, market demands, and consumer preferences. They conduct research and analysis to identify emerging fashion trends and translate them into innovative designs that resonate with the brand's target market. They attend fashion shows, trade events, and showrooms to stay informed about the latest developments in the fashion industry and identify potential collaborations or partnerships. The Fashion Director's role extends beyond design and aesthetics. They also contribute to the financial success of the brand by making strategic decisions regarding pricing, production, and marketing. They analyze market trends, consumer feedback, and sales data to inform their decisions and drive the brand's profitability. They work closely with the sales and marketing teams to create effective marketing campaigns that promote the brand and generate sales. In summary, the Fashion Director is a pivotal figure in the fashion industry, responsible for shaping the creative direction and success of a fashion brand. Their expertise in design, trend forecasting, and business acumen enable them to make informed decisions that drive the brand's aesthetic, profitability, and market relevance.

Fashion Distributor

A fashion distributor is a company or individual that is responsible for distributing fashion products to retailers or directly to consumers. They play a crucial role in the fashion industry, as they help connect fashion designers and manufacturers with their target audience. The primary role of a fashion distributor is to ensure that fashion products reach the right market at the right time. They work closely with fashion designers, manufacturers, and retailers to create a seamless distribution process. This involves managing the logistics of transporting fashion products from the production facility to the retail store or directly to the consumer.

Fashion Documentary

A fashion documentary, in the context of fashion design, refers to a non-fiction film or video that explores various aspects of the fashion industry, including the history, design processes, cultural influences, and societal impact. This genre of documentary aims to provide an in-depth and informative look into the fashion world, capturing the creative journey, struggles, and achievements of fashion designers, models, photographers, and other key players in the industry. It documents their experiences, perspectives, and contributions, presenting a comprehensive narrative of the evolution of fashion. Fashion documentaries often feature interviews with prominent figures in the industry, showcasing their expertise and shedding light on their unique creative processes. They provide insights into the inspirations behind fashion collections, the materials and techniques employed, and the challenges faced during the design and production phases. Additionally, fashion documentaries highlight the cultural and societal influences that shape fashion trends. They explore the interplay between fashion, art, music, politics, and popular culture, allowing viewers to connect the dots and understand the wider impact of fashion on society. These documentaries also delve into the historical significance of fashion, tracing its roots and examining how it has evolved over time. They explore iconic fashion moments, movements, and designers that have revolutionized the industry, leaving a lasting impact. Moreover, fashion documentaries serve as a platform for showcasing emerging talents and unconventional approaches to design. They give voice to underrepresented designers, highlighting their unique perspectives, contributions, and challenges faced within the fashion industry. In summary, fashion documentaries provide a captivating and informative glimpse into the world of fashion design. They present a rich tapestry of creativity, history, culture, and societal impact, allowing viewers to deepen their understanding and appreciation for the art of fashion.

Fashion Draping

Fashion draping is a technique used in fashion design that involves manipulating and pinning fabric directly on a dress form or live model to create three-dimensional garments. It allows designers to visualize and experiment with different silhouettes, shapes, and design elements before cutting and sewing the fabric. The process of fashion draping begins by draping a basic fabric block, typically made from muslin or calico, on the dress form or model. The fabric is carefully pinned, tucked, and folded to create the desired shape and structure. The designer uses their creativity and knowledge of garment construction to mold the fabric and make adjustments to achieve the desired fit and style. During the draping process, the designer pays attention to the grainlines of the fabric, ensuring that they follow the body's natural curves and lines. The fabric is manipulated to create movement, volume, and drapes that flatter the body shape and enhance the design aesthetics. Once the initial draping is complete, the designer may make further adjustments by using additional pins or marking the fabric with chalk to indicate seams, dart placements, or style lines. These markings act as guidelines for the next stage of garment construction. After the draping process, the fabric is carefully removed from the dress form or model, and a flat pattern is created by tracing or transferring the draped fabric onto paper or muslin. This flat pattern serves as a blueprint for cutting the final fabric and sewing the garment together. Fashion draping is an essential skill for fashion designers as it allows them to sculpt and visualize their designs in three-dimensional form. It provides a hands-on approach to design development, enabling designers to experiment with different shapes, proportions, and details before committing to the final garment construction. The technique of fashion draping combines artistic flair with technical expertise, resulting in unique and well-fitted garments that are both aesthetically pleasing and functional.

Fashion E-Commerce Platforms

Fashion E-Commerce

Fashion E-commerce refers to the buying and selling of fashion products, including clothing, accessories, and footwear, through online platforms. It is a digital marketplace where fashion designers, brands, and retailers can showcase and sell their products to a global audience. In the context of fashion design, E-commerce has revolutionized the way designers reach customers and sell their creations. It provides a platform for designers to establish their brand presence, display their collections, and connect with potential buyers without the limitations of physical retail stores. Fashion E-commerce platforms typically feature a user-friendly interface that allows customers to browse through different products, filter their search based on specific criteria such as size, color, or style, and make purchases with ease. These platforms often provide detailed product descriptions, high-quality images, and customer reviews to help customers make informed decisions. For fashion designers, E-commerce offers various advantages. Firstly, it allows designers to reach a wider audience beyond their local or regional markets. Through digital platforms, designers can attract customers from different parts of the world, expanding their customer base and increasing sales potential. Additionally, E-commerce provides designers with a cost-effective way to sell their products. Setting up an online store requires minimal investment compared to establishing a physical retail outlet. Designers can save on expenses such as rent, utilities, and staffing, allowing them to offer competitive prices for their products. Fashion E-commerce also enables designers to gather valuable data and insights about their customers' preferences and purchasing behavior. Through analytics tools, designers can track sales trends, identify popular products, and understand customer demographics, which can inform future design decisions and marketing strategies. In conclusion, Fashion E-commerce has significantly transformed the fashion design industry. It has provided designers with a global platform to showcase and sell their creations, expanded their customer reach, and provided a cost-effective and data-driven approach to running a fashion business.

Fashion Editor

A fashion editor is a key role in the field of fashion design, responsible for overseeing and curating the visual content of a fashion publication or brand. They play a crucial role in shaping the direction and aesthetic of a publication or brand, working closely with designers, photographers, stylists, and other creative professionals. The primary role of a fashion editor is to select and style garments, accessories, and other fashion items for editorial shoots, fashion shows, and campaigns. They collaborate with the creative team to develop concepts and themes, ensuring that the visuals align with the brand's or publication's overall vision and target audience. As a fashion editor, one must have a keen eye for trends, understanding the current and upcoming fashion movements and styles. They are responsible for conducting research and staying up-to-date with industry news to provide insights and guidance to the creative team. They attend fashion shows, tradeshows, and industry events to scout and source garments and accessories. An essential part of a fashion editor's role is to oversee the entire production process of fashion editorials or campaigns. This includes concept development, model selection, location scouting, and coordinating the work of photographers, stylists, hair and makeup artists, and set designers. They ensure that the execution of the creative vision is cohesive and visually striking. In addition to editorial shoots and campaigns, a fashion editor also has a hand in the selection and curation of fashion content for editorial features, articles, and interviews. They work closely with writers and photographers to create engaging and visually appealing fashion spreads that tell a compelling story. To be a successful fashion editor, one must possess strong communication, organization, and leadership skills. They need to have an in-depth knowledge of fashion history, designers, and brands, as well as a understanding of the current market trends and consumer preferences. In summary, a fashion editor is a vital figure in the fashion industry who is responsible for overseeing and curating the visual content of a fashion publication or brand. They collaborate with a team of creative professionals to develop concepts and themes, select and style garments and accessories, and ensure that the overall aesthetic aligns with the brand's or publication's vision. They also play a key role in the production and curation of fashion editorials and features.

Fashion Editorial

A fashion editorial is a visual narrative that showcases the latest trends and designs in the world of fashion. It is a form of fashion journalism that is typically presented in print publications, such as magazines, or online through fashion websites and blogs. The purpose of a fashion editorial is to inspire and inform readers about current fashion trends, designers, and styles. It is a way for designers, stylists, and photographers to showcase their work and express their creative vision through images and accompanying text.

Fashion Education Summit

A Fashion Education Summit is an event that brings together professionals, educators, students, and industry leaders from the fashion design field to share knowledge, ideas, and expertise. The summit serves as a platform for discussions, workshops, and presentations that aim to enhance the understanding and practice of fashion design education. During a Fashion Education Summit, participants engage in various activities such as panel discussions, keynote speeches, and interactive sessions. These activities cover a wide range of topics related to fashion education, including curriculum development, teaching methodologies, industry trends, and technological advancements. The summit provides opportunities for attendees to learn from each other's experiences, exchange best practices, and explore innovative approaches to fashion design education. One of the key objectives of a Fashion Education Summit is to foster collaboration and networking among professionals in the fashion industry. Participants have the chance to connect with like-minded individuals, form partnerships, and build relationships that can lead to future collaborations and career opportunities. The summit also serves as a platform for industry leaders to identify emerging talent and engage with aspiring fashion designers. Furthermore, a Fashion Education Summit plays a crucial role in promoting the importance of fashion design education and its impact on the industry. Through discussions and presentations, participants gain insights into the evolving nature of the fashion industry and the skills and knowledge required to succeed in this field. This awareness helps educators and institutions in developing relevant and updated curricula that meet industry demands and prepare students for successful careers in fashion design.

Fashion Education And Mentorship

Fashion Embroidery

Fashion embroidery refers to the technique of decorating garments or accessories with intricate and detailed designs using thread or yarn. It is a form of ornamentation that adds visual interest, texture, and a touch of luxury to the fabric. The process of fashion embroidery involves the careful placement of stitches on a fabric surface to create various patterns, motifs, or images. These stitches can be made by hand or with the help of a machine, depending on the complexity of the design and the desired outcome. The thread or yarn used for embroidery can be of different colors, thicknesses, and textures, allowing for endless creative possibilities. Embroidery has been a part of fashion for centuries, with its origins dating back to ancient civilizations. It was initially done by hand, using needles and threads made from natural fibers such as silk or wool. Over time, embroidery techniques and tools have evolved, making it easier and faster to create intricate designs. Today, fashion embroidery is widely used in both haute couture and ready-to-wear fashion. It can be found on a range of garments and accessories, including dresses, skirts, blouses, jackets, handbags, shoes, and even hats. Embroidery adds a sense of craftsmanship and individuality to these items, making them stand out in a sea of mass-produced fashion. The designs used in fashion embroidery can vary greatly, from simple floral motifs to complex scenes or abstract patterns. They can be inspired by various sources, such as nature, art, culture, or personal experiences. Fashion designers often collaborate with skilled embroiderers or embroidery houses to bring their vision to life, creating truly unique pieces that capture the essence of their brand. In addition to its decorative purpose, fashion embroidery can also serve functional roles. It can reinforce seams or patches, add structure to a garment, or enhance its drape and movement. Embroidered details can create focal points, draw attention to specific areas, or even flatter the wearer's body shape. Fashion embroidery is a versatile and timeless technique that continues to inspire and captivate both designers and fashion enthusiasts alike. Its intricate and delicate craftsmanship elevates garments and accessories, making them works of art that celebrate the beauty of thread and fabric.

Fashion Entrepreneur

A fashion entrepreneur is an individual who creates and operates a business in the fashion industry, leveraging their creativity, business acumen, and industry knowledge to develop and market fashionable clothing, accessories, or other fashion-related products. As a fashion entrepreneur, the individual is responsible for every aspect of their business, from designing and producing the products to marketing and selling them. They are often involved in the entire process, from concept development to retail distribution.

Fashion Ethical Fashion

Ethical fashion, in the context of fashion design, refers to the practice of creating clothing and accessories in a way that considers and respects the social, environmental, and economic impact of the fashion industry. From a social perspective, ethical fashion emphasizes fair labor practices and safe working conditions for garment workers. It aims to ensure that workers are paid a fair wage and have access to proper training and support. Ethical fashion also promotes the empowerment and well-being of workers, especially those in marginalized communities or developing countries. From an environmental standpoint, ethical fashion strives to minimize its ecological footprint. This involves reducing waste and pollution throughout the production process, using sustainable materials and processes, and prioritizing recycling and upcycling. Ethical fashion designers may also incorporate renewable energy sources and minimize water consumption in their operations. Furthermore, ethical fashion addresses the economic impact of the fashion industry by promoting responsible and transparent supply chains. This means sourcing materials from ethical suppliers who prioritize sustainability and social responsibility. Ethical fashion designers also strive to build long-term relationships with their suppliers, fostering fair trade practices and supporting local economies. Overall, ethical fashion designers are committed to creating garments and accessories that uphold a set of values centered around social justice, environmental sustainability, and economic responsibility. They are constantly seeking innovative ways to improve the sustainability and ethics of their practices, challenging the norms of the fast fashion industry, and leading the way towards a more responsible and conscious fashion future.

Fashion Ethics Lecture

The Fashion Ethics Lecture explores the moral and ethical considerations that arise in the field of fashion design. It aims to analyze the social, environmental, and economic implications of fashion choices while promoting sustainable and responsible practices within the industry. Throughout the lecture, various dimensions of fashion ethics are discussed, including labor rights, animal welfare, cultural appropriation, and environmental sustainability. By examining these aspects, fashion designers are encouraged to critically assess their creative processes, supply chains, and marketing strategies, with the ultimate goal of minimizing harm and maximizing ethical behavior.

Fashion Ethics

Fashion Ethics refers to the set of moral principles and values that govern the actions and decisions made by fashion designers in their design process as well as in the production and marketing of their fashion products. It involves considering the social, environmental, and economic impacts of fashion design and manufacturing, and taking responsibility for the consequences of these actions. Fashion designers need to be mindful of the ethical implications of their choices, such as the use of materials, labor practices, cultural appropriation, and environmental sustainability.

Fashion Event Planning

Fashion event planning refers to the process of organizing and managing events related to fashion design. These events could include fashion shows, runway presentations, fashion weeks, or new collection launches. The primary goal of fashion event planning is to create a platform for fashion designers to showcase their work and for industry professionals to network and discover new talent. The role of a fashion event planner is to coordinate all aspects of the event, from conceptualization to execution. This involves selecting a suitable venue, managing event logistics such as seating arrangements and lighting, and coordinating with designers, models, hair and makeup artists, and other stakeholders. A fashion event planner must also take into consideration factors such as budget, target audience, and the overall theme or concept of the event. One key aspect of fashion event planning is the fashion show, which serves as the centerpiece of the event. A fashion show is a carefully choreographed presentation of the designer's collection, usually featuring models walking on a runway or stage. The fashion event planner is responsible for coordinating all elements of the fashion show, including selecting the models, arranging their lineup, and ensuring that the flow of the show is smooth and seamless. In addition to the fashion show, a fashion event may also include other activities such as panel discussions, networking sessions, or pop-up shops. These additional components of the event serve to enrich the experience for attendees and provide further opportunities for designers to connect with industry professionals and potential buyers. Overall, fashion event planning is a crucial element of the fashion industry as it serves as a platform for designers to showcase their talent and for industry professionals to discover new trends and talent. By carefully organizing and managing fashion events, fashion event planners play a vital role in creating opportunities for designers and fostering the growth of the industry as a whole.

Fashion Event Sponsorship

Fashion event sponsorship refers to the financial or in-kind support provided by a brand, company, or individual to a fashion event or show. This support allows the sponsor to gain exposure and visibility among the target audience of the event while also helping to cover the costs and logistics of organizing the fashion event. In the context of fashion design, fashion event sponsorship plays a crucial role in bringing together designers, models, industry professionals, and fashion enthusiasts. These events provide a platform for showcasing new collections, promoting upcoming trends, and fostering creative collaborations.

Fashion Exhibition

A fashion exhibition is an event where fashion designers showcase their latest collections and creations to a select audience, typically including industry professionals, media, buyers, and fashion enthusiasts. It is a platform for designers to display their artistic vision, express their unique style, and captivate the audience with their innovative designs. At a fashion exhibition, designers present their collections through carefully curated runway shows or static displays. Runway shows involve models walking down a designated catwalk, showcasing the garments, accessories, and overall styling. Static displays, on the other hand, involve mannequins or dress forms where the garments are exhibited in a set design or vignette. These visual presentations allow attendees to closely examine every detail and appreciate the craftsmanship behind each piece.

Fashion Fabric Library

A fashion fabric library is a collection of textile samples used by fashion designers to explore and select fabrics for their designs. It serves as a resource for sourcing and referencing different types of fabrics, textures, colors, patterns, and prints. The fashion fabric library plays a crucial role in the design process, as it allows designers to physically examine and compare the properties of various fabrics. This helps them make informed decisions regarding the choice of fabric for a particular garment or collection. In a fashion fabric library, each sample is typically labeled with relevant information such as the fabric composition, weight, width, care instructions, and sometimes even the manufacturer or supplier details. This information helps designers assess the suitability of a fabric for their specific design requirements and also aids in the production process. The fabric samples in a fashion fabric library can vary in size, with some being small swatches and others larger panels. They may be organized and categorized based on different criteria, such as fabric type (cotton, silk, wool, etc.), weave structure (plain, twill, satin, etc.), or seasonality (summer, winter, etc.). Some libraries may also include sample books or catalogs, which showcase a wider range of fabrics from various manufacturers. When designing a new collection or individual garments, fashion designers often refer to the fabric library to draw inspiration and explore different possibilities. They can examine how a fabric drapes, stretches, or holds its shape and visualize how it would look and feel when used in a specific design. This hands-on approach to fabric selection allows designers to better understand the material's potential and make design decisions that complement the fabric's properties. The fashion fabric library is not only valuable for designers but also for those involved in the production process, such as pattern makers, sample makers, and manufacturers. It ensures consistent communication and understanding between all stakeholders by providing a tangible reference for the desired fabric choices and specifications.

Fashion Fabrication

Fashion Fabrication refers to the process of creating custom clothing and accessories using various materials and techniques. It involves the manipulation of fabrics, trims, and other components to construct garments that are unique and tailored to the wearer's preferences and specifications. In the world of fashion design, fabrication is an essential step in the production process. Designers use their creative flair and technical skills to transform raw materials into finished products that embody their vision and reflect current trends and styles.

Fashion Fair

A Fashion Fair is an event that showcases the latest trends and designs in the fashion industry. It serves as a platform for designers, brands, and fashion enthusiasts to come together and celebrate the artistry and creativity of fashion. The Fashion Fair typically takes place in a designated venue, such as a convention center or exhibition hall. It can be organized by fashion houses, fashion councils, or event management companies. The fair may have a specific theme or focus, such as haute couture, sustainable fashion, or emerging designers. One of the main features of a Fashion Fair is the fashion show. Models walk down the runway, showcasing the collections of various designers. These shows allow designers to present their latest creations to a wide audience, including buyers, journalists, and fashion influencers. The runway presentations often incorporate music, lighting, and choreography to create a captivating and immersive experience. In addition to fashion shows, a Fashion Fair may include exhibition spaces or stalls where brands and designers can display their products. These spaces allow attendees to interact with the designs, see the materials used, and ask questions about the collections. It provides an opportunity for designers to meet potential buyers, establish new partnerships, and generate interest in their brand. Another vital component of a Fashion Fair is the networking aspect. Designers, industry professionals, and fashion enthusiasts gather at the fair, creating opportunities for collaboration and networking. It allows designers to connect with buyers, suppliers, and potential investors. Fashion enthusiasts can meet like-minded individuals, share ideas, and learn from industry experts through panel discussions, workshops, and seminars that are often part of the fair's program. A Fashion Fair is not only a platform to promote and celebrate fashion but also a market where fashion professionals and consumers come together. It is an event that drives the fashion industry forward, introducing new trends, fostering innovation, and providing a platform for emerging designers to showcase their talent. Overall, a Fashion Fair is a vibrant and dynamic event that is essential in the world of fashion design.

Fashion Fashion Accelerator

A Fashion Fashion Accelerator is a program or organization that supports and nurtures emerging fashion designers, providing them with the necessary resources and guidance to accelerate their careers in the fashion industry. These accelerators typically offer a range of services and support systems to help designers develop their brands and expand their businesses. This can include mentorship, networking opportunities, access to industry professionals, funding, workspace, and educational workshops.

Fashion Fashion Advertising

Fashion advertising is a form of marketing communication that promotes and showcases fashion products and brands to a targeted audience. It is a strategic and creative process aimed at influencing consumer perceptions and behavior towards fashion items and trends. Within the context of fashion design, advertising plays a crucial role in creating brand awareness and establishing brand identity. It involves various channels and mediums, such as print media (magazines, newspapers), digital platforms (websites, social media), television, and outdoor advertisements, to deliver the fashion message to consumers. The main objective of fashion advertising is to increase product visibility, generate interest, and ultimately drive sales. The process of fashion advertising begins with extensive market research and target audience analysis. Designers and brands need to understand the preferences, lifestyles, and values of their target consumers in order to create effective advertising campaigns. This research informs the development of creative concepts, visuals, and copywriting that align with the brand image and the desires of the target audience. Once the advertising strategy is established, fashion designers collaborate with advertising agencies, photographers, models, stylists, and other professionals to bring their vision to life. These collaborations involve creating visually appealing and emotionally compelling imagery that captures the essence of the brand and the fashion product. The final advertisement may focus on showcasing individual pieces, demonstrating their versatility, or highlighting the overall aesthetic of the brand. In addition to visuals, fashion advertising also relies on persuasive language to communicate product features, benefits, and unique selling propositions. Copywriting is often used to create narratives, evoke emotions, or convey lifestyle aspirations associated with the fashion brand. Through carefully crafted taglines, slogans, and descriptions, designers aim to captivate the audience and persuade them to consider purchasing the showcased fashion items. Fashion advertising is not limited to promoting products, but also extends to building brand image and reputation. It enables designers to establish a specific brand identity and differentiate themselves from competitors. Through consistent messaging, visual cues, and storytelling, fashion brands create a distinct persona and establish a connection with their target audience. This helps in building brand loyalty and fostering long-term relationships with consumers.

Fashion Fashion Apprenticeship

A Fashion Apprenticeship is a formal training program in the field of fashion design, aimed at providing individuals with the necessary skills and knowledge to pursue a career in the industry. It is a structured learning experience that combines theory and practical training, under the guidance of experienced professionals in the fashion field. The main objective of a Fashion Apprenticeship is to develop and enhance the creative skills of aspiring fashion designers, while also providing them with a comprehensive understanding of the fashion industry. The program typically covers a wide range of topics, including design principles, garment construction, fabric selection, pattern making, and fashion illustration. During a Fashion Apprenticeship, apprentices have the opportunity to work closely with industry experts, gaining hands-on experience and exposure to real-world fashion projects. They are involved in all aspects of the design process, from conceptualizing ideas to creating prototypes and final garments. In addition to practical training, apprentices also attend classroom lectures and workshops, where they learn about fashion history, trend forecasting, marketing, and business aspects of the industry. The program also emphasizes the importance of sustainability and ethical practices in fashion design. Throughout the Fashion Apprenticeship, apprentices are encouraged to develop their own unique design style and aesthetic, while also honing their technical skills. They are given opportunities to showcase their work through fashion shows, exhibitions, and industry events, thereby building a portfolio of their designs. Upon successful completion of the Fashion Apprenticeship, apprentices have the necessary skills and knowledge to pursue a variety of career paths in the fashion industry. They can work as fashion designers, assistant designers, pattern makers, garment technologists, or even start their own fashion labels. In summary, a Fashion Apprenticeship is a comprehensive training program that equips individuals with the skills, knowledge, and experience needed to thrive in the competitive field of fashion design.

Fashion Fashion Association

The Fashion Fashion Association (FFA) is an organization dedicated to the advancement and promotion of the fashion design industry. FFA serves as a platform for collaboration, knowledge sharing, and networking among fashion designers, industry professionals, and fashion enthusiasts. As a primary objective, FFA aims to provide resources and support to fashion designers at various stages of their careers. This includes offering workshops, seminars, and mentorship programs to help designers develop their skills, expand their knowledge, and navigate the complexities of the fashion industry. FFA also organizes fashion shows, exhibitions, and competitions, providing opportunities for designers to showcase their talent, gain exposure, and establish connections with potential clients and collaborators. Furthermore, FFA actively engages in advocacy and awareness campaigns to promote sustainable and ethical practices within the fashion industry. With a focus on social and environmental responsibility, the association encourages designers to create collections that prioritize fair labor practices, use eco-friendly materials, and minimize waste. FFA works closely with organizations, institutions, and policy-makers to shape industry standards and promote positive change. Collaboration is a key pillar of FFA's activities. The association fosters partnerships between designers, fashion brands, retailers, and manufacturers, facilitating the creation of innovative and marketable fashion products. By connecting designers with industry professionals, FFA helps to bridge the gap between creativity and business, enabling designers to reach a wider audience and achieve commercial success. In summary, the Fashion Fashion Association plays a vital role in supporting and empowering fashion designers. Through its various initiatives, programs, and events, FFA strives to elevate the fashion industry, promote sustainable practices, and create opportunities for designers to thrive and make meaningful contributions to the field of fashion design.

Fashion Fashion Branding

Fashion branding, in the context of fashion design, refers to the process of creating a distinct and recognizable identity for a fashion brand. It involves strategically establishing and promoting the brand's image, values, and personality to differentiate it from its competitors and attract the target audience. A successful fashion branding encompasses various components such as the brand name, logo, tagline, typography, color palette, and overall visual identity. These elements work together to create a cohesive and compelling brand identity that resonates with consumers and conveys the brand's unique style and message.

Fashion Fashion Business

Fashion design is a form of art and business that involves the creation and production of clothing and accessories. It is the process of applying specific design aesthetics and techniques to create original and innovative garments that reflect current trends and individual style. In the fashion industry, fashion design serves as the foundation for the creation of new and exciting collections each season. Fashion designers draw inspiration from various sources such as historical eras, different cultures, nature, and art, and then incorporate these influences into their designs. They use their creativity, technical skills, and knowledge of fabric, color, and construction to bring their ideas to life. A fashion designer begins by conducting thorough research to identify popular styles, colors, and trends. They then sketch out their ideas, creating detailed and accurate drawings that showcase the overall design, silhouette, and details of the garment. These sketches serve as a visual blueprint for the creation of the final product. Once the design is finalized, the fashion designer selects the appropriate fabrics, trims, and embellishments to bring the concept to reality. They create patterns and prototypes, which are tested and adjusted to ensure proper fit and comfort. The designer works closely with patternmakers, cutters, and sewers to oversee the production process, ensuring that the final product meets their vision. Fashion design is not limited to clothing alone. It also includes the creation of accessories, such as shoes, bags, and jewelry, which complement and enhance the overall look. Designers often collaborate with specialists in these particular areas to ensure that their designs are executed with the highest level of craftsmanship and quality. Successful fashion designers possess a keen artistic eye, strong business acumen, and an understanding of consumer preferences. They must keep up with the ever-changing fashion landscape, stay ahead of trends, and anticipate the needs and desires of their target market. Fashion design requires a delicate balance between creativity and commerce, as designers must create innovative and visually appealing collections that also resonate with consumers and generate profit for the business.

Fashion Fashion Buying

Fashion buying is a crucial aspect of the fashion design industry, encompassing the strategic planning, selection, and procurement of merchandise to be sold in retail stores. It involves analyzing market trends, understanding consumer preferences, and making informed decisions to maximize profitability and meet customer demands. At its core, fashion buying requires a deep understanding of the target market and the ability to anticipate and respond to consumers' ever-changing tastes and preferences. Buyers carefully analyze data and research to identify emerging trends and popular styles, ensuring that the merchandise they select reflects the current fashion landscape.

Fashion Fashion CEO

A Fashion Fashion CEO is an executive position in the fashion industry, responsible for overseeing the strategic direction and operations of a fashion design company. This role involves leading a team of designers, merchandisers, and other professionals to create and market fashionable clothing, accessories, and other products. The Fashion Fashion CEO is typically responsible for developing and implementing the company's vision and mission, as well as setting goals and objectives to drive growth and profitability. They analyze market trends and consumer preferences to develop innovative designs that appeal to target customers. In addition to the creative aspect of fashion design, the Fashion Fashion CEO also focuses on the business side of the industry. They are responsible for budgeting, financial planning, and resource allocation to ensure the company's financial success. They establish relationships with suppliers, manufacturers, and retailers to ensure efficient production and distribution of the fashion products. The Fashion Fashion CEO also plays a crucial role in building and maintaining the company's brand image. They develop marketing strategies and campaigns to promote the fashion brand to a wider audience. They collaborate with fashion influencers, celebrities, and media outlets to increase brand visibility and credibility. This executive position requires exceptional leadership and management skills. The Fashion Fashion CEO must inspire and motivate their team to deliver high-quality designs and products. They provide guidance and feedback to designers, ensuring that the creative vision aligns with the overall brand identity. Furthermore, the Fashion Fashion CEO must stay updated with the latest fashion trends, industry developments, and technological advancements. They attend fashion shows, trade fairs, and networking events to connect with industry professionals and gain insights into emerging trends and opportunities. Overall, the Fashion Fashion CEO plays a critical role in shaping the success and growth of a fashion design company. They combine creativity, business acumen, and leadership skills to drive innovation, build a strong brand, and deliver stylish and desirable fashion products to consumers.

Fashion Fashion CFO

A Fashion CFO, or Chief Financial Officer, is a senior executive in the fashion industry who is responsible for overseeing the financial operations of a fashion company. They play a crucial role in the management and strategic decision-making process of the company by providing financial analysis and guidance to the CEO and other executives. The Fashion CFO's main responsibilities include managing the company's financial resources, monitoring the financial health of the business, and providing accurate and timely financial reports to the management team. They work closely with other departments such as design, production, and marketing to ensure that financial goals and objectives are aligned with the overall business strategy.

Fashion Fashion CMO

A fashion CMO, or Chief Marketing Officer, is a senior executive position in the fashion industry that is responsible for overseeing the marketing and promotional strategies of a fashion brand or company. This role involves developing and implementing marketing plans, managing brand positioning, and ensuring the company's messaging and communication efforts align with its overall brand identity and objectives. As a key member of the executive team, the fashion CMO plays a crucial role in shaping the brand's image and driving its growth and success. They are responsible for analyzing market trends, consumer behavior, and competitive landscapes to identify opportunities for growth and develop impactful marketing strategies that resonate with the target audience.

Fashion Fashion COO

A Fashion COO, also known as a Chief Operating Officer in the fashion industry, is a senior executive responsible for overseeing and managing the day-to-day operations of a fashion design company. This role is crucial in ensuring the smooth and efficient functioning of the business, making strategic decisions, and driving overall growth and profitability. The Fashion COO's main responsibilities include strategic planning, process optimization, resource management, and performance evaluation. They work closely with the Chief Executive Officer (CEO) and other top-level executives to establish organizational goals, formulate business strategies, and develop operational plans to achieve them. In terms of strategic planning, the Fashion COO collaborates with the CEO to define the company's vision, mission, and values. They analyze market trends, consumer preferences, and competitive landscape to identify opportunities and threats, and then formulate strategies to capitalize on the former and mitigate the latter. These strategies may involve new product development, expansion into new markets, or adoption of innovative technologies. Process optimization is another key responsibility of the Fashion COO. They streamline the company's operations by identifying inefficiencies, bottlenecks, and other areas of improvement. This includes implementing lean manufacturing principles, enhancing supply chain management, and optimizing production processes to minimize costs and maximize productivity. The Fashion COO also ensures compliance with industry regulations and ethical practices. Resource management is a critical aspect of the Fashion COO's role. They oversee the allocation of financial, human, and technological resources to various departments and projects, ensuring they are utilized effectively and efficiently. This involves budgeting, cost control, talent acquisition, and performance management. The Fashion COO works closely with the finance and human resources departments to align resource allocation with the company's strategic goals. Performance evaluation is another essential responsibility of the Fashion COO. They monitor and analyze key performance indicators (KPIs) to assess the company's overall performance and identify areas of improvement. This includes analyzing sales data, production reports, and customer feedback. Based on these evaluations, the Fashion COO devises strategies and action plans to address any performance gaps and improve operational efficiency. Overall, a Fashion COO plays a pivotal role in driving the success of a fashion design company. They bring together strategic thinking, operational expertise, and leadership skills to ensure the business operates smoothly, efficiently, and profitably in an ever-changing industry.

Fashion Fashion Calendar

Fashion Calendar is a vital tool in the field of fashion design that serves as a comprehensive reference for the scheduling and organization of various fashion-related events. It provides a systematic framework for planning and executing fashion shows, presentations, trade shows, fashion weeks, and other significant industry events. The primary purpose of a Fashion Calendar is to facilitate effective communication and coordination between designers, brands, retailers, buyers, media, and other stakeholders involved in the fashion industry. It ensures that all the key events and activities within the fashion community are integrated and synchronized, allowing for maximum exposure and optimal utilization of resources. A Fashion Calendar typically covers a span of one year and is released well in advance, enabling industry professionals to plan their schedules accordingly and align their activities with the proposed dates. It typically includes the dates, times, and locations of various fashion shows, trade fairs, market weeks, showroom appointments, press days, and other related events. In addition to the scheduling aspect, a Fashion Calendar also includes relevant contact information, such as the PR agencies and showrooms associated with each event, which allows designers and brands to reach out and collaborate with the appropriate contacts. Moreover, it often incorporates supplementary details like theme, guest list, dress code, and any specific guidelines or requirements for participation. Due to the dynamic and fast-paced nature of the fashion industry, a Fashion Calendar is subject to ongoing updates and revisions throughout the year. New events may be added, or existing ones may be rescheduled or canceled. To stay informed and up to date, fashion professionals depend on regular updates and notifications from fashion councils, event organizers, media outlets, and other reliable sources. Overall, a Fashion Calendar acts as a centralized and comprehensive resource that plays a crucial role in the efficient planning, execution, and promotion of fashion-related events. It streamlines the fashion industry's activities, fosters collaboration and synergy, and enhances the visibility and success of fashion brands and designers.

Fashion Fashion Career

Fashion design is a highly creative and artistic profession that involves the design, development, and production of clothing and accessories. It is a career field that requires a combination of technical skills, keen attention to detail, and a deep understanding of aesthetic principles. A fashion designer is primarily responsible for creating original designs that reflect the latest trends and cater to the target audience's needs and preferences. They work closely with clients, manufacturers, and retailers to bring their designs to life. The fashion design process begins with research and concept development. Designers gather inspiration from various sources such as art, culture, history, and current fashion trends. They then sketch their ideas, experimenting with different silhouettes, colors, and fabrics. Once the initial sketches are finalized, designers create prototypes or samples using muslin or other inexpensive materials. These samples are then fitted and adjusted to ensure a perfect fit and the desired look. The final design is then translated into patterns, which are used to cut and sew the actual garment. In addition to designing garments, fashion designers also create accessories such as handbags, shoes, and jewelry. They may collaborate with other professionals, such as textile designers, to develop unique fabrics or prints for their collections. A successful career in fashion design requires a combination of creativity, technical skills, and business acumen. Designers must stay updated with the latest fashion trends and market demands. They need to possess strong communication and teamwork skills to effectively collaborate with various stakeholders in the industry. Furthermore, fashion designers need to be able to work under tight deadlines and handle the pressures of the fast-paced fashion industry. They must continuously innovate and adapt their designs to cater to changing consumer preferences. In conclusion, fashion design is a multifaceted career that blends artistic talent, technical expertise, and a deep understanding of the fashion industry. It offers exciting opportunities for individuals passionate about creativity, style, and innovation.

Fashion Fashion Casting

Fashion casting is a process within the field of fashion design that involves selecting models to showcase a designer's collection or a particular fashion event. It is an integral part of the fashion industry, as models play a crucial role in presenting the designer's vision to the audience. The casting process involves evaluating various factors such as the models' appearance, body shape, charisma, and ability to embody the brand's ethos. The purpose of fashion casting is to find models who align with the aesthetic and brand identity of the designer. The casting director or team responsible for the casting process carefully selects models who can bring the designer's clothing to life on the runway or in promotional materials. These models should possess the ability to capture the attention of the audience and create a strong impact.

Fashion Fashion Conference

A Fashion Conference is an event in the field of fashion design that brings together professionals, experts, and enthusiasts to discuss and explore various aspects of the fashion industry. It serves as a platform for sharing knowledge, ideas, and insights, as well as fostering networking and collaboration opportunities among participants. The primary objective of a fashion conference is to facilitate dialogue and exchange of information related to the latest trends, techniques, and innovations in fashion design. This includes discussions on topics such as fashion forecasting, textile technology, sustainable practices, marketing strategies, and brand development. Through presentations, panel discussions, workshops, and exhibitions, participants have the opportunity to gain valuable insights into the current and future landscape of the fashion industry. Fashion conferences also play a crucial role in promoting and nurturing talent within the fashion community. They often provide a platform for emerging designers to showcase their work and receive feedback from industry professionals. This exposure not only helps in building their confidence but also opens doors for potential collaborations and business opportunities. In addition to knowledge sharing, a fashion conference also serves as a catalyst for networking and relationship-building within the industry. Participants have the opportunity to connect with like-minded individuals, including fashion designers, stylists, buyers, retailers, influencers, and media representatives. These interactions create opportunities for collaborations, partnerships, and even employment within the industry. Moreover, fashion conferences often focus on critical issues in the industry, such as sustainability and ethical practices. They provide a platform for discussions on how the fashion industry can become more conscious of its environmental impact and promote responsible fashion practices. This includes exploring sustainable sourcing and production techniques, promoting fair labor practices, and reducing waste. Overall, a fashion conference is an essential event in the field of fashion design that brings together industry professionals, experts, and enthusiasts to share knowledge, discuss trends, foster collaboration, and address critical issues within the industry. It is an ideal platform for staying updated with the latest trends, networking with industry professionals, and gaining insights into the future of fashion design.

Fashion Fashion Council

The Fashion Fashion Council is an influential organization within the fashion industry that works to promote and support fashion designers, brands, and businesses. It functions as a governing body that sets standards and guidelines for the fashion design industry, ensuring professionalism and creativity.The Fashion Fashion Council plays a crucial role in shaping the direction of the fashion industry by organizing events, exhibitions, and fashion shows. Their events serve as platforms for designers to showcase their collections and for industry professionals to network and discover emerging talent.

Fashion Fashion Design

Fashion design refers to the art and profession of creating clothing and accessories that are visually appealing, functional, and in line with current fashion trends. It involves a combination of creativity, technical skills, and knowledge of the fashion industry. Fashion designers conceptualize and produce garments, footwear, accessories, and even costumes for various occasions and purposes. Fashion design encompasses the entire process of creating clothing, starting from the initial idea or inspiration and ending with the finished product. This process involves several stages, including research, sketching, pattern making, fabric selection, and garment construction. Fashion designers utilize their creativity to develop unique designs and strive to create pieces that are both original and commercially viable.

Fashion Fashion Designer Showcase

Fashion Designer Showcase is a platform in the field of fashion design that allows designers to exhibit and present their creations to a selected audience, such as fashion industry professionals, media, or potential buyers. It serves as a showcase for the designer's unique style, creativity, and craftsmanship. During a Fashion Designer Showcase, designers have the opportunity to display their latest collections through various mediums such as runway shows, presentations, exhibitions, or pop-up shops. The event aims to capture the essence and vision of the designer, highlighting their artistic abilities and brand identity. It provides a platform for designers to communicate their inspirations, storytelling, and innovative techniques to the attendees.

Fashion Fashion Distribution

Fashion distribution in the context of fashion design refers to the process of delivering fashion products to the final consumer through various channels and methods. It encompasses the entire supply chain from the creation and production of garments to their availability in retail stores or through online platforms. This distribution process involves several key players, including fashion designers, manufacturers, wholesalers, retailers, and logistics companies. Each of these entities plays a crucial role in ensuring that fashion products are efficiently and effectively delivered to the target market. At the initial stage, fashion designers create unique and innovative designs based on market research and trend forecasting. These designs are then transformed into actual garments through the manufacturing process. Manufacturers are responsible for producing the garments in large quantities while adhering to design specifications and quality standards. Once the garments are produced, they are typically sold to wholesalers who purchase them in bulk. Wholesalers act as intermediaries between the manufacturers and retailers, buying large quantities of fashion items at a discounted price and then sell them to retailers at a markup. They provide an important link in the distribution chain by aggregating products from multiple manufacturers and offering a wide selection to retailers. Retailers, such as department stores, boutiques, and online platforms, are the final intermediaries between the fashion designers and the end consumers. They determine the assortment of fashion products to be stocked based on customer demand and market trends. Retailers are responsible for marketing, merchandising, and selling the fashion items to the target market through their physical stores or e-commerce platforms. In recent years, the rise of e-commerce has revolutionized fashion distribution by providing a new platform for designers and retailers to reach consumers directly. Online marketplaces and websites enable fashion brands to bypass the traditional retail channels and connect with customers worldwide. This direct-to-consumer approach has opened up new opportunities and challenges in terms of logistics, supply chain management, and customer experience. Overall, fashion distribution is a complex and dynamic process that involves multiple stakeholders working together to deliver fashion products to the end consumers. It requires effective coordination and collaboration at every stage of the supply chain to ensure that fashion items are available in the right place, at the right time, and in the right quantity.

Fashion Fashion Documentary

A fashion fashion documentary refers to a type of documentary film that focuses specifically on the field of fashion design and its various components. It aims to provide an in-depth exploration and analysis of the fashion industry, its evolution over time, and the designers, trends, and cultural influences that have shaped it. These documentaries typically showcase the creative process behind fashion design, including the inspiration, research, experimentation, and craftsmanship involved in creating a collection or a single garment. They may feature interviews with renowned fashion designers, models, stylists, photographers, and other industry professionals, offering insights into their perspectives, experiences, and expertise. In addition to delving into the creative aspect, fashion fashion documentaries also examine the business side of the industry. They may explore topics such as the impact of globalization, sustainability, ethical production, marketing strategies, and the role of technology in fashion design and consumption. By shedding light on these aspects, these documentaries aim to give viewers a comprehensive understanding of the multifaceted nature of the fashion industry. Furthermore, fashion fashion documentaries often showcase fashion shows, runway presentations, and fashion weeks from around the world. They provide a glimpse into the world of high fashion, highlighting the glitz, glamour, and cultural significance associated with these events. These visual spectacles not only celebrate the artistry and craftsmanship of fashion, but also offer a platform for designers to showcase their work to a global audience. Overall, a fashion fashion documentary serves as a valuable resource for fashion enthusiasts, students, industry professionals, and anyone interested in gaining a deeper understanding of the world of fashion design. Through a combination of captivating visuals, interviews, and storytelling techniques, these documentaries provide a comprehensive and insightful exploration of the fashion industry, its history, trends, and the creative individuals who shape its future.

Fashion Fashion E-Commerce

Fashion e-commerce refers to the buying and selling of fashion products and services over the internet. It involves the use of online platforms, websites, and apps to showcase and sell fashion items such as clothing, accessories, footwear, and beauty products. In the context of fashion design, fashion e-commerce has revolutionized the way fashion designers and brands showcase and sell their creations. It enables fashion designers to reach a wider audience, both domestically and internationally, without the limitations of physical stores.

Fashion Fashion Education

Fashion education, in the context of fashion design, refers to the academic and practical training provided to individuals aspiring to pursue a career in the fashion industry. It encompasses a comprehensive curriculum that equips students with the necessary skills, knowledge, and techniques required for success in the field of fashion design. The primary goal of fashion education is to develop a strong foundation in design principles, construction techniques, and creative expression. This involves a combination of theoretical instruction, hands-on training, and real-world experiences to help students articulate their unique design visions and execute them effectively. Within a fashion education program, students learn about the history and evolution of fashion, gaining an understanding of the social, cultural, and economic influences that shape the industry. They also study various aspects of design, such as pattern-making, draping, sewing, and textile manipulation, to develop technical proficiency and craftsmanship. In addition to design skills, fashion education also focuses on fostering creativity and innovation. Students are encouraged to explore their own aesthetic sensibilities, experiment with different materials, and push the boundaries of traditional design conventions. They learn to develop concepts, conduct research, and create mood boards to inform their design process and generate original ideas. Furthermore, a comprehensive fashion education program emphasizes the importance of practical experience and industry exposure. Students are often provided with opportunities to work on real fashion projects, collaborate with professional designers and brands, and participate in internships or fashion shows. These hands-on experiences help students develop their professional networks, gain a deeper understanding of the industry, and refine their design skills in a real-world setting. In conclusion, fashion education is a crucial stepping stone for individuals interested in pursuing a career in fashion design. Through a blend of theory, hands-on training, and industry exposure, it equips students with the necessary skills, knowledge, and creative mindset required to succeed in the dynamic and competitive fashion industry.

Fashion Fashion Entrepreneurship

Fashion entrepreneurship refers to the act of creating, managing, and scaling a successful business within the fashion industry. It involves the application of entrepreneurial principles and strategies to the world of fashion design, production, and retail. Fashion entrepreneurs identify opportunities in the market, develop innovative products or services, and build sustainable and profitable businesses. a fashion entrepreneur is not only a designer but also a businessperson who understands and navigates the complex and ever-changing landscape of the fashion industry. They possess a unique combination of creativity, business acumen, and a deep understanding of consumer behavior and market trends. Fashion entrepreneurship encompasses various aspects, including fashion design, sourcing materials, manufacturing, branding, marketing, and distribution. A fashion entrepreneur needs to have a clear vision and a strong sense of aesthetic to create unique and desirable products that resonate with consumers. One crucial aspect of fashion entrepreneurship is identifying and understanding the target market. This involves conducting market research, analyzing consumer preferences and trends, and identifying gaps or opportunities in the market. By understanding their target audience, fashion entrepreneurs can create products that meet their needs and desires, ultimately ensuring the success and profitability of their business. In addition to product development, fashion entrepreneurs must develop effective marketing and branding strategies to differentiate themselves from competitors and attract customers. They need to establish a unique brand identity and communicate their brand story effectively through various channels, such as social media, advertising, and public relations. Successful fashion entrepreneurs also need to build strong networks within the fashion industry, including relationships with suppliers, manufacturers, retailers, and other industry professionals. These relationships are vital for sourcing quality materials, securing production capabilities, and accessing distribution channels. Overall, fashion entrepreneurship is the process of envisioning, creating, and managing a fashion business that brings innovative and desirable products to market. It requires a combination of artistic talent, business skills, and an entrepreneurial mindset to navigate the competitive and ever-evolving fashion industry.

Fashion Fashion Ethics

Fashion Fashion Ethics refers to the principles and values that guide the ethical decisions and actions of fashion designers in the creation, production, and distribution of clothing and accessories. As a field of study, Fashion Fashion Ethics explores the moral and social responsibilities of fashion designers, as well as the impact of their choices on the environment, labor conditions, and consumer well-being. It aims to promote a more sustainable, fair, and conscious fashion industry.

Fashion Fashion Executive

A fashion executive, in the context of fashion design, refers to a high-level professional who oversees and manages various aspects of fashion brands and companies. This role is responsible for making key strategic decisions and ensuring the successful execution of creative designs, marketing campaigns, and overall brand development. Fashion executives hold an influential position within the industry and play a crucial role in shaping and promoting the brand's image and reputation. As a fashion executive, one of the primary responsibilities is to develop and implement effective business strategies to drive growth and profitability. This involves analyzing market trends, consumer behavior, and competitor activities to identify market opportunities and potential risks. Fashion executives must have a deep understanding of the target customer base and be able to develop innovative strategies to attract and retain customers. In addition, fashion executives collaborate closely with creative teams, including designers, stylists, and merchandisers, to ensure that the brand's vision is effectively communicated through its products and collections. They oversee the entire design process, from concept development to production, and ensure that quality standards are met. Fashion executives also work closely with manufacturers and suppliers to streamline operations and ensure timely delivery of products. Another crucial aspect of a fashion executive's role is marketing and brand management. They develop and execute marketing campaigns that effectively communicate the brand's unique selling proposition and appeal to the target audience. This includes planning and organizing fashion shows, events, and other promotional activities to generate brand awareness and drive sales. Fashion executives also play a vital role in building and maintaining relationships with industry stakeholders, such as retailers, wholesalers, and media. They negotiate contracts and partnerships, establish distribution channels, and collaborate with influencers and celebrities to boost brand visibility. Additionally, fashion executives monitor the financial performance of the brand, set budgets, and analyze sales data to make informed business decisions. In summary, a fashion executive is a senior professional who leads and manages fashion brands and companies. They are responsible for developing and implementing business strategies, overseeing the design process, managing marketing and brand activities, and maintaining industry relationships. Their role is integral to the success and growth of a fashion brand.

Fashion Fashion Exhibition

A fashion exhibition refers to an organized event or showcase where fashion designers present their latest collections and designs to a targeted audience, such as industry professionals, fashion enthusiasts, buyers, and media. During a fashion exhibition, designers have the opportunity to display their creativity, craftsmanship, and unique fashion aesthetics through various mediums, including garments, accessories, installations, and interactive displays. These exhibitions often serve as a platform for designers to communicate their design concept, brand story, and the inspiration behind their collections. The main purpose of a fashion exhibition is to highlight and promote the work of established and emerging designers, fostering industry connections, and generating publicity and recognition for their brands. It provides an avenue for designers to gain exposure, attract potential clients and buyers, and potentially secure financial backing or collaborations. Typically, fashion exhibitions are curated and organized by industry professionals, curators, or fashion organizations. These professionals carefully select and curate the designs and garments to create a visually compelling and cohesive narrative throughout the exhibition space. Fashion exhibitions may be held in a variety of settings, including galleries, museums, trade shows, or even outdoor spaces. The exhibition layout and design are crucial elements in creating an immersive and engaging experience for visitors, allowing them to connect with the designer's vision and understand the context of the collection. Visitors to a fashion exhibition can expect to see a range of designs, from ready-to-wear pieces to couture creations. They may also have the opportunity to interact with the designers, attend panel discussions, or even witness live fashion performances or installations. In conclusion, a fashion exhibition serves as a significant platform for designers to showcase their talent, creativity, and unique fashion vision. It creates a space for industry professionals, fashion enthusiasts, and the media to discover new talents, trends, and innovations within the fashion industry.

Fashion Fashion Fabric Sourcing

Fashion fabric sourcing refers to the process of finding and obtaining suitable fabrics for fashion design. It involves researching, identifying, and selecting fabrics that meet the specific requirements and aesthetic goals of a fashion collection. In fashion design, fabric selection plays a crucial role in achieving the intended design vision and ensuring the quality and functionality of the final garment. Fabric sourcing involves considering various factors such as fiber content, weave, weight, color, pattern, texture, and finish. The first step in fabric sourcing is conducting research to understand the latest trends, industry innovations, and customer preferences. This helps designers stay updated and informed about the available options in the market. Once the desired fabric characteristics have been identified, designers can begin the search for suitable suppliers and manufacturers. During the sourcing process, designers may reach out to fabric suppliers, attend trade shows, or explore online platforms to find potential fabric options. They may also collaborate with textile experts or sample makers to obtain fabric swatches or create prototypes for evaluation and testing. When evaluating fabrics, designers consider not only the aesthetic appeal but also the functional aspects. They assess factors such as durability, drape, stretch, breathability, and care requirements to ensure the fabric's suitability for the intended garment type and usage. Another important aspect of fabric sourcing is considering sustainability and ethical sourcing practices. Designers are increasingly prioritizing environmentally friendly and socially responsible fabrics, aiming to reduce the fashion industry's impact on the environment and workers. Once the ideal fabric options have been identified, designers proceed with negotiating prices, minimum order quantities, and delivery timelines with the chosen suppliers. They may also request fabric samples or color cards for final selection. In conclusion, fabric sourcing is a critical step in fashion design, encompassing the research, selection, and acquisition of fabrics that align with the design vision, quality requirements, and sustainability goals of a fashion collection.

Fashion Fashion Fair

Fashion Fashion Fair is a highly anticipated event in the fashion industry that showcases the latest trends and designs from various fashion designers and brands. It serves as a platform for designers to display their collections and attract potential buyers, media coverage, and industry professionals. During Fashion Fashion Fair, fashion designers present their collections in the form of runway shows or exhibitions. These shows often have a specific theme or concept, which helps to create a cohesive and visually appealing presentation. The collections are created and curated by designers who have a deep understanding of current fashion trends, consumer demands, and their own design aesthetic. Fashion Fashion Fair is not only limited to clothing but also includes accessories like jewelry, shoes, handbags, and other fashion-related products. This gives designers the opportunity to showcase their creativity in various aspects of fashion design. The fair attracts a wide range of attendees, including fashion buyers, retailers, journalists, fashion enthusiasts, and industry professionals. It provides a platform for networking, establishing business relationships, and exploring collaborations. Fashion Fashion Fair also plays a crucial role in building brand awareness and promoting new designers or brands in the fashion industry. The fair is usually organized by a fashion council, association, or event management company. These organizers are responsible for selecting the participating designers, managing the logistics of the event, promoting the fair, and ensuring a seamless experience for both the participants and attendees. Fashion Fashion Fair is not only a platform for established designers but also an opportunity for emerging talents to gain recognition in the industry. Many designers use this platform to launch their careers and establish themselves in the competitive world of fashion. Overall, Fashion Fashion Fair is a significant event in the fashion industry that brings together designers, buyers, and industry professionals. It serves as a catalyst for innovation, creativity, and business opportunities in the world of fashion design.

Fashion Fashion Finance

Fashion design is the art of applying design, aesthetics, and natural beauty to clothing and its accessories. It is influenced by cultural and social attitudes and has evolved over time and place. Fashion designers work in a range of ways in designing clothing and accessories, such as bracelets and necklaces. Because of the time required to bring a garment onto the market, designers must at times anticipate changes to consumer tastes. Fashion finance refers to the financial aspects and strategies involved in the fashion industry. It encompasses various financial activities, including budgeting, financial planning, investments, and financial analysis specifically tailored to the fashion sector. Fashion finance professionals ensure that all financial components of fashion design and production are running smoothly and effectively, focusing on profit maximization, cost control, and financial stability.

Fashion Fashion Forecasting

Fashion forecasting is a strategic and creative process used in the fashion industry to predict upcoming trends and styles. It involves researching and analyzing a variety of factors such as cultural, social, economic, and technological influences to anticipate the next big fashion movement. By studying consumer preferences, historical data, and market trends, fashion forecasters can identify emerging styles and predict the direction of the fashion industry. The primary goal of fashion forecasting is to provide valuable insights and guidance to fashion designers, buyers, and retailers. Designers rely on fashion forecasting to inform their creative process, ensuring their collections are relevant and appeal to target consumers. Buyers and retailers use fashion forecasting to make informed decisions about which styles to stock, which brands to invest in, and which trends to promote.

Fashion Fashion Garment Construction

Fashion garment construction is the process of creating wearable garments in the fashion industry. It involves the assembly of various fabric pieces, such as cutting, sewing, and finishing, to transform them into the final product. This process requires a high level of skill in pattern making, fabric manipulation, and sewing techniques. The first step in garment construction is pattern making, which involves creating a blueprint or template for the garment. This is done by taking measurements and developing a pattern that will ensure a proper fit. The pattern is then used to cut the fabric into the desired shape and size. It is essential to pay attention to grain lines and fabric pattern placement during this process to ensure that all the pieces align correctly. Once the fabric pieces are cut, they are assembled together through sewing. This is where the garment begins to take shape. Different sewing techniques are used depending on the type of garment and the desired outcome. These techniques include basic stitches like straight stitch and zigzag stitch, as well as more complex techniques like gathering, pleating, and topstitching. Throughout the assembly process, it is important to pay attention to the garment's structure and fit. Darts, tucks, and pleats may be added to create shape and contour to the body. The garment should also allow for ease of movement and comfort for the wearer. This requires careful consideration of seam allowances and the use of appropriate closures, such as zippers, buttons, or hooks and eyes. Finishing touches are added to the garment to give it a polished look. This includes hemming the edges, applying trims or embellishments, and adding any necessary closures. The final garment should be visually appealing, well-constructed, and able to withstand regular wear and tear. Overall, fashion garment construction is a complex and intricate process that requires a combination of creativity, technical skill, and attention to detail. It is the foundation of the fashion industry, allowing designers to bring their vision to life and create wearable, stylish pieces for consumers to enjoy.

Fashion Fashion HR

Fashion HR, short for Fashion Human Resources, refers to the specialized field within the fashion industry that focuses on managing and coordinating the human capital of fashion companies. It combines the principles of human resource management with the unique requirements and demands of the fashion design world. Fashion HR professionals play a key role in recruiting, hiring, and retaining talented individuals for various roles in fashion companies, including designers, stylists, merchandisers, production staff, and sales associates. They are responsible for ensuring that the right people with the right skills and qualifications are hired to meet the company's objectives and contribute to its overall success. One of the primary tasks of Fashion HR is to stay current with the latest fashion trends, industry developments, and emerging talent. By having a deep understanding of the fashion industry, Fashion HR professionals are able to identify individuals who possess the creativity, innovation, and passion necessary to thrive in the fashion design field. In addition to recruitment, Fashion HR is also responsible for managing employee performance, training and development, compensation and benefits, and employee relations. They create and implement policies and procedures that promote a positive and inclusive work environment, encourage employee engagement and satisfaction, and ensure compliance with employment laws and regulations. Furthermore, Fashion HR professionals are involved in strategic workforce planning and talent management. They collaborate with top-level management to anticipate future hiring needs, assess the existing talent pool, and develop strategies to attract and retain highly skilled individuals. They also assist in succession planning, identifying potential leaders within the organization and grooming them for future leadership positions. In summary, Fashion HR is a crucial function within the fashion industry that focuses on effectively managing the human capital of fashion companies. It encompasses various tasks such as recruitment, performance management, training and development, compensation and benefits, and strategic workforce planning. By leveraging their knowledge of the fashion industry, Fashion HR professionals ensure that the right people are in place to drive innovation, creativity, and success in the dynamic world of fashion design.

Fashion Fashion Illustration

Fashion Fashion Illustration refers to the art of visually representing clothing, accessories, and fashion trends through drawings or sketches. It plays a crucial role in the design and communication processes within the fashion industry. An essential tool for fashion designers, fashion illustration allows for the exploration and visualization of creative ideas. It provides a platform for designers to translate their thoughts, concepts, and inspirations into visual representations, helping them to refine their designs and bring them to life.

Fashion Fashion Incubator

The Fashion Fashion Incubator is a specialized program or organization that supports and nurtures emerging fashion designers and entrepreneurs in developing and growing their own fashion brands. Within the fashion industry, incubators have become a vital resource for designers looking to launch their own labels, providing a supportive environment to develop their creative ideas, business acumen, and entrepreneurial skills. These incubators offer a range of resources and services tailored to the needs of fashion designers, such as mentorship, workspace, access to equipment and technology, and opportunities for collaboration and networking. The primary objective of a fashion incubator is to help designers navigate the complex and competitive fashion industry, providing them with the knowledge, tools, and support to transform their ideas into successful businesses. Through mentorship programs, designers can receive guidance from industry experts who can offer insights into various aspects of fashion design, including sourcing manufacturers, marketing strategies, and retail distribution. This guidance not only helps designers avoid potential pitfalls but also accelerates their growth and increases their chances of success. In addition to mentorship, fashion incubators often provide designers with access to shared workspaces or studios, where they can work on their designs, create prototypes, and collaborate with other like-minded individuals. These shared spaces foster a sense of community and collaboration, encouraging designers to exchange ideas, collaborate on projects, and learn from one another. This collaborative environment can be especially beneficial for designers who are just starting out, as it provides them with a support network of peers who understand the unique challenges and opportunities of the fashion industry. Fashion incubators also play a crucial role in connecting designers with potential investors, buyers, and retailers. They often organize events, showcases, and presentations where designers can showcase their work to industry professionals and potential customers. This exposure can help designers gain visibility, secure funding, and establish relationships with key players in the fashion industry. In conclusion, the Fashion Fashion Incubator is a valuable resource for emerging fashion designers, offering them mentorship, workspace, and networking opportunities to help them navigate the competitive fashion industry and turn their creative ideas into successful businesses.

Fashion Fashion Industry

The fashion industry is a dynamic, creative, and highly influential sector that encompasses the design, production, distribution, and promotion of clothing and accessories. It is an ever-evolving industry that sets trends and shapes the way individuals express themselves through style and personal appearance. Fashion designers play a crucial role in this industry as they are responsible for creating innovative and aesthetically appealing designs that resonate with target consumers. The fashion industry can be broadly categorized into two main sectors: haute couture and ready-to-wear. Haute couture refers to high-end, custom-made clothing that is meticulously crafted and tailored to perfection. It is often showcased on prestigious runways and worn by a select clientele. On the other hand, ready-to-wear (also known as prêt-à-porter) encompasses mass-produced clothing that is manufactured and sold in standard sizes to the general public. Ready-to-wear collections are designed to be more affordable, accessible, and reflect the latest fashion trends. In addition to fashion design, the industry encompasses numerous other disciplines, including fashion merchandising, textile manufacturing, fashion journalism, and retail management. Fashion merchandisers are responsible for selecting and sourcing clothing and accessories from designers and manufacturers and bringing them to the market. They analyze consumer trends, conduct market research, and collaborate with designers to create visually appealing displays and promote products effectively. Textile manufacturing plays a vital role in the fashion industry as it involves the production of fabrics, prints, and materials used in clothing and accessory production. This includes processes such as spinning, weaving, dyeing, and finishing. Fashion journalists and critics provide insights and analysis on the latest fashion trends, runway shows, and designer collections through various media channels, including magazines, newspapers, and online platforms, influencing consumer choices and shaping public opinion. Overall, the fashion industry is a complex and multifaceted sector that involves various creative and business aspects. It represents a fusion of art, culture, commerce, and self-expression, continuously evolving to meet the demands and desires of consumers worldwide.

Fashion Fashion Innovation

Fashion innovation refers to the introduction of new and creative ideas, techniques, materials, and technologies in the field of fashion design. It involves the continuous exploration and adaptation of novel concepts and practices to create innovative and unique fashion products. Fashion designers strive to push the boundaries of traditional fashion norms and challenge conventional design approaches through innovation. They seek to break away from established norms and create avant-garde and progressive designs that capture the attention and imagination of consumers.

Fashion Fashion Institutes

Fashion Institutes are educational institutions that offer programs and courses focused on the study and practice of fashion design. These institutes are dedicated to training and preparing students for a successful career in the fashion industry. The primary goal of fashion institutes is to provide students with the necessary knowledge, skills, and techniques required to excel in the field of fashion design. They offer a comprehensive curriculum that covers various aspects of fashion, including design principles, garment construction, patternmaking, textile selection, fashion illustration, and fashion history. By studying these subjects, students gain a deep understanding of the fundamentals of fashion design and develop their creative abilities. In addition to theoretical knowledge, fashion institutes also emphasize practical training. Students are given ample opportunities to apply their learning through hands-on projects, workshops, and internships. These practical experiences allow them to refine their technical skills and build a professional portfolio, which is essential for showcasing their talent to potential employers in the fashion industry. Moreover, fashion institutes foster a supportive and collaborative learning environment. Students have the opportunity to work with fellow fashion enthusiasts and industry professionals, which helps them develop their networking and teamwork skills. Collaboration also encourages the exchange of ideas and the exploration of new perspectives, fostering innovation in fashion design. Furthermore, fashion institutes often host fashion shows, exhibitions, and industry events that provide students with valuable exposure to the real-world fashion industry. These events allow students to showcase their designs to industry experts, potential employers, and even the general public. The feedback and recognition received during these events play a crucial role in shaping students' careers and opening doors to future opportunities in fashion. In conclusion, fashion institutes play a vital role in shaping the next generation of fashion designers. By providing a comprehensive education, practical training, networking opportunities, and exposure to the fashion industry, these institutions empower students to pursue successful careers in the dynamic and competitive world of fashion design.

Fashion Fashion Internship

A fashion internship is an opportunity for individuals interested in fashion design to gain practical experience and knowledge in the industry. It is a temporary position, typically lasting a few months, where interns work closely with professionals in the fashion industry, such as designers, stylists, or production managers. During a fashion internship, interns are exposed to various aspects of the fashion industry and have the chance to work on real-world projects. They may assist with designing clothing or accessories, creating sketches or patterns, conducting research on current fashion trends, or assisting with fashion shows or photo shoots.

Fashion Fashion Journalism

Fashion journalism is a specialized field within the fashion industry that focuses on the reporting, analysis, and critical evaluation of fashion trends, styles, designers, and events. It serves as a bridge between the fashion industry and the general public, providing information and insights into the ever-changing world of fashion. At its core, fashion journalism involves the collection and dissemination of information related to fashion. This includes conducting interviews with designers, models, and industry experts, attending and reporting on fashion shows and events, and analyzing the latest fashion trends and styles. Through various forms of media, such as print, online publications, television, and social media, fashion journalists play a crucial role in shaping public opinion and influencing consumer behavior.

Fashion Fashion Law

Fashion law refers to the legal rules and regulations that govern the fashion industry, specifically focusing on the protection and enforcement of intellectual property rights, contract law, and other legal issues relevant to the design, production, distribution, and promotion of fashion products. The primary objective of fashion law is to safeguard the intellectual property of designers and brands, ensuring that their creations are protected from unauthorized copying or counterfeiting. This includes copyright protection for original designs, trademarks for brand names and logos, and design patents for unique ornamental aspects of fashion items. Fashion law also encompasses the legal mechanisms that designers can utilize to prevent others from infringing on their intellectual property rights, such as cease and desist letters, lawsuits for damages, and injunctions to stop the sale or production of counterfeit goods. In addition to intellectual property, fashion law also deals with contract law, as designers often enter into agreements with manufacturers, distributors, and retailers for the production and sale of their fashion products. These contracts govern various aspects, including licensing, distribution rights, royalties, and exclusivity arrangements. Fashion law ensures that these contracts are legally binding and provides a means for resolving disputes that may arise between parties. Furthermore, fashion law encompasses consumer protection laws, which seek to safeguard the rights and interests of consumers when purchasing fashion products. These laws may govern issues such as false advertising, product labeling, size labeling, and warranties or guarantees for fashion items. Fashion law also addresses ethical and sustainability concerns within the industry, encouraging transparency and responsible practices in the production and sourcing of materials and labor. Overall, fashion law plays a crucial role in protecting the interests of designers, brands, and consumers, providing a legal framework for the fashion industry to operate within. It ensures fair competition, encourages innovation, and promotes responsible practices, all while maintaining the delicate balance between creativity and legal rights in the world of fashion design.

Fashion Fashion Leadership

Fashion leadership in the context of fashion design refers to the ability of a designer or fashion brand to set trends, influence the industry, and lead the way in terms of style and innovation. It involves taking a proactive approach to creating new and exciting fashion concepts, pushing boundaries, and inspiring others in the industry and beyond. A fashion leader is someone who is ahead of the curve, constantly thinking outside the box, and challenging the status quo. They have a deep understanding of the fashion industry, including current trends, consumer preferences, and market demands. By staying informed and observing what is happening in the world of fashion, leaders are able to identify emerging trends and anticipate what will resonate with consumers in the future. Fashion leadership is not limited to individual designers or brands; it can also be exhibited by fashion influencers, tastemakers, and celebrities who have a significant impact on the fashion choices of others. These individuals have the power to shape public opinion and drive sales, making them instrumental in defining what is considered fashionable. Being a fashion leader requires vision, creativity, and a strong sense of personal style. It involves taking risks and being unafraid to experiment with new ideas, fabrics, colors, and silhouettes. Fashion leaders understand that innovation and originality are key to standing out in a crowded market and capturing the attention of consumers. Furthermore, fashion leadership involves understanding the importance of sustainability and ethical practices in the fashion industry. Leaders strive to promote responsible and conscious fashion, incorporating eco-friendly materials and production processes into their designs. In summary, fashion leadership encompasses the ability to influence and shape the fashion industry through trend-setting, innovation, and a deep understanding of market dynamics. It requires staying ahead of the curve, pushing boundaries, and inspiring others within the industry. By demonstrating creativity, vision, and a commitment to sustainability, fashion leaders can make a lasting impact on the world of fashion.

Fashion Fashion Lecture

Fashion Fashion Licensing

Fashion fashion licensing is a business arrangement in the context of fashion design where a fashion brand grants another company the right to use their brand name, logo, designs, and other intellectual property in connection with the production and sale of fashion-related products. This licensing agreement allows the licensee (the company receiving the rights) to benefit from the brand recognition and reputation of the fashion brand, while the licensor (the fashion brand) receives royalties or licensing fees in return. Through fashion fashion licensing, the licensee gains access to the expertise, creativity, and established reputation of the fashion brand, enabling them to produce and market fashion products that align with the brand's aesthetic and target market. This arrangement allows the licensee to tap into a ready-made consumer base and benefit from the brand's existing marketing efforts and promotional activities.

Fashion Fashion Logistics

Fashion logistics refers to the process of managing the flow of fashion goods from the sourcing of raw materials to the delivery of finished products to the end consumer. It involves the coordination and organization of various activities, including procurement, production, inventory management, transportation, and distribution. At the heart of fashion logistics is the goal of ensuring that the right products are available in the right place, at the right time, and in the right quantities. This requires careful planning, efficient execution, and effective communication across different stages of the supply chain. The fashion design industry operates in a fast-paced environment, where trends change rapidly and consumer demands fluctuate. As a result, fashion logistics plays a crucial role in supporting the dynamic nature of the industry and ensuring that fashion brands can respond quickly to market demands. Raw material procurement is an important aspect of fashion logistics. It involves identifying and sourcing high-quality materials that meet the design specifications and requirements of the fashion brand. This includes fabrics, trims, accessories, and other components necessary for the production of garments and accessories. Once the raw materials are secured, the production process begins. Fashion logistics encompasses the planning and management of production activities, which include cutting, sewing, and finishing of garments. It also involves quality control measures to ensure that the final products meet the brand's standards and customer expectations. Inventory management is another critical component of fashion logistics. It involves keeping track of stock levels, monitoring product availability, and planning for reordering or replenishment. Effective inventory management minimizes the risk of stockouts or overstocking, thus optimizing the use of resources and reducing costs. Transportation and distribution are vital stages in fashion logistics. They involve the movement of finished products from production facilities to retail stores or directly to customers. This requires selecting the most appropriate modes of transportation, such as air, sea, or land, and coordinating the logistics of shipping, customs clearance, and delivery. In summary, fashion logistics is the backbone of the fashion design industry, ensuring the efficient and timely delivery of fashion goods to customers. It encompasses a range of activities, from raw material procurement to production, inventory management, and transportation. By effectively coordinating and managing these processes, fashion brands can meet consumer demands, stay competitive, and thrive in the fast-paced world of fashion. """"

Fashion Fashion Lookbook

A fashion lookbook is a curated collection of visual images and accompanying descriptions that showcase a fashion designer's latest creations, inspirations, and styling ideas. It serves as a comprehensive visual reference or catalog to highlight the designer's vision and aesthetic. Similar to a portfolio, a fashion lookbook is an essential marketing tool used by designers to present their work to potential clients, buyers, and the general public. It typically features professional photographs of models or mannequins wearing the designer's garments in various settings or poses, effectively illustrating how the pieces can be styled and worn. The photos are often accompanied by brief descriptions, including fabric details, color options, sizes, and pricing information. The purpose of a fashion lookbook is to communicate the key elements of a designer's collection, such as the theme, mood, and creative concept, to a wider audience. By visually presenting the garments in a cohesive and visually appealing manner, a lookbook helps establish the designer's brand identity and creates a visual narrative that resonates with the target audience. Furthermore, a fashion lookbook serves as a source of inspiration and reference for stylists, fashion editors, and fashion enthusiasts, who can utilize the imagery and styling ideas for their own projects or personal styling choices. It provides a comprehensive overview of the designer's current season or latest collection, allowing consumers to gain insight into the designer's unique design philosophy and artistic vision. Designers often collaborate with photographers, stylists, models, hair and makeup artists, and other creative professionals to bring their lookbook vision to life. The selection of locations, props, and models are carefully considered to effectively convey the desired aesthetic and message. In addition to print format, lookbooks are frequently shared digitally through websites, social media platforms, and digital publications, increasing their accessibility and reach to a global audience. In conclusion, a fashion lookbook is a visual catalog that showcases a fashion designer's latest collection through carefully curated images and descriptions. It serves as a marketing tool, brand identity-establishing tool, source of inspiration, and reference for industry professionals and consumers alike.

Fashion Fashion Management

Fashion Fashion Management is a specialized branch of management that focuses on the planning, organization, and coordination of activities within the fashion industry. It combines elements of both business management and fashion design to ensure the successful development, production, and promotion of fashion products. At its core, Fashion Fashion Management involves overseeing various aspects of the fashion design process, including trend analysis, product development, sourcing materials, manufacturing, marketing, retailing, and distribution. It also encompasses the management of human resources, financial resources, and operations to ensure efficiency and profitability within the fashion business. One of the primary roles of Fashion Fashion Management is to identify and anticipate consumer preferences and market trends. This involves conducting market research, analyzing fashion forecasts, and staying updated on industry news to inform strategic decision-making. By understanding the needs and desires of consumers, Fashion Fashion Managers can guide the design team in creating fashion products that will resonate with the target audience. Furthermore, Fashion Fashion Management plays a crucial role in coordinating the production process. This includes establishing relationships with suppliers, negotiating contracts, and overseeing the procurement of materials. Fashion Fashion Managers are responsible for ensuring that the production process is efficient, timely, and cost-effective, while maintaining quality standards. Once the fashion products are ready for the market, Fashion Fashion Management focuses on developing effective marketing and promotional strategies. This involves creating branding strategies, managing social media platforms, organizing fashion shows, and collaborating with retailers to showcase and sell the fashion products. By implementing strategic marketing initiatives, Fashion Fashion Managers aim to increase brand awareness, attract customers, and drive sales. In addition to the creative aspects of fashion design, Fashion Fashion Management is also concerned with the financial aspects of running a fashion business. Fashion Fashion Managers are responsible for budgeting, cost analysis, and financial forecasting to ensure the profitability and sustainability of the fashion brand. They also oversee inventory management, pricing strategies, and sales analysis to optimize revenue and minimize costs. In summary, Fashion Fashion Management is a multidisciplinary field that combines elements of fashion design and business management. It involves overseeing the entire fashion design process, from trend analysis to product development, manufacturing, marketing, and retailing. Fashion Fashion Managers play a vital role in ensuring the success and profitability of fashion brands by coordinating various aspects of the business and aligning them with consumer preferences and market trends.

Fashion Fashion Manufacturing

Fashion manufacturing refers to the process of producing clothing, accessories, or other fashion products on a large scale. It involves a series of steps from the initial design concept to the final production and distribution of the goods. In fashion design, the manufacturing process begins with the creation of design sketches or digital renditions. These designs are typically based on fashion trends, market research, and the target audience. Once the designs are finalized, they are transformed into patterns or templates that will be used to create the garments or accessories. The next step in fashion manufacturing is sourcing the materials and trims required for production. This may involve working with suppliers to procure fabrics, buttons, zippers, and other components necessary for the construction of the products. Quality control is an essential aspect of this stage, ensuring that the materials meet the necessary standards for durability and aesthetics. After the materials are obtained, the production process begins. This typically involves cutting the fabric according to the patterns and assembling the pieces together through sewing or other techniques. Skilled workers, such as pattern makers, cutters, and seamstresses, are employed to execute these tasks with precision and attention to detail. Once the garments or accessories are assembled, they undergo a series of finishing processes, such as pressing, steaming, and quality checks. This is done to ensure that the final products are of high quality, free from any defects or flaws. Any necessary alterations or adjustments are made at this stage to achieve the desired fit and appearance. Finally, the fashion products are packaged and prepared for distribution. This may involve labeling, tagging, and packaging the items according to specific requirements. The products are then shipped to retailers, wholesalers, or directly to consumers through online platforms. In summary, fashion manufacturing encompasses the entire process of bringing fashion designs to life on a larger scale. It involves the stages of design, material sourcing, production, finishing, and distribution. Attention to detail, quality control, and adherence to current fashion trends are key elements of successful fashion manufacturing.

Fashion Fashion Marketing

Fashion marketing in the context of fashion design is the strategic and creative process of promoting and selling fashion products to target consumers. It involves understanding and analyzing current fashion trends, as well as consumer behavior and preferences, in order to develop and implement effective marketing strategies. Fashion marketers play a crucial role in the fashion industry by bridging the gap between designers and consumers. They collaborate with designers to identify the target audience for a particular fashion collection and develop marketing campaigns that effectively communicate the brand's message. This includes creating promotional materials such as advertisements, lookbooks, and social media content. Furthermore, fashion marketing encompasses various activities such as market research, brand management, public relations, and retail management. Market research helps fashion marketers identify consumer insights and market opportunities, allowing them to make informed decisions about product development and marketing strategies. Brand management involves maintaining and enhancing the brand image and reputation, ensuring consistency across all marketing communication channels. Fashion marketers also work closely with public relations teams to create buzz and generate media coverage for fashion events, product launches, and collaborations. In addition, fashion marketing involves managing retail operations and distribution channels. This includes selecting retail partners, creating visual merchandising displays, and analyzing sales data to identify trends and opportunities for growth. Overall, fashion marketing is a dynamic and multifaceted field that requires a deep understanding of the fashion industry, consumer behavior, and marketing principles. It combines creativity, analytical skills, and strategic thinking to effectively promote fashion products and drive sales.

Fashion Fashion Masterclass

A fashion masterclass refers to a comprehensive educational program or workshop for individuals interested in fashion design. It is designed to provide participants with in-depth knowledge and practical skills necessary to succeed in the fashion industry. The masterclass typically covers various aspects of fashion design, including conceptualization, sketching, pattern making, garment construction, and portfolio development. The aim of a fashion masterclass is to offer aspiring fashion designers the opportunity to enhance their creativity, refine their technical skills, and gain a deeper understanding of the fashion design process. Through hands-on exercises, demonstrations, and expert guidance, participants are able to develop their own unique style and aesthetic while staying abreast of current fashion trends and industry practices. During a fashion masterclass, participants may be introduced to the fundamental principles of design, such as color theory, proportion, and silhouette. They may also learn about different fabrics, their properties, and how to select the most suitable materials for their designs. In addition, participants are likely to be taught various techniques for garment construction, including cutting, sewing, and finishing. One of the key benefits of attending a fashion masterclass is the opportunity to receive feedback and critique from industry professionals. Participants may have their work reviewed by experienced fashion designers who can provide valuable insights and advice for improvement. This feedback enables participants to refine their designs and gain a better understanding of how their creations are perceived in the fashion market. Furthermore, a fashion masterclass often includes sessions on industry-related topics, such as fashion marketing, branding, and retailing. Participants may learn about the importance of market research, trend forecasting, and effective communication strategies in promoting their fashion designs. They may also gain insights into the business side of the fashion industry and discover potential career opportunities. In conclusion, a fashion masterclass is an intensive educational program that equips individuals with the knowledge, skills, and guidance required to excel in the field of fashion design. It provides a platform for aspiring fashion designers to explore their creativity, gain practical experience, and receive expert feedback. By participating in a fashion masterclass, individuals can enhance their chances of success in the competitive and ever-evolving world of fashion.

Fashion Fashion Mentorship

A fashion mentorship is a structured and focused relationship between a more experienced fashion professional (the mentor) and a less experienced fashion designer (the mentee), in which the mentor provides guidance, advice, and support to help the mentee develop their skills, knowledge, and professional network in the fashion industry. The mentorship is typically a mentor-led program designed to facilitate the mentee's growth and development as a fashion designer. The mentor serves as a role model and provides insight into the industry, sharing their own experiences, successes, and challenges. They offer feedback on the mentee's work, helping them refine their design skills and develop their personal style and aesthetic. The fashion mentorship relationship can take various forms, including one-on-one mentorship, group mentorship, or even virtual mentorship through online platforms. The duration of the mentorship can vary, ranging from a few months to several years, depending on the goals and objectives of the mentor and mentee. The fashion mentorship is not limited to design skills and creative development; it also encompasses professional development. The mentor advises the mentee on career opportunities, job search strategies, and how to navigate the fashion industry. They may provide guidance on portfolio development, resume building, and interview preparation. Through the mentorship, the mentee gains access to the mentor's professional network, expanding their own connections within the fashion industry. This can lead to potential job opportunities, collaborations, and introductions to key industry professionals. Overall, a fashion mentorship is a valuable opportunity for a less experienced fashion designer to receive personalized guidance and support from a more experienced professional. It accelerates their growth and development in both their creative and professional journey, helping them establish a strong foundation for a successful career in the fashion industry.

Fashion Fashion Merchandising

Fashion merchandising is a discipline in the field of fashion design that involves the planning, buying, and selling of fashion products. It encompasses the business side of the fashion industry, combining elements of marketing, sales, and merchandising to create a successful fashion retail operation. The role of a fashion merchandiser is multifaceted and requires a combination of creativity, analytical skills, and business acumen. They are responsible for analyzing market trends, consumer preferences, and sales data to develop strategies for buying and selling fashion products. By understanding the target market and anticipating consumer demands, fashion merchandisers are able to curate a selection of products that will resonate with customers and drive sales. One of the key functions of fashion merchandising is assortment planning. This involves determining the mix of products that will be offered by a fashion retailer, taking into account factors such as price range, brand selection, and style variety. The goal is to create a balanced assortment that appeals to the target market while also maximizing profitability and inventory turnover. In addition to assortment planning, fashion merchandisers are also responsible for buying products from fashion designers and manufacturers. This involves negotiating contracts, placing orders, and managing the supply chain to ensure that products are delivered on time and in the desired quantities. Merchandisers must be knowledgeable about fashion trends, fabrics, and production techniques in order to make informed buying decisions and maintain strong relationships with suppliers. Once the products are purchased, fashion merchandisers play a crucial role in promoting and selling them. They collaborate with marketing teams to develop visual merchandising strategies, create compelling product displays, and manage the overall store environment. By effectively showcasing the fashion products, merchandisers aim to attract customers, highlight key styles, and drive sales. Overall, fashion merchandising is an essential component of the fashion industry, bridging the gap between design and retail. It requires a combination of creative vision, analytical skills, and business expertise to successfully bring fashion products to market and meet the demands of consumers.

Fashion Fashion Model Agency

A fashion model agency is a company that represents fashion models and connects them with clients in the fashion industry. It serves as an intermediary between the models and the clients, facilitating the hiring process and managing the professional relationships. The main role of a fashion model agency is to scout and discover new talent, as well as manage and promote the careers of existing models. This involves finding potential models through various means, such as attending fashion shows, reviewing portfolios, or conducting open castings. Once a model is signed with the agency, they become part of the agency's roster and are available for bookings. Fashion model agencies play a vital role in the fashion design industry by providing a centralized platform for models and clients to connect. They act as a bridge between designers, photographers, stylists, brands, and other industry professionals, making it easier for them to find suitable models for their projects. When a client requires models for a fashion show, editorial shoot, commercial campaign, or any other fashion-related project, they reach out to a fashion model agency to inquire about available models. The agency then presents a selection of models from their roster that best match the client's requirements, considering factors such as age, measurements, look, and experience. Once a model is chosen for a job, the agency handles the contractual and logistical aspects, ensuring that the model's schedule is coordinated, transportation arrangements are made, and all necessary agreements are in place. They also negotiate the model's fees and rights, acting as a representative to secure the best possible terms for their clients. Additionally, fashion model agencies provide guidance and support to their models, helping them develop their careers and navigate the industry. This can include providing advice on personal branding, portfolio development, networking, and even financial management. The agency acts as a mentor and advocate for the models, ensuring their well-being and professional growth. Overall, a fashion model agency is an essential entity in the fashion design ecosystem, facilitating the collaboration between models and clients, and contributing to the industry's creativity and success.

Fashion Fashion Mood Board

A fashion mood board is a visual tool used by fashion designers to convey and explore ideas for a specific collection or garment. It serves as a creative collage that captures the desired aesthetic, color palette, materials, and overall theme of the design concept. The purpose of a fashion mood board is to inspire and guide the design process, helping designers to visualize their ideas and communicate them effectively with others. By gathering images, swatches, and other visual elements, designers can conceptualize their vision and develop a cohesive and coherent collection.

Fashion Fashion Networking

Fashion Networking is an essential aspect of the fashion design industry. It refers to the process of establishing and maintaining professional relationships with individuals and organizations within the fashion industry. These connections and collaborations are crucial for fashion designers to gain exposure, access resources, and establish their brand in the competitive fashion world. Networking in the context of fashion design involves actively engaging with other professionals such as designers, stylists, retailers, manufacturers, photographers, models, and influencers. It is a reciprocal process where individuals support and promote each other's work to create a mutually beneficial network. Networking can take place through various channels, including industry events, trade shows, fashion weeks, social media platforms, and professional organizations.

Fashion Fashion Panel

In the context of fashion design, a fashion panel refers to a group or panel of experts who provide opinions, critiques, and insights into the latest trends, styles, and designs in the fashion industry. These experts typically include fashion designers, stylists, journalists, influencers, buyers, and other professionals who have extensive knowledge and experience in the field of fashion. The main purpose of a fashion panel is to evaluate and analyze the current fashion landscape, including runway shows, fashion publications, fashion weeks, and other fashion-related events. They offer their expertise and perspectives on various aspects of fashion, such as colors, fabrics, silhouettes, patterns, and accessories. The opinions and critiques provided by the fashion panel are highly influential and play a significant role in shaping the direction of the fashion industry. Their insights are often sought after by fashion designers, retailers, and fashion enthusiasts alike, as they provide a deeper understanding of the latest trends and help inform decision-making processes. Through their discussions and analyses, fashion panels contribute to the development of new ideas and inspire designers in their creative process. They assess the success and potential of different fashion trends, offering valuable feedback to designers, brands, and retailers. This feedback aids in making informed decisions regarding product development, production, marketing, and merchandising strategies. In addition to evaluating current trends, fashion panels also predict future trends, helping to influence and guide the direction of the fashion industry. By analyzing consumer behavior, cultural shifts, and market research, they provide invaluable insights into what may be popular and desirable in the coming seasons. Overall, fashion panels play a crucial role in the fashion industry by providing expert opinions, critiques, and trend predictions. Their expertise and insights inform the decisions of designers, brands, and retailers, shaping the fashion landscape and influencing consumer preferences.

Fashion Fashion Pattern Making

Pattern making is an essential aspect of fashion design. It involves the creation of templates or patterns that serve as a blueprint for constructing garments. These patterns are based on specific measurements and are used to cut out fabric pieces that, when sewn together, create the desired garment. The process of pattern making begins with a fashion designer's sketch or concept. The designer communicates their vision through drawings, including details on the silhouette, seams, darts, and other design elements. The pattern maker then takes these sketches and uses them as a reference to translate the design into a three-dimensional form. Accuracy is crucial in pattern making as any errors or miscalculations can result in ill-fitting garments. The pattern maker uses specialized tools such as a ruler, French curve, and a set square to ensure precise measurements and curves. They also consider the properties of the chosen fabric, taking into account factors such as stretch, drape, and grainline. Pattern making involves various stages. Initially, the pattern maker creates a basic block or sloper, which is a simple pattern that represents the fundamental shape of a garment. This block can then be modified and manipulated to create different styles and designs. To do this, the pattern maker adds or removes fullness, reshapes seams and darts, and adjusts proportions to achieve the desired fit and design aesthetic. Once the pattern is finalized, it is marked with notches, seam allowances, and other construction details to guide the sewing process. These markings ensure that the fabric pieces align correctly during assembly, resulting in a professionally finished garment. The pattern maker may also create separate patterns for lining, interlining, and other components that add structure and support to the garment. Pattern making is a critical skill for fashion designers, as it enables them to bring their designs to life. It requires a deep understanding of garment construction, body proportions, and fabric behavior. By creating accurate and well-drafted patterns, fashion designers can ensure that their garments fit well and look aesthetically pleasing, setting the foundation for a successful collection.

Fashion Fashion Photography

Fashion photography is a specialized form of photography that focuses on showcasing clothing, accessories, and fashion trends. It is an essential component of the fashion industry, as it plays a crucial role in creating visual representations of fashion designs for advertising and editorial purposes. The main objective of fashion photography is to capture the beauty and uniqueness of fashion garments, accessories, and fashion models in visually compelling ways. It involves the collaboration of a team of professionals, including photographers, stylists, makeup artists, hairstylists, and models, who work collectively to bring the designer's vision to life through photographs. A fashion photographer's role is to interpret the designer's vision and create captivating images that evoke emotions and highlight the essence of the fashion design. They use their technical skills, creativity, and knowledge of fashion trends to capture the aesthetics, details, and textures of the garments. The photographer carefully considers lighting, composition, and angles to enhance and emphasize the fashion elements being photographed. Additionally, fashion photography also plays a crucial role in conveying brand messages and creating brand identities. It helps in promoting fashion designers, fashion brands, and fashion trends by creating visually appealing images that capture the attention of the target audience. Through the selection of appropriate locations, props, and models, fashion photographs aim to evoke a certain mood or ambiance that aligns with the desired brand image. Moreover, fashion photography extends beyond capturing still images. It encompasses various genres such as editorial, advertising, catalog, and runway photography. Editorial fashion photography is often found in fashion magazines and is known for its artistic and storytelling approach. Advertising fashion photography focuses on promoting fashion products in print ads and commercials. Catalog photography aims to showcase the details and features of fashion products, while runway photography captures the energy and movement of fashion shows. Fashion photography is constantly evolving, influenced by changing fashion trends, technological advancements, and cultural shifts. It plays a vital role in the fashion industry by creating visually captivating images that inspire, inform, and influence consumers. Through creative expression and mastery of technical skills, fashion photography brings fashion designs to life and contributes to shaping the visual language of the fashion world.

Fashion Fashion Podcast

A fashion podcast is a digital audio or video program that focuses on discussing various topics related to fashion design. It offers a platform for fashion enthusiasts, designers, industry experts, and influencers to share their knowledge, insights, and experiences with a wider audience. These podcasts typically feature interviews with fashion designers, stylists, models, and other fashion industry professionals. They delve into topics such as the latest trends, fashion history, sustainable fashion, styling tips, industry news, and emerging designers. Some podcasts also cover related areas like beauty, lifestyle, and culture, which are often interconnected with the world of fashion.

Fashion Fashion Pop-Up Shop

A pop-up shop is a temporary retail space that is set up to sell a specific product or showcase a brand for a limited period of time. In the context of fashion design, a fashion pop-up shop is a temporary physical store that offers a unique and immersive shopping experience for customers to interact with a specific fashion brand or collection. Unlike traditional retail stores that have a permanent location, a fashion pop-up shop allows designers or brands to create a temporary presence in different locations, such as high-traffic areas, trendy neighborhoods, or during fashion events. This temporary nature of the pop-up shop adds an element of exclusivity and urgency to the shopping experience, as customers know that they need to visit the shop within a limited timeframe.

Fashion Fashion Promotion

Fashion promotion refers to the activities and strategies used to create awareness and generate interest in fashion products or brands. It encompasses various marketing techniques and communication channels that are employed to promote and sell fashion design collections, clothing, accessories, or trends. The aim of fashion promotion is to create a favorable image of the brand or product, increase brand visibility, and ultimately drive sales. It involves a range of activities, including advertising, public relations, events, digital marketing, social media campaigns, visual merchandising, and retail promotions. Advertising plays a major role in fashion promotion, as it allows brands to reach a wider audience and communicate their key messages. Fashion brands often create visually compelling advertisements for various media platforms, such as magazines, billboards, television, and online platforms. These advertisements feature models or celebrities wearing the brand's clothing or accessories, showcasing the style, quality, and uniqueness of the products. Public relations (PR) is another crucial aspect of fashion promotion. PR activities involve managing relationships with the media, fashion influencers, and celebrities. Through press releases, fashion shows, and collaborations, PR professionals aim to generate positive media coverage, increase brand exposure, and create a buzz around the brand or collection. Events are also commonly used in fashion promotion. Fashion shows, trade fairs, launch parties, and store events provide opportunities for brands to showcase their latest designs, engage with customers, and create memorable experiences. These events often attract media attention and generate substantial publicity for the brand. In the digital era, fashion promotion has expanded to include various online channels. Brands use websites, social media platforms, influencers, and fashion blogs to connect with their target audience, share content, and promote their products. Social media campaigns and collaborations with popular influencers or celebrities are effective ways to create a buzz and generate interest in fashion brands and collections. Visual merchandising is the art of presenting fashion products in an appealing way to attract and engage customers. Brands design their store layouts, window displays, and product placements to create a visually pleasing and cohesive brand image, enticing customers to enter the store and make a purchase. Retail promotions, such as discounts, special offers, or loyalty programs, also play a role in fashion promotion by incentivizing customers to buy the products.

Fashion Fashion Public Relations

Fashion Fashion Public Relations, also known as fashion PR, is a specialized field within the fashion industry that focuses on managing the communication and image of fashion brands, designers, and events. It involves building and maintaining relationships with the media, influencers, celebrities, and the public to generate positive publicity and enhance brand reputation. The primary goal of fashion PR is to create awareness and buzz around a brand or a designer's collection. It involves strategizing and implementing various communication tactics to reach the target audience and build brand visibility. This includes creating press releases, organizing fashion shows, coordinating photo shoots, and managing social media presence. Fashion PR professionals work closely with fashion journalists, editors, stylists, and bloggers to secure media coverage for their clients. They pitch story ideas, send sample products or garments for editorial shoots, and arrange interviews and features in print and digital publications. These efforts help to promote a brand's latest collections, collaborations, events, and brand initiatives. In addition to traditional media, fashion PR also focuses on influencer marketing and celebrity endorsements. PR professionals identify and collaborate with influencers and celebrities who align with the brand's image and target demographic. They may provide them with free products or garments to wear, feature them in brand campaigns, or invite them to attend fashion shows and events. The aim is to leverage their influence and reach to gain exposure and credibility for the brand. Fashion PR also plays a crucial role in managing crises and reputation management. PR professionals monitor media coverage, social media conversations, and online reviews to ensure any negative publicity is addressed promptly and effectively. They may issue public statements, organize press conferences, or engage in damage control strategies to protect the brand's reputation. Overall, Fashion Fashion Public Relations is an integral part of the fashion industry, responsible for shaping and managing the public image of fashion brands and designers. Through strategic communication and relationship-building efforts, fashion PR professionals help to generate excitement, drive sales, and establish a brand's credibility and relevance in the ever-evolving fashion landscape.

Fashion Fashion Research

Fashion Design is the art and craft of designing clothing and accessories that reflect cultural, social, and individual aesthetics. It involves the creation of unique and innovative designs, taking into account the latest trends, materials, and construction techniques. Fashion designers use their creativity and technical skills to conceptualize, sketch, and create prototypes of garments, which are then brought to life through the process of production. At its core, fashion design is a form of self-expression that allows individuals to communicate their identity and personality through clothing. It encompasses various elements such as color, silhouette, texture, and pattern, which are carefully chosen to create visually appealing and harmonious outfits. Fashion designers also consider the practicality and functionality of their designs, ensuring that they are comfortable and suitable for different body types and occasions. In addition to creating garments, fashion designers often collaborate with other professionals in the industry, such as stylists, photographers, and models, to effectively showcase their designs. They stay up-to-date with fashion trends and market demands, conducting extensive research to understand consumer preferences and lifestyle choices. This research plays a vital role in the design process, as it helps designers create collections that are both market-relevant and forward-thinking. Overall, fashion design is a multifaceted discipline that combines creativity, technical skills, and an understanding of cultural and societal influences. It is constantly evolving and adapting to reflect the changing dynamics of the fashion industry and the world at large. Through their designs, fashion designers have the power to shape and influence trends, challenge conventions, and make a statement, making fashion an integral part of our daily lives.

Fashion Fashion Retail Store

A fashion retail store is a physical or online establishment where customers can browse, try on, and purchase a variety of fashion items such as clothing, footwear, accessories, and jewelry. These stores typically stock a range of brands and designers, catering to different styles, trends, and budgets. At a fashion retail store, customers can explore a curated selection of fashion products, allowing them to find pieces that suit their personal preferences and express their individuality. These stores provide a platform for both established and emerging designers to showcase their creations and make them accessible to a wider consumer base.

Fashion Fashion Retail

Fashion retail refers to the process of selling clothes, accessories, and other fashion-related items to consumers. It involves various activities such as purchasing, merchandising, marketing, and selling fashion products in physical stores or through online platforms. The fashion retail industry is dynamic and constantly changing, influenced by factors like trends, customer preferences, and market demands. Fashion designers play a crucial role in this industry as they create new designs and collections that appeal to consumers and drive sales for fashion retailers. Fashion design is the art of applying design principles and aesthetics to create garments and accessories. It involves conceptualizing, sketching, and creating prototypes to bring unique and fashionable ideas to life. Fashion designers utilize their creativity, knowledge of textiles and materials, and understanding of current trends to design products that meet the demands and desires of consumers. Fashion retailers collaborate with fashion designers to source and stock their designs in their stores or online platforms. They work to create a seamless shopping experience for consumers by curating a diverse range of fashion products that cater to different tastes, sizes, and budgets. The role of fashion retail goes beyond just selling products. It includes activities like inventory management, pricing, and promotion to ensure profitability and customer satisfaction. Good fashion retail involves effective marketing strategies, visual merchandising, and customer service practices to attract and retain customers. In the modern era, fashion retail has expanded to include e-commerce platforms, allowing customers to shop for fashion products online. This has opened up new opportunities for both retailers and designers to reach a wider audience and increase sales. In conclusion, fashion retail is the process of selling fashion products to consumers, where fashion designers and retailers collaborate to offer a diverse range of fashionable items. It requires a deep understanding of consumer preferences, market trends, and effective management practices to ensure success in the fashion industry.

Fashion Fashion Retailing

Fashion retailing refers to the business activities involved in selling fashion products to consumers. It encompasses the processes of sourcing, merchandising, marketing, and selling fashion items through various channels, such as physical stores, e-commerce platforms, and mobile applications. At its core, fashion retailing revolves around understanding the preferences and needs of consumers and delivering fashionable products that align with their tastes. This requires a deep understanding of current fashion trends, consumer demographics, and buying behaviors.

Fashion Fashion Runway

The fashion runway is a platform where fashion designers showcase their latest collections through a live fashion show. It is an essential part of the fashion industry as it allows designers to reach a larger audience and gain recognition for their work. The fashion runway is typically a long, narrow stage that serves as a catwalk for models to showcase the designer's creations. It is often set up in a specific location, such as a fashion week event or a high-profile fashion show, where industry professionals, buyers, and media representatives are in attendance. During a fashion show, models walk down the runway, displaying the designer's garments to the audience. The runway provides an opportunity for designers to present their unique vision and creativity through the styling, fabrics, and silhouettes of their collections. Designers carefully plan and choreograph the fashion show, considering factors such as music, lighting, and overall atmosphere to create a memorable experience for the audience. The length and layout of the runway may vary depending on the venue and the designer's preferences. Fashion runways also play a significant role in setting trends and influencing the fashion industry. The collections showcased on the runway often set the tone for upcoming seasons, dictating what styles and designs will be popular in the future. The audience, including fashion editors, buyers, and celebrities, observe the runway shows to identify new trends and select pieces for editorial spreads or retail stores. In addition to its promotional aspect, the fashion runway serves as a platform for designers to express their artistic vision and create a narrative around their collections. It allows them to showcase their craftsmanship, attention to detail, and ability to push boundaries in terms of design and aesthetics. The fashion runway provides an immersive experience for both the audience and the designers. It is a moment of anticipation, as the audience eagerly awaits the next look and the designer's grand finale. Through the runway, fashion designers can establish their brand, gain exposure, and leave a lasting impression on the fashion industry.

Fashion Fashion Sales

Fashion Fashion Sales refers to the process of selling fashion products, such as clothing, accessories, or footwear, through various channels and strategies in order to maximize profit and increase brand visibility. It involves a combination of marketing, merchandising, and sales techniques to attract customers and persuade them to make a purchase. In the world of fashion design, Fashion Fashion Sales plays a crucial role in the success of a brand or designer. It encompasses a wide range of activities, including but not limited to personal selling, online retail, wholesale distribution, and promotional campaigns. The goal is to reach a target audience and create a demand for the products being offered. Personal selling is one of the key components of Fashion Fashion Sales. It involves sales representatives or brand ambassadors engaging directly with customers, either in stores or at events, to provide information about the brand and its products. This form of sales allows for a personalized and interactive experience, where customers can ask questions, receive styling advice, and try on items before making a purchase. Online retail has become an essential aspect of Fashion Fashion Sales, especially with the rise of e-commerce. Brands and designers now have the opportunity to reach a global audience and sell their products directly through their own websites or online marketplaces. This requires effective digital marketing strategies, user-friendly online platforms, and efficient logistics and fulfillment processes. Wholesale distribution is another important channel in Fashion Fashion Sales. This involves selling fashion products in bulk to retailers, who then sell them to the end consumers. Wholesale sales require strong relationships with buyers, effective product merchandising, and competitive pricing. It is a way for brands and designers to expand their reach and increase their sales volume. Promotional campaigns are a crucial part of Fashion Fashion Sales, as they help create brand awareness and generate interest in the products being offered. This can include advertising in traditional media, such as magazines or billboards, as well as utilizing digital marketing channels, such as social media platforms or influencer collaborations. The goal is to create a buzz around the brand and its products, ultimately leading to increased sales.

Fashion Fashion Sample Making

Fashion sample making is a crucial process in fashion design that involves the creation of prototypes or samples of a garment or accessory. It serves as a visual and physical representation of the designer's vision and helps translate their ideas into tangible products. Sample making is an essential step in the design and production cycle, allowing for experimentation, refinement, and validation of the design concept before mass production. During the sample making process, skilled patternmakers, seamstresses, and technicians work closely with the fashion designer to bring the design to life. The process typically starts with the creation of a pattern, which serves as the blueprint for the garment. The pattern is then used to cut fabric pieces, which are then sewn together to create the initial sample. This sample is often referred to as a toile or muslin, and it is made from inexpensive fabric that mimics the weight and drape of the final fabric. Once the initial sample is made, it is reviewed by the designer and their team. They assess the fit, proportions, and overall aesthetic of the garment. Adjustments and modifications are often made at this stage to perfect the design. The sample may undergo multiple fittings and alterations until it meets the designer's vision and requirements. In addition to fit and aesthetics, sample making also allows for the evaluation of the garment's construction and functionality. The sample is tested for durability, comfort, and ease of movement to ensure that it performs well in real-life scenarios. It also helps determine the feasibility of the design for mass production, as technical aspects such as fabric consumption, production time, and cost can be assessed during this stage. Once the sample is approved, it serves as a reference for the production team to follow. They use the approved sample as a guide to create the final garments in multiple sizes and quantities. The sample making process is critical in fashion design as it bridges the gap between the designer's concept and the production of market-ready products. It allows for refinement, experimentation, and validation of the design, ensuring that the final product meets the designer's vision and the requirements of the target market.

Fashion Fashion Scholarships

A fashion scholarship is a monetary award or grant given to individuals who are pursuing a career in fashion design or related disciplines. It is offered by various organizations, institutions, and individuals to support aspiring fashion designers and help them achieve their educational and professional goals. The purpose of fashion scholarships is to promote and recognize talent in the fashion industry and provide financial assistance to students who demonstrate exceptional skills, creativity, and dedication to their craft. These scholarships aim to enable students to pursue their education at renowned fashion schools, colleges, or universities, covering a range of expenses such as tuition fees, books, materials, and living costs.

Fashion Fashion Season

A fashion season refers to a specific period within the fashion industry in which designers and brands showcase their latest collections and trends to buyers, press, and consumers. These seasons are typically divided into four main categories: spring/summer, fall/winter, resort/cruise, and pre-fall. During a fashion season, designers and fashion houses present their collections through various mediums such as runway shows, presentations, lookbooks, or digital platforms. The purpose of these showcases is to introduce new designs, styles, and silhouettes that reflect the current trends and aesthetic preferences. The spring/summer season represents the warmer months of the year, featuring lightweight fabrics, bold colors, and vibrant prints. It is a time when designers experiment with fresh and airy designs, incorporating elements such as floral patterns, pastel hues, and flowy silhouettes. Fall/winter season, on the other hand, is characterized by heavier fabrics, deeper tones, and more layered ensembles. This season often showcases cozy knitwear, tailored outerwear, and rich textures. Designers focus on warmth, comfort, and functionality in their collections to adapt to the colder climate. The resort/cruise season, also referred to as pre-summer, emphasizes vacation-ready clothing. It typically features versatile pieces that can be worn not only during holidays but also in warm climates throughout the year. This season is known for resortwear, swimwear, and casual yet chic looks suitable for beach destinations. Pre-fall season serves as a transitional period between summer and fall, incorporating elements from both seasons. Designers often present pieces that can be worn during the change in weather, offering versatility with lightweight layering options, neutral colors, and versatile silhouettes. Fashion seasons play a vital role in the industry as they set the trends and influence consumers' purchasing decisions. They provide an opportunity for designers to showcase their creativity and craftsmanship, while also allowing buyers and fashion enthusiasts to discover new styles and plan their wardrobes accordingly.

Fashion Fashion Seminar

A fashion seminar in the context of fashion design is an educational event that brings together professionals, experts, and aspiring individuals in the fashion industry to discuss and explore various aspects of fashion. It provides a platform for exchanging knowledge, sharing experiences, and fostering creative thinking within the fashion community. The main objective of a fashion seminar is to facilitate the learning and development of participants by offering them valuable insights into the latest trends, techniques, and innovations in fashion design. Through presentations, panel discussions, workshops, and interactive sessions, attendees gain exposure to different perspectives and broaden their understanding of the industry.

Fashion Fashion Show Gala

A Fashion Show Gala is a highly anticipated event in the fashion industry that showcases the latest designs and trends of fashion designers. It is a grand affair where designers, models, celebrities, and fashion enthusiasts come together to celebrate and appreciate the artistry and creativity of fashion. The primary objective of a Fashion Show Gala is to present the designer's collection to a wider audience, including potential buyers, retailers, and fashion influencers. It serves as a platform for designers to promote their brand and establish themselves in the industry. The gala is usually organized by fashion houses or event management companies in collaboration with sponsors and partners. The Fashion Show Gala is meticulously planned and executed to create a captivating and immersive experience for the attendees. It typically features a runway or catwalk where models showcase the designer's garments one by one. The runway is designed with lights, music, and props to complement the theme and aesthetic of the collection. The event begins with a red carpet entrance, where designers, models, and celebrities make their appearance, dressed in their finest attire. The attendees, including media personnel and VIP guests, get a chance to interact with the designers and get a closer look at the garments. The show is divided into segments, each representing a different collection or theme by various designers. The order and flow of the show are carefully choreographed to create a seamless transition between the different segments. The models walk down the runway, showcasing each garment with poise and confidence, while the audience admires the craftsmanship and innovation of the designs. Apart from the runway, a Fashion Show Gala may also include live performances, art installations, and guest speakers to enhance the overall experience. The event often culminates in an after-party or reception, where attendees can mingle, network, and celebrate the success of the show. In conclusion, a Fashion Show Gala is a prestigious event that provides a platform for fashion designers to showcase their creativity and designs to a wider audience. It is an opportunity to establish their brand, connect with potential buyers, and make a lasting impression in the fashion industry.

Fashion Fashion Sketching

Fashion sketching is a fundamental tool used in fashion design to visually represent and explore ideas, concepts, and designs. It involves the creation of detailed and proportionate drawings of garments and fashion accessories on paper. Through fashion sketching, designers are able to communicate their creative vision and design concepts to others, including clients, manufacturers, and fellow designers. These sketches provide a clear visual representation of the desired silhouette, style, and details of a particular garment or accessory.

Fashion Fashion Sourcing

Fashion Fashion Startups

A fashion startup is a newly established company in the fashion industry that aims to disrupt traditional fashion practices through innovation and technology. It is an entrepreneurial endeavor that focuses on introducing unique and innovative fashion concepts, designs, products, or services to the market. These startups typically operate on a small scale with limited resources, but they aspire to make a big impact in the industry. They leverage technology, creativity, and entrepreneurial spirit to challenge the status quo and bring fresh perspectives to the fashion world.

Fashion Fashion Styling

Fashion styling is a process of visually enhancing and creating an aesthetic image through the careful selection and arrangement of clothing, accessories, and props. It involves analyzing and understanding the client's or brand's desired image or message and then utilizing various garments and elements to convey that message effectively. The primary role of a fashion stylist is to curate and create outfits that represent the client's unique style and personality, while also considering current fashion trends and the occasion or event at hand. This involves having a deep understanding of different fabrics, colors, patterns, and cuts, as well as an eye for creating well-balanced and visually pleasing compositions. During the styling process, the fashion stylist may collaborate with fashion designers, photographers, makeup artists, and hairstylists to create a cohesive and harmonious overall look. They may also be responsible for sourcing and selecting clothing and accessories from fashion showrooms, boutiques, and online platforms. In addition to working with individual clients, fashion stylists also play a crucial role in editorial fashion shoots, advertising campaigns, fashion shows, and celebrity styling. They are responsible for conceptualizing and executing creative themes or concepts through their styling choices, ensuring that the final visual representation aligns with the intended message or story. Furthermore, fashion styling extends beyond just selecting clothing and accessories. It often involves paying attention to detail by ensuring proper fit, altering garments if necessary, and being knowledgeable about various fashion brands and their distinct aesthetic. A fashion stylist should have a keen sense of fashion history and trends, as well as the ability to predict and anticipate future trends. In conclusion, fashion styling is a multifaceted process that involves creating visually appealing and cohesive outfits or looks for individuals or brands. It requires a deep understanding of fashion, trends, and aesthetics, as well as strong creative and organizational skills. A successful fashion stylist can transform a person or brand's image, leaving a lasting impact on the fashion industry.

Fashion Fashion Summit

A Fashion Fashion Summit is a highly anticipated event in the fashion design industry that brings together experts, designers, and fashion enthusiasts to discuss and explore the latest trends, challenges, and innovations in the world of fashion. It serves as a platform for networking, exchange of ideas, and fostering collaborations among professionals in the field. The Fashion Fashion Summit is typically organized by renowned fashion organizations, institutions, or industry leaders with the aim of fostering sustainable practices, ethical production, and responsible consumption in the fashion industry. The summit offers a unique opportunity for all participants to engage in thought-provoking discussions, interactive sessions, and workshops on various aspects of fashion design.

Fashion Fashion Supply Chain

The fashion supply chain refers to the network and processes involved in the design, production, and distribution of fashion products. It encompasses all the stages from the initial conception of a design to its eventual availability for purchase by consumers. The first stage of the fashion supply chain is the design phase, where fashion designers create innovative and aesthetically pleasing designs based on market trends, consumer preferences, and their creative vision. These designs are then transformed into patterns and prototypes, which serve as the foundation for the production process. Next, the production phase involves sourcing raw materials, such as fabrics and accessories, and manufacturing the garments or accessories according to the design specifications. This may involve multiple steps, such as fabric cutting, sewing, and quality control, to ensure that the final product meets the desired standards of quality and craftsmanship. Once the products are ready for distribution, they move into the logistics and distribution phase of the fashion supply chain. This involves the transportation of the products from the production facilities to distribution centers or directly to retail stores. From there, the products are made available for purchase by consumers either in physical stores or through e-commerce platforms. Throughout the fashion supply chain, various stakeholders play important roles. Fashion brands and designers collaborate with manufacturers, suppliers, and logistics providers to bring their designs to life and make them accessible to consumers. Retailers and fashion outlets act as intermediaries, showcasing and marketing the products to attract customers. The fashion supply chain is a complex and dynamic system that requires collaboration, coordination, and efficient management to ensure the timely delivery of fashion products to the market. It is influenced by factors such as changing consumer demands, global sourcing strategies, and sustainability concerns. In conclusion, the fashion supply chain is the process through which fashion designs are transformed into tangible products and made available for purchase by consumers. It encompasses design, production, and distribution stages, involving various stakeholders and requiring effective management to meet market demands.

Fashion Fashion Sustainability

Fashion sustainability refers to the practice of designing, producing, and consuming fashion items in a way that minimizes negative impacts on the environment, society, and economy. It involves considering the entire lifecycle of a fashion product, from the sourcing of raw materials to its disposal, and aims to reduce waste, pollution, and unethical practices. In fashion design, sustainability is about creating garments that are not only aesthetically pleasing but also ethically and environmentally responsible. This includes using sustainable materials, such as organic cotton, hemp, or recycled fabrics, which have a lower impact on the environment compared to conventional textiles. Additionally, sustainable fashion design promotes the use of environmentally friendly production processes, such as natural dyeing methods or water-saving techniques, to reduce pollution and resource depletion. Furthermore, sustainable fashion design considers the social aspect of production, ensuring fair and safe working conditions for garment workers. This entails collaborating with ethical manufacturers and suppliers who prioritize fair wages, worker health and safety, and human rights. It also involves supporting and promoting local artisans and traditional craftsmanship to sustain cultural diversity and social cohesion. By adopting sustainable practices, fashion designers contribute to a more sustainable and circular fashion ecosystem. They aim to extend the lifespan of garments through design strategies such as modularity, durability, and repairability. This means creating timeless and versatile pieces that can be restyled or repaired, reducing the need for constant consumption and ultimately decreasing waste. Overall, fashion sustainability in the realm of design is about rethinking the way fashion is created, consumed, and perceived. It prioritizes the well-being of the environment, society, and economy, aiming to create a more responsible and resilient fashion industry.

Fashion Fashion Symposium

The Fashion Fashion Symposium is an event that brings together professionals and enthusiasts in the field of fashion design to discuss and explore various aspects of the industry. It serves as a platform for sharing knowledge, ideas, and experiences, and aims to inspire and engage individuals with a passion for fashion. During the Fashion Fashion Symposium, experts from different areas of fashion design, including designers, stylists, photographers, and educators, come together to present their work, insights, and perspectives. The symposium typically includes a series of panel discussions, presentations, workshops, and exhibitions, providing attendees with a well-rounded and immersive experience.

Fashion Fashion Tailoring

Fashion tailoring is a specialized skill within the field of fashion design that involves the creation and alteration of garments to fit a client's body shape and personal preferences. It combines elements of art, craftsmanship, and technical expertise to create clothing that is not only visually appealing but also comfortable and well-fitting. The process of fashion tailoring begins with taking accurate measurements of the client's body, including the bust, waist, hips, and inseam. These measurements serve as the foundation for creating a pattern, which is a template used to cut the fabric and sew the garment. The pattern is customized to the client's specific measurements and can be adjusted to accommodate any unique body proportions. Once the pattern is created, the tailor selects the appropriate fabric and begins cutting the pieces according to the pattern. This step requires precision and attention to detail to ensure that the fabric is cut accurately and symmetrically. After cutting the fabric, the tailor sews the garment together, following the pattern instructions and employing various sewing techniques. This stage involves joining the individual fabric pieces using stitches or specialized machinery, such as a sewing machine or serger. The tailor must possess a thorough understanding of different sewing techniques and be skilled in using various tools and equipment. In addition to assembling the garment, fashion tailoring also involves fitting the garment to the client's body. This process typically includes multiple fittings and adjustments to ensure that the garment fits correctly and flatters the client's body shape. The tailor may need to make alterations to the garment, such as taking in or letting out seams, shortening or lengthening hemlines, or adjusting the fit of sleeves or waistbands. Overall, fashion tailoring plays a crucial role in the fashion industry by transforming flat pieces of fabric into wearable garments that accentuate the wearer's body shape and style. It requires a combination of technical skill, artistic vision, and attention to detail to create garments that are both aesthetically pleasing and functional.

Fashion Fashion Technology

Fashion technology refers to the incorporation of advanced techniques, materials, and processes in the creation and production of fashion designs. It encompasses the use of various technologies, such as computer-aided design (CAD) software, digital printing, and virtual reality, to enhance the efficiency and creativity of the fashion industry. With the rapid advancements in technology, fashion designers have been able to experiment with new materials, textures, and patterns that were previously unattainable. Through the development of innovative techniques, fashion technology has revolutionized the way garments are designed, manufactured, and marketed.

Fashion Fashion Textile Design

Fashion textile design is a specialized field within the broader realm of fashion design that focuses specifically on the creation and development of unique textiles or fabrics used in garments and accessories. It involves a combination of artistic creativity and technical knowledge to design, produce, and manipulate textiles in a way that enhances the overall aesthetic and functionality of the final fashion product.A fashion textile designer is responsible for researching current trends, identifying new materials, and experimenting with various textile techniques to develop innovative fabrics that align with the envisioned fashion collection. They work closely with fashion designers to understand their design concept and translate it into fabric designs that complement and enhance the overall garment or accessory.In the initial stages of the design process, fashion textile designers draw inspiration from various sources such as nature, historical references, cultural influences, or even contemporary art movements. They take these inspirations and create hand-drawn or digital sketches to develop unique patterns, color palettes, and textures that reflect the desired aesthetic. Using their technical knowledge, they also consider factors like fabric composition, weight, and drape to ensure the textiles meet both the aesthetic and functional requirements of the design.Once the textile designs are finalized, fashion textile designers collaborate with textile mills or manufacturers to produce the fabrics on a larger scale. They oversee the production process to ensure that the fabrics are being manufactured to their specifications and quality standards. They may also be involved in dyeing, printing, or finishing processes to add further dimension to the fabrics.One of the key aspects of fashion textile design is the ability to constantly innovate and stay updated with the latest advancements in textile technologies and sustainable practices. Designers need to be knowledgeable about the properties and characteristics of different fibers, weaving and knitting techniques, printing methods, and dyeing processes to create textiles that are not only visually appealing but also durable and eco-friendly.In summary, fashion textile design is a specialized field that focuses on creating unique and innovative textiles for the fashion industry. It requires a blend of artistic creativity, technical expertise, and a deep understanding of fashion trends and market demands to develop textiles that enhance the overall aesthetic and functionality of fashion garments and accessories.

Fashion Fashion Trade Show

A Fashion Trade Show is a specialized event in the fashion industry that brings together designers, brands, retailers, and other professionals to showcase and promote their latest collections, products, and services. At a Fashion Trade Show, participants set up booths or stands to display their designs, garments, accessories, or other fashion-related items. These booths are typically designed in an appealing and visually attractive manner to attract the attention of attendees, who may include buyers, fashion journalists, stylists, influencers, and other industry insiders. The main purpose of a Fashion Trade Show is to provide a platform for fashion professionals to network, establish business relationships, and create opportunities for collaboration. It allows designers and brands to connect with potential buyers, retailers, and distributors, who may be interested in showcasing their products in their stores or online platforms. Additionally, it offers a chance for designers to receive feedback, gain exposure, and generate sales leads. During a Fashion Trade Show, designers and brands may organize fashion shows or runway presentations to showcase their collections. These fashion shows are often attended by industry professionals and media representatives, providing a platform for designers to generate buzz and generate media coverage. Furthermore, Fashion Trade Shows often feature seminars, workshops, and panel discussions on various topics related to the fashion industry. These educational and informative sessions allow participants to learn from industry experts, gain insights into current trends, and discuss challenges and opportunities within the fashion business. Fashion Trade Shows are usually held in major fashion capitals or exhibition centers around the world, such as New York, Paris, Milan, London, and Tokyo. They can range in size and scale, from small regional events to large international trade shows that attract participants from all corners of the globe. Overall, Fashion Trade Shows play a vital role in the fashion industry by providing a platform for designers, brands, and retailers to showcase their latest creations, establish connections, and stay up-to-date with the latest trends and developments in the fashion world.

Fashion Fashion Trends Analysis

A fashion trend analysis in the context of fashion design refers to the process of evaluating and examining the current and emerging trends in the fashion industry. It involves observing and analyzing the preferences, styles, and choices of designers, fashion influencers, and consumers to understand the direction in which fashion is moving. The analysis of fashion trends is crucial for fashion designers as it helps them make informed decisions about the design, production, and marketing of their collections. By staying updated on the latest trends, designers can create designs that align with consumer preferences, making their products more commercially viable.

Fashion Fashion Webinar

A fashion fashion webinar is a virtual presentation or workshop conducted through a web-conferencing platform that focuses on various aspects of fashion design. It aims to educate and inspire aspiring fashion designers, industry professionals, or fashion enthusiasts about the latest trends, techniques, and strategies in the fashion industry. During a fashion fashion webinar, experts in the field of fashion design may present and discuss a wide range of topics, such as fashion forecasting, garment construction, pattern-making, styling, branding, marketing, and more. These webinars provide participants with the opportunity to learn from experienced professionals and gain valuable insights into the ever-evolving world of fashion.

Fashion Fashion Workshop

A fashion workshop refers to a creative space where fashion designers collaborate, experiment, and engage in hands-on activities to develop their design skills and create new fashion concepts. It is a place where aspiring and established fashion designers come together to learn, share knowledge, and exchange ideas. At a fashion workshop, designers have the opportunity to participate in various activities and workshops that enhance their understanding of fashion design techniques, fabric manipulation, pattern-making, and garment construction. These workshops often include demonstrations, practical sessions, and discussions conducted by experienced industry professionals, enhancing the learning experience and providing valuable insights into the fashion industry. The main objective of a fashion workshop is to foster creativity, encourage innovation, and inspire designers to explore new ideas and push boundaries in their designs. It serves as a platform for designers to expand their skills, experiment with different materials and techniques, and refine their personal aesthetic. Through collaboration and interaction with fellow designers, participants can gain fresh perspectives and broaden their creative horizons. Moreover, fashion workshops also play a significant role in nurturing emerging talent and providing opportunities for aspiring fashion designers to gain practical experience and exposure in the industry. They often serve as a launching pad for new designers to showcase their work and establish connections with industry professionals, buyers, and influential figures in the fashion world. Overall, a fashion workshop is a dynamic and inspiring environment that serves as a catalyst for innovation, creativity, and growth within the fashion design industry. By providing a space for experimentation, skill development, and collaboration, it empowers designers to push boundaries, refine their craft, and contribute to the ever-evolving world of fashion.

Fashion Fast Fashion

The term "fast fashion" refers to a business model and a trend in the fashion industry characterized by the rapid production and consumption of low-cost garments inspired by the latest fashion trends. Fast fashion brands are known for their ability to swiftly produce and distribute new designs, effectively imitating the styles seen on designer runways and celebrity red carpets. Fast fashion brands are able to keep up with the ever-changing trends by constantly monitoring the fashion world, observing the designs showcased by high-end brands, and quickly reproducing them at a fraction of the cost. This allows them to offer consumers affordable versions of the latest runway looks in a matter of weeks, often with an incredibly short production cycle.

Fashion Faux Fur

Fashion faux fur refers to a type of synthetic fur that is commonly used in the fashion industry as an alternative to real animal fur. It is designed to replicate the luxurious and soft texture of real fur while remaining cruelty-free and environmentally friendly. Fashion designers use faux fur as a versatile and sustainable material in their collections. The faux fur fabric is typically made from a variety of synthetic fibers, such as polyester or acrylic, that closely mimic the look and feel of natural fur. These fibers are often woven or knitted together to create a soft and fluffy texture that can be used to make a wide range of clothing items, accessories, and home decor pieces.

Fashion Footwear

Fashion footwear is an essential component of the fashion industry, encompassing a wide range of footwear styles designed to complement and enhance an individual's overall fashion ensemble. It is a category of footwear that combines both functionality and aesthetic appeal, designed with the latest fashion trends in mind. Fashion footwear plays a crucial role in completing an outfit, adding a touch of style, and making a fashion statement. It goes beyond basic functionality, as it is crafted with attention to detail, incorporating various materials, textures, colors, and embellishments to create visually appealing and fashion-forward designs. Fashion footwear is not limited to a specific gender, age group, or occasion but caters to a diverse range of preferences and fashion sensibilities.

Fashion Forecasting

Fashion forecasting is a strategic analysis and prediction of upcoming fashion trends, based on a thorough understanding of historical data, cultural influences, consumer behavior, and market research. It plays a crucial role in the fashion industry by providing designers, retailers, and manufacturers with valuable insights to make informed decisions about their collections and merchandise. Through fashion forecasting, professionals analyze various elements such as color palettes, fabric choices, silhouettes, patterns, and accessories to anticipate the direction in which fashion trends are likely to evolve. By closely observing fashion shows, street style, social media, and other sources of inspiration, forecasters interpret emerging style cues and translate them into tangible trends that can be easily understood by the industry. One key aspect of fashion forecasting is trend analysis, which involves studying fashion cycles and movements, as well as identifying emerging micro-trends that might influence the broader fashion landscape. This involves looking at historical fashion references, cultural shifts, global events, and societal changes to understand how they might impact fashion preferences and consumption patterns. In addition to trend analysis, fashion forecasting also encompasses market analysis, where professionals evaluate consumer demographics, psychographics, and spending habits to identify target markets and anticipate their needs and desires. By understanding the profile of target customers, forecasters can predict what types of products, styles, and price points will resonate with them, enabling designers and brands to cater to their preferences and capture market share. Fashion forecasting is a collaborative process that involves a wide range of experts, including trend analysts, forecasters, designers, merchandisers, buyers, and retail experts. By working together, these professionals can pool their insights and knowledge to create accurate forecasts that align with market demand and consumer tastes.

Fashion Formal Wear

Fashion formal wear refers to clothing and attire that is specifically designed for formal occasions and events. It is a category of dress that is elevated in sophistication and elegance, often associated with black tie and white tie dress codes. Formal wear is characterized by its refined and polished aesthetic, tailored fit, and attention to detail. When designing fashion formal wear, designers pay careful attention to the choice of materials, construction techniques, and silhouettes. Fabrics such as silk, satin, velvet, and chiffon are commonly used to create luxurious and opulent garments. The use of intricate details such as beading, embroidery, lace, and sequins adds a touch of glamour and sophistication to the designs. The silhouette of formal wear varies depending on the specific occasion, but it generally gravitates towards a more structured and fitted style. For men, formal wear often includes tailored suits or tuxedos with crisp shirts, bowties or neckties, and polished dress shoes. Women's formal wear, on the other hand, may consist of elegant gowns, cocktail dresses, or pantsuits, paired with high heels and statement accessories. In terms of color, formal wear traditionally features darker shades such as black, navy, and deep jewel tones. However, modern interpretations of formal wear have expanded the color palette to include lighter hues and metallics, allowing for more diverse and creative choices. Ultimately, fashion formal wear is designed to make a bold and sophisticated statement. It is meant to elevate the wearer's style, exuding confidence, class, and elegance. By carefully considering materials, construction techniques, and attention to detail, fashion designers create formal wear that embodies the spirit of special occasions and helps individuals feel their best when dressing for these momentous events.

Fashion Fundraiser

A fashion fundraiser is a charitable event or initiative that aims to raise funds for a specific cause or organization, using fashion design as the main medium of expression and avenue for generating donations. Fashion fundraisers typically involve the collaboration of fashion designers, brands, models, influencers, and other industry professionals who contribute their skills, time, and resources to support the fundraising efforts. The primary objective of a fashion fundraiser is to combine philanthropy with the world of fashion, leveraging the power of creativity and style to make a positive impact on society. The event can take various forms, including fashion shows, exhibitions, auctions, galas, or online campaigns that promote designer fashion items or collections as a means to generate revenue for a chosen cause.

Fashion Fundraising Event

A fashion fundraising event is a formal gathering organized by a fashion designer or fashion-related organization with the aim of raising funds for a specific cause or charity. The event typically involves a fashion show, where the designer showcases their latest collection or a curated selection of garments. Guests are usually required to purchase tickets to attend the event, with the proceeds going towards the designated cause or charity. The fashion show itself is the main highlight of the event, featuring professional models wearing the designer's creations on a runway. The garments on display can range from ready-to-wear pieces to high-end couture, depending on the designer's aesthetic and target audience. The fashion show may be accompanied by live music, lighting effects, and stage decorations to create a captivating atmosphere. Besides the fashion show, a fashion fundraising event may also include other activities to entertain and engage the attendees. This can include live performances, silent auctions, raffles, or even pop-up shops where guests can purchase items directly from the designer. These additional elements serve to further encourage donations and generate excitement among the attendees. The purpose of a fashion fundraising event extends beyond showcasing the designer's talent and generating revenue. It allows the fashion designer or fashion-related organization to use their platform and influence to raise awareness and support for a cause they believe in. The chosen cause may be related to social issues, health concerns, or other charitable initiatives. By organizing and hosting a fashion fundraising event, the designer can make a positive impact on society and contribute to bringing about positive change. In conclusion, a fashion fundraising event is a formal gathering that combines fashion, entertainment, and charity. It allows fashion designers and fashion-related organizations to raise funds and awareness for a specific cause through a fashion show and other engaging activities. It serves as a platform for designers to showcase their work while also making a positive impact on society.

Fashion Fur

Fashion fur refers to the use of animal fur in clothing and accessory designs within the context of the fashion industry. It involves the incorporation of fur, typically obtained from animals such as minks, rabbits, foxes, and chinchillas, into various fashion items, including coats, jackets, hats, and handbags. Designers often utilize fashion fur to add a luxurious and glamorous element to their creations. The use of fur can enhance the aesthetic appeal, texture, and overall design of a fashion piece, providing it with a distinctive and sophisticated look. Fashion fur is known for its warmth, durability, and natural beauty, which make it a popular choice among designers and consumers.

Fashion Gala

A Fashion Gala is an extravagant event in the world of fashion design that brings together designers, models, industry professionals, and fashion enthusiasts to showcase the latest trends, collections, and designs. It is a platform where creativity, innovation, and style collide to create a mesmerizing experience for all attendees. At a Fashion Gala, fashion designers present their fashion collections through runway shows. These shows are carefully choreographed performances that exhibit the designer's vision and artistic expression. Models strut down the runway, showcasing the garments with confidence and grace, while the audience observes and admires the designs in awe.

Fashion Garment Construction

Fashion garment construction refers to the process of creating clothing or garments by combining various materials and sewing techniques. It involves the assembly of fabric pieces, the addition of trims and finishes, and the creation of structured elements such as darts, pleats, and seams. This process begins with the development of a garment pattern, which is a blueprint or template for cutting the fabric pieces. The pattern is usually created based on a design sketch or concept, and it specifies the shape and size of each fabric piece required to construct the garment. Once the pattern is ready, the fabric is carefully selected and prepped for cutting. This may involve washing, ironing, and laying out the fabric to ensure that it is free of any wrinkles or imperfections. The pattern pieces are then placed on the fabric and marked before being cut out using fabric shears or a rotary cutter. After cutting, the fabric pieces are sewn together using a variety of sewing techniques such as straight stitches, zigzag stitches, and decorative stitches. The seams are finished to prevent fraying and to create a neat and professional appearance. This can be done by serging the edges, using a zigzag stitch, or by folding and pressing the seam allowances. In addition to seams, other elements such as darts, pleats, and gathers may be incorporated into the construction of a garment to create shape and volume. These techniques involve folding and stitching the fabric in specific ways to create fullness or to create a more tailored fit. Once the main construction is complete, trims and finishes are added to enhance the garment's design and functionality. This may include attaching buttons, zippers, or other closures, as well as adding decorative elements such as lace, embroidery, or appliques. Fashion garment construction requires a high level of skill and attention to detail. It involves combining artistic creativity with technical knowledge to bring a design concept to life. Through this process, the designer transforms a flat piece of fabric into a three-dimensional garment that can be worn and enjoyed.

Fashion Glam Style

Fashion Glam Style is a genre of fashion design that focuses on creating luxurious and sensual looks with an emphasis on opulence, sophistication, and extravagance. It is characterized by its bold and dramatic aesthetic, featuring high-end fabrics, intricate details, and glamorous embellishments. The Fashion Glam Style draws inspiration from various sources, including vintage fashion, Hollywood glamour, and haute couture. It evokes a sense of elegance and grandeur, often incorporating elements such as sequins, feathers, lace, and fur. The garments are tailored to highlight the female form, embracing curves and creating a seductive silhouette. Key components of Fashion Glam Style include evening gowns, cocktail dresses, and glamorous separates. Evening gowns are typically floor-length and designed to make a statement, featuring plunging necklines, cut-outs, and thigh-high slits. Cocktail dresses are shorter in length but still exude a sense of sophistication and allure. Other key pieces include tailored blazers, high-waisted trousers, and fitted bodysuits. The color palette of Fashion Glam Style is often rich and vibrant, incorporating bold hues such as deep reds, royal blues, and metallic tones. Black is also a staple color, adding a touch of elegance and timelessness to the overall look. The use of prints and patterns is minimal, as the focus is on the luxurious nature of the fabrics and the craftsmanship of the garments. When it comes to accessorizing, Fashion Glam Style embraces statement pieces. This includes large and elaborate jewelry, such as chandelier earrings, oversized cocktail rings, and layered necklaces. Handbags and clutches are often embellished or adorned with luxurious materials such as satin or velvet. Footwear options range from high-heeled pumps to embellished sandals and boots. In conclusion, Fashion Glam Style is a fashion design genre that embodies luxury, sophistication, and sensuality. It is characterized by its bold and glamorous aesthetic, featuring opulent fabrics, intricate details, and statement accessories. This style allows individuals to express their confidence and embrace their inner diva.

Fashion Gloves

Fashion gloves are accessories designed to cover and protect the hands while also adding a stylish touch to an outfit. These gloves are made from various materials such as leather, fabric, or synthetic materials and come in a wide range of styles and designs to complement different fashion ensembles. Fashion gloves serve both functional and aesthetic purposes. They provide protection from cold weather conditions, keeping the hands warm and comfortable. Additionally, they act as a barrier between the skin and potentially harsh elements, such as wind and rain. For individuals who spend a significant amount of time outdoors, fashion gloves offer a practical solution to maintain hand health and prevent discomfort. In the world of fashion design, gloves are considered an essential accessory that can elevate the overall look and feel of an outfit. They have the power to transform a simple ensemble into a sophisticated and fashionable statement. Designers incorporate gloves into their collections to add an element of elegance, drama, or whimsy, enhancing the visual appeal of their creations. When it comes to fashion gloves, the design options are limitless. Long gloves that extend up to the elbow or even the upper arm exude a sense of formality and glamour, often associated with high-class events and evening wear. Shorter gloves, such as wrist-length or fingerless gloves, offer a more casual and sporty vibe, perfect for everyday wear or accessorizing street-style-inspired outfits. Embellishments and details play a significant role in enhancing the aesthetic appeal of fashion gloves. From delicate lace and intricate embroidery to studs, buckles, and fur trims, these elements add texture, visual interest, and a unique touch to the gloves. The choice of fabric or material can also influence the overall design, with leather gloves exuding a sleek and edgy vibe, while fabric gloves convey a softer and more romantic feel. Overall, fashion gloves are integral in creating a cohesive and stylish look. These accessories not only protect the hands but also serve as a canvas for self-expression, allowing individuals to showcase their personal style and creativity through the various designs, materials, and details available.

Fashion Graduation Show

A fashion graduation show is a culminating event that showcases the work of graduating fashion design students. It is typically held at the end of their academic program and serves as a platform for these students to exhibit their final collections to a wider audience, including industry professionals, peers, and the general public. The purpose of a fashion graduation show is to highlight the creativity, skills, and innovative ideas of the graduating students. It provides them with an opportunity to apply their theoretical knowledge and practical skills acquired throughout their studies, and demonstrate their individual design aesthetics and unique styles. During a fashion graduation show, each participating student presents their collection through a carefully choreographed runway presentation. The collections often revolve around a central theme or concept, which the designer has developed and explored during their research and design process. The runway show allows the audience to experience the designer's vision come to life as models confidently strut down the catwalk, showcasing the garments and accessories that make up their collection. In addition to the runway presentation, a fashion graduation show may also include static displays or exhibitions, where individual garments or portfolios are showcased in a more stationary setting. This allows viewers to closely examine the construction, details, and craftsmanship of each design, as well as gain insight into the designer's design process and inspirations. Furthermore, a fashion graduation show often serves as a networking platform for graduating students and industry professionals. It offers an opportunity for aspiring fashion designers to establish connections, receive feedback on their work, and potentially forge partnerships or secure employment opportunities. Many industry insiders, such as fashion journalists, buyers, and recruiters, attend these shows to scout emerging talent and discover potential future collaborators or employees. In conclusion, a fashion graduation show is a significant event in the fashion industry that celebrates the achievements of graduating fashion design students. It showcases their creative abilities, allows them to express their unique styles, and provides an opportunity to connect with industry professionals. Overall, it is a momentous occasion that marks the beginning of their journey as professional fashion designers.

Fashion Grunge Style

The fashion grunge style is a fashion design movement that emerged in the early 1990s and is characterized by its fusion of elements from grunge music and the fashion industry. It is a rebellious, anti-conformist style that rejects traditional fashion norms and embraces a more rugged, unconventional aesthetic. At its core, the fashion grunge style is defined by its disheveled, "undone" look. It embraces a deliberately messy and unpolished appearance, often incorporating oversized and ill-fitting clothing, layers, and mismatched patterns. The style draws inspiration from the grunge music scene, which was known for its raw and gritty sound, and translates that aesthetic into fashion. One of the key elements of the fashion grunge style is the use of distressed and worn-out materials. This includes ripped jeans, tattered t-shirts, and frayed fabrics. The idea is to create a sense of authenticity and nonchalance, as if the wearer doesn't care about their appearance. The clothing often has a worn-in, vintage quality, with faded colors and washed-out prints. The fashion grunge style also incorporates elements of androgyny and gender non-conformity. It blurs the lines between traditionally masculine and feminine clothing, often featuring oversized sweaters, flannel shirts, combat boots, and Doc Martens. The style celebrates individualism and rejects societal expectations of how one should dress based on their gender. Accessories play a key role in the fashion grunge style as well. Chunky combat boots, studded belts, chokers, and fishnet stockings are commonly used to complete the look. The overall aesthetic is edgy and anti-establishment, with references to subversive and countercultural movements. In conclusion, the fashion grunge style is a rebellion against conventional fashion norms, characterized by its disheveled and unconventional aesthetic. It draws inspiration from the grunge music scene of the early 1990s and incorporates elements of distressed materials, androgyny, and anti-establishment accessories. It celebrates individualism and rejects societal expectations, creating a unique and edgy fashion statement.

Fashion Hairstyling

Fashion hairstyling is the art and technique of creating hairstyles that complement and enhance a particular fashion design aesthetic. It involves the creative manipulation of hair to achieve a desired look that harmonizes with the overall concept and vision of the fashion collection. The role of fashion hairstyling is to contribute to the overall visual impact of a fashion presentation, whether it is on the runway, in a photoshoot, or in a fashion editorial. It requires a deep understanding of fashion trends, the ability to interpret a designer's vision, and the technical skills to execute various hairstyles.

Fashion Hat

A fashion hat is a head covering that is designed and worn for its aesthetic value in the context of fashion design. It is a versatile accessory that can complement or enhance an individual's outfit, adding a touch of style and personality to their overall look. Unlike utilitarian hats that serve primarily functional purposes, such as protection from the sun or cold weather, fashion hats focus on making a fashion statement. They are created with creativity and imagination, incorporating various materials, colors, patterns, and embellishments to create unique and eye-catching designs.

Fashion Haute Couture

Fashion Haute Couture is a term that refers to high-end, individually tailored fashion creations made by highly skilled fashion designers. It is the epitome of luxury and exclusivity in the fashion industry. Haute Couture garments are meticulously crafted using the highest quality fabrics and materials, often embellished with intricate handwork such as embroidery, beading, and lacework. These pieces are made to measure, ensuring a perfect fit for the client.

Fashion History Exhibition

A Fashion History Exhibition is a curated presentation of garments, accessories, and other fashion-related artifacts that showcase the evolution of fashion through different eras and styles. This exhibition provides a comprehensive overview of the historical context, fashion trends, and societal influences that have shaped the world of fashion. The purpose of a Fashion History Exhibition is to educate and enlighten visitors about the significant milestones, key designers, and transformative moments in the history of fashion. By examining the garments and accessories on display, visitors can gain an understanding of how fashion has continually evolved, reflecting cultural, political, and economic changes throughout history. Each exhibit is carefully curated to present a chronological narrative, highlighting key periods such as the Renaissance, Baroque, Rococo, Victorian, Art Deco, and many others. Within each period, specific styles, silhouettes, and materials are showcased to provide a comprehensive understanding of the fashion of that time. Fashion History Exhibitions seek not only to present the aesthetics of fashion but also to reflect on the social and cultural contexts in which fashion plays a significant role. By examining the garments and accessories worn by different social classes, genders, and ethnicities throughout history, visitors can gain insights into power dynamics, social norms, and identity expression through fashion. In addition to garments, Fashion History Exhibitions may also include photographs, illustrations, videos, and interactive displays to enhance the visitors' experience and provide a more immersive exploration of fashion history. These exhibits may also feature collaborations with contemporary designers, who reinterpret historical garments or showcase their own creations influenced by past styles. Overall, a Fashion History Exhibition serves as a visual and educational reminder of the rich and complex history of fashion. It invites visitors to appreciate the craftsmanship, innovation, and artistic expression that have made fashion an integral part of our cultural heritage. It also encourages visitors to reflect on the societal impact of fashion and its ongoing evolution in the modern world. Fashion History Exhibition is an immersive and captivating experience that brings together the past, present, and future of fashion, allowing visitors to appreciate its beauty, diversity, and enduring influence.

Fashion History

Fashion history refers to the study of clothing and adornment styles throughout different eras and cultures. It analyzes the social, cultural, and historical factors that influenced the development and evolution of fashion over time. Through the study of fashion history, fashion designers gain insight into past fashion trends and silhouettes, allowing them to draw inspiration and create innovative designs that reflect a contemporary interpretation of certain periods or styles. By understanding the influences of the past, fashion designers can create designs that are both contemporary and timeless.

Fashion Hosiery

A fashion hosiery refers to the specialized legwear that is designed to complement and enhance an individual's outfit, adding a stylish and fashionable touch to their overall look. It is an essential component of fashion design, offering a wide range of options to create unique and trendsetting ensembles. Hosiery includes various types of leg coverings such as stockings, tights, pantyhose, socks, and leggings. These garments are typically made from a combination of fabrics such as nylon, spandex, polyester, cotton, and wool, ensuring a comfortable fit and durability. Fashion hosiery is known for its versatility, as it can be worn for both formal and casual occasions, allowing individuals to express their personal style and creativity. Stockings are a traditional form of hosiery that covers the leg from the toes to the upper thighs. They are often made of sheer or semi-sheer materials, accentuating the natural skin tone and giving a more elegant and sophisticated appearance. Tights, on the other hand, are similar to stockings but cover the entire leg, providing more coverage and warmth. They are available in a variety of thicknesses, colors, and patterns, allowing fashion enthusiasts to experiment with different looks. Pantyhose combines the features of stockings and tights, extending from the waist to the toes. They provide a smoother and more streamlined silhouette, making them ideal for wearing with skirts, dresses, or office attire. Pantyhose often come in skin tones to create a natural look, but they are also available in a wide range of fashion-forward colors and designs. Socks and leggings are another category of hosiery that can add a fashionable twist to an outfit. Socks come in various lengths, from ankle to knee-high, and can be adorned with intricate patterns, textures, and embellishments. Leggings, on the other hand, are footless and extend from the waist to the ankles. They are made from stretchy materials, providing a comfortable and form-fitting option that can be paired with dresses, tunics, or oversized sweaters. In the realm of fashion design, hosiery plays a crucial role in completing a look. It can be used to create contrast, texture, or a bold statement, allowing individuals to express their individuality. Fashion hosiery is a versatile accessory that can elevate any outfit, adding a touch of sophistication, glamour, or playfulness depending on the desired effect.

Fashion House

A fashion house is a company or brand that designs, produces, and sells high-end clothing and accessories. It is a prominent player in the fashion industry and is known for its distinct style, creativity, and innovation. A fashion house typically has a team of highly skilled designers who are responsible for creating unique and fashionable designs. These designs are then produced in limited quantities and sold at premium prices. The fashion house may also collaborate with other designers or artists to create special collections or limited edition pieces. One of the key elements of a fashion house is its brand identity. It is crucial for a fashion house to create and maintain a strong brand image that resonates with its target customers. This includes having a recognizable logo, a distinctive design aesthetic, and a consistent brand message. In addition to designing and producing clothing, a fashion house may also offer a range of other products and services. This may include accessories such as bags, shoes, and jewelry, as well as fragrances, cosmetics, and even home goods. These additional products help to further reinforce the brand's identity and appeal to a wider customer base. A fashion house often showcases its collections through fashion shows or presentations, where the latest designs are displayed on the runway. These events are attended by industry professionals, celebrities, and fashion enthusiasts, and serve as a platform to generate buzz and publicity for the brand. Furthermore, a fashion house may have its own retail stores or boutiques, where customers can directly purchase its products. It may also have a presence in department stores or luxury retailers, both offline and online, to reach a broader audience. Additionally, collaborations with other brands or designers can help to expand the fashion house's reach and exposure. In conclusion, a fashion house is a prestigious and influential player in the fashion industry. It is renowned for its design expertise, craftsmanship, and luxury products. With its unique style and brand identity, a fashion house sets trends and influences the fashion landscape.

Fashion Icon

A fashion icon is a person who has a significant influence on the fashion industry through their distinctive and influential personal style. They are recognized for their ability to set trends and inspire others with their fashion choices, often becoming a source of inspiration for designers, brands, and consumers. What sets a fashion icon apart is their ability to effortlessly showcase their individuality, creativity, and personal taste through their clothing, accessories, and overall style aesthetic. Their fashion choices are often daring, innovative, and thought-provoking, pushing the boundaries of traditional fashion norms and leading the way for new trends.

Fashion Illustration

Fashion Illustration is a form of artistic expression that captures and showcases the creative vision of a fashion designer. It involves translating ideas, concepts, and designs into visual representations using various artistic techniques and mediums. The primary purpose of fashion illustration is to communicate the designer's concept and design details to others involved in the garment production process, such as pattern makers, cutters, and manufacturers. This visual representation serves as a guide for creating the actual garment with accurate proportions, shaping, and construction techniques. Through a fashion illustration, a designer can convey the style, silhouette, fabric choice, and overall aesthetic of a garment. This allows for effective communication and collaboration between the designer and other stakeholders, ensuring that the final product aligns with the intended design vision. Fashion illustrators often use a combination of traditional and digital mediums to depict their designs. Traditional techniques may include pencil, ink, watercolor, and markers, while digital tools like graphic tablets and software programs offer additional flexibility and the ability to create intricate details and textures. A fashion illustration can range from a simple, gestural sketch to a highly detailed rendering. It may showcase a single garment or an entire collection, presented on human figures or mannequins. The choice of style and technique depends on the designer's preference and the purpose of the illustration, whether it is for concept development, presentation, or publication. In addition to its practical function, fashion illustration is also valued for its artistic expression and aesthetic appeal. It captures the essence of fashion, often incorporating elements of movement, texture, and fabric drape to bring the designs to life on paper or digital platforms. This artistic element allows the viewer to appreciate and connect with the designer's creativity and vision. In conclusion, fashion illustration is a visual representation of a fashion designer's ideas and designs, serving as a means of communication and collaboration in the garment production process. It combines artistic expression, technical accuracy, and aesthetic appeal to showcase the style, silhouette, and overall aesthetic of a garment or collection.

Fashion Incubator

A fashion incubator is a business platform or program that provides support, resources, and mentorship to emerging fashion designers and entrepreneurs, helping them to launch and establish their own fashion brands. The main purpose of a fashion incubator is to cultivate and nurture talented individuals in the fashion industry, offering them access to industry professionals, educational workshops, networking opportunities, and production facilities. This type of program typically operates within a specific timeframe, ranging from several months to a few years, during which participants receive intensive guidance and assistance to develop their fashion collections and business plans. By offering a comprehensive range of services, fashion incubators aim to empower and prepare emerging designers for the challenges of the fashion market. The support provided can include guidance in areas such as fashion design, product development, branding, marketing, sales, and financial management. One of the key advantages of participating in a fashion incubator is the access to a network of industry experts and mentors who can provide valuable insights and guidance. These mentors often have extensive experience in the fashion industry and can offer advice on important aspects such as production, sourcing materials, pricing, and building relationships with retailers and buyers. In addition to mentorship, fashion incubators often provide resources such as studio space, equipment, and manufacturing facilities. This allows designers to have a physical space where they can create their collections, carry out fittings, and develop prototypes. By sharing resources and expenses, participants can minimize costs and overcome some of the financial barriers often faced by emerging designers. Overall, a fashion incubator serves as a launchpad for emerging fashion designers, providing them with the tools, knowledge, and support necessary to establish and grow their own fashion brands. Through mentorship, resources, and networking opportunities, designers can gain a competitive edge in the industry and increase their chances of success.

Fashion Industry Conference

A Fashion Industry Conference is a formal gathering or meeting organized within the context of fashion design, where professionals from various sectors of the industry come together to exchange knowledge, insights, and ideas related to the latest trends, techniques, and challenges in fashion design, production, marketing, and retail. During a Fashion Industry Conference, experts share their experiences, research findings, and innovative approaches through presentations, panel discussions, workshops, and networking events. These gatherings aim to create a platform for industry professionals, designers, entrepreneurs, educators, and researchers to connect, collaborate, and stay updated with the evolving landscape of the fashion industry.

Fashion Industry Gala

A fashion industry gala is a prestigious event that celebrates and showcases the artistry and creativity of fashion design. It brings together industry professionals, fashion enthusiasts, celebrities, and influencers to commemorate the achievements of designers and brands, and to promote their latest collections. The gala serves as a platform for designers to present their work in a grand and theatrical manner. Fashion shows, often the highlight of the event, feature models strutting down the runway wearing the latest designs, meticulously curated to reflect the designer's vision and aesthetics. These shows captivate the audience with their choreographed display of fashion, combining music, lights, and stunning outfits to create a captivating experience. The gala also provides an opportunity for designers to network and engage with industry insiders, potential buyers, and investors. It is a space where new collaborations are formed, deals are negotiated, and business relationships are fostered. Designers have the chance to showcase their talent, seek feedback, and gain exposure, which can be vital for their career trajectory and brand recognition. Besides the fashion shows, a fashion industry gala often includes various activities and attractions. These may include pop-up boutiques where attendees can shop for designer merchandise, interactive displays where guests can experience the design process firsthand, and art installations that further emphasize the artistic nature of fashion. Additionally, guest speakers, panel discussions, and workshops may be organized to shed light on current trends, industry challenges, and emerging design techniques. The dress code for a fashion industry gala is typically formal and glamorous, encouraging attendees to don their most exquisite attire. Celebrities adorn themselves in high-end designer outfits, often leading to iconic fashion moments that are widely discussed and photographed. The red carpet, a key feature of the gala, becomes a spectacle of sartorial elegance, where attendees' fashion choices become the focal point of media attention, influencing trends and inspiring fashion enthusiasts around the world.

Fashion Industry Insider

The fashion industry insider refers to an individual who possesses in-depth knowledge, experience, and expertise in the dynamic realm of fashion design. With their impeccable sense of style, trend forecasting abilities, and meticulous attention to detail, fashion industry insiders play a crucial role in shaping the ever-evolving landscape of fashion. These insiders are at the forefront of the fashion world, staying on top of the latest trends, styles, and consumer preferences. They possess an innate understanding of fabrics, color palettes, and garment construction, enabling them to create innovative and visually appealing designs. Fashion industry insiders often collaborate with renowned fashion houses, brands, or start their own labels, infusing their unique vision and creativity into their collections. Moreover, fashion industry insiders are involved in every stage of the design process. From sketching initial concepts to sourcing materials, they ensure that their designs not only meet the highest aesthetic standards but are also functional and practical. They possess a keen eye for detail, ensuring that every stitch, seam, and embellishment is flawlessly executed. Additionally, fashion industry insiders are highly skilled at forecasting upcoming trends. They monitor global fashion weeks, runway shows, and street style to identify emerging styles and predict future fashion directions. By analyzing consumer behavior and market demands, they are able to develop collections that resonate with the target audience. Furthermore, fashion industry insiders are adept at creating diverse and inclusive designs. They acknowledge the importance of representing various body types, cultures, and backgrounds through their collections. By embracing diversity, they contribute to a more inclusive fashion industry that caters to a wide range of individuals. In conclusion, fashion industry insiders are indispensable figures in the world of fashion. Their expertise and creativity shape the industry and influence the way we dress. With their ability to forecast trends, attention to detail, and passion for creating unique designs, fashion industry insiders set the benchmark for innovation and style in the fashion world.

Fashion Industry Leader

A Fashion Industry Leader is a person who holds a significant position within the fashion design field and is recognized for their expertise, influence, and impact on the industry as a whole. They are individuals who have made significant contributions to shaping trends, driving innovation, and setting standards within the fashion world. As a leader in the fashion industry, their role is multifaceted and encompasses a range of responsibilities. They are responsible for overseeing the creative direction of a brand or fashion house, providing strategic guidance, and making decisions that shape the overall aesthetic and image of the brand. They are often involved in the design process, working closely with designers to ensure that collections align with the brand's vision and resonate with consumers. In addition to their creative responsibilities, a Fashion Industry Leader is also involved in managing the business side of fashion. They work closely with executives and stakeholders to develop and implement business strategies, establish partnerships, and drive financial growth. They have a deep understanding of market trends, consumer behavior, and the competitive landscape, which enables them to make informed decisions that drive success for the brand. Furthermore, a Fashion Industry Leader plays a crucial role in setting and upholding industry standards. They influence the fashion community by setting trends, establishing best practices, and advocating for diversity, sustainability, and ethical practices within the industry. They use their platform to promote positive change and shape the future of fashion. Overall, a Fashion Industry Leader is an influential figure who has achieved a significant level of success and recognition within the fashion design field. They possess a unique combination of creative vision, business acumen, and industry knowledge that allows them to lead, inspire, and shape the fashion industry as a whole.

Fashion Industry Pioneer

A fashion industry pioneer refers to an individual or organization that plays a significant role in introducing innovative ideas, trends, or styles in the field of fashion design. They are the trailblazers who push the boundaries of creativity and set new directions for the fashion industry. These pioneers often challenge the status quo, bringing fresh perspectives and unconventional approaches to the design process. They are known for their ability to think outside the box, pushing the limits of fashion and creating a lasting impact on the industry.

Fashion Industry Regulations

The fashion industry regulations refer to a set of guidelines and rules that govern the production, distribution, and marketing of fashion items, ensuring compliance with ethical, environmental, and safety standards. These regulations aim to protect the rights of workers, consumers, and the environment while promoting fair trade and sustainable practices. The regulations in the fashion industry cover various aspects, including labor standards, product safety, labeling requirements, intellectual property rights, and environmental impact. Labor standards regulations ensure that workers involved in the manufacturing process receive fair wages, work under safe and healthy conditions, and are not subjected to exploitative practices such as child labor or forced labor. Product safety regulations ensure that fashion items meet certain quality standards and do not pose any health or safety risks to consumers. This includes regulations related to the use of hazardous chemicals, flammability standards, and product testing requirements. Labeling requirements regulations dictate that fashion items must provide accurate information about their composition, country of origin, and care instructions. This helps consumers make informed purchasing decisions and enables them to identify products that align with their values, such as sustainability or the use of cruelty-free materials. Intellectual property rights regulations protect designers' original creations from unauthorized copying or imitation. These regulations encompass copyright protection, trademark rights, and design patents, ensuring that designers can benefit from their creative work and discourage the production of counterfeit goods. Environmental impact regulations in the fashion industry aim to minimize the negative effects of production and consumption on the environment. This includes regulations regarding waste management, water usage, energy efficiency, and the use of sustainable materials. These regulations encourage fashion brands to adopt more eco-friendly practices and reduce their carbon footprint.

Fashion Industry Visionary

A fashion industry visionary is an individual who possesses exceptional foresight and creative ability within the fashion design field. They possess a deep understanding of the fashion industry, its trends, and its history, allowing them to envision and shape the future of fashion. These individuals have the ability to predict upcoming fashion trends, identifying what will be popular and in-demand in the future. They use their insight to guide their own designs and influence the direction of the fashion industry as a whole. Their visionary approach allows them to introduce fresh concepts, innovative techniques, and groundbreaking styles that push the boundaries of fashion design.

Fashion Influencer Partnerships

Fashion influencer partnerships refer to collaborative relationships between fashion influencers and brands or designers in the field of fashion design. These partnerships involve influencers promoting and endorsing specific products, collections, or fashion brands through their social media platforms, blogs, or other online channels. Influencer partnerships have become an integral part of the fashion industry, as they provide a valuable means of reaching target audiences and increasing brand awareness. Fashion influencers, who are individuals with a significant following and influence in the fashion community, have the ability to shape and influence consumer opinions, trends, and purchasing decisions. Through these partnerships, brands and designers can tap into the influencers' loyal audience base and leverage their influence to create buzz around their products or collections. Influencers typically create content featuring the brand's products or collections, such as outfit posts, fashion hauls, or styling tips. They provide visual representations and personal recommendations that resonate with their followers. Moreover, influencer partnerships allow brands and designers to benefit from the influencers' expertise and unique perspectives. Influencers often have a deep understanding of the fashion industry, trends, and consumer preferences. They can offer valuable insights and feedback during the design and development process, helping brands create products that align with the latest fashion trends and meet the needs of their target audience. These partnerships also provide an opportunity for brands and designers to tap into new markets and expand their reach. Influencers often have a diverse and global audience, allowing brands to connect with potential customers who may not have been previously aware of their existence. By collaborating with influencers from different regions or demographics, brands can tailor their marketing efforts and product offerings to different markets. In conclusion, fashion influencer partnerships are collaborative relationships between fashion influencers and brands or designers. They involve influencers promoting and endorsing specific products or collections through their online platforms, providing valuable exposure, brand awareness, and reaching target audiences. These partnerships also allow brands to benefit from influencers' expertise, tap into new markets, and create products that align with the latest fashion trends and consumer preferences.

Fashion Influencer

A fashion influencer is an individual who has a significant impact on the fashion industry through their personal style, social media presence, and ability to shape trends. They have a keen eye for fashion and possess the ability to curate and showcase unique and inspiring looks. As trendsetters, fashion influencers have the power to influence consumer behavior and shape the fashion landscape. They often collaborate with brands, designers, and retailers to promote their products and collections, creating buzz and driving sales. Fashion influencers have a strong following on various social media platforms, including Instagram, YouTube, and TikTok, where they share their outfit ideas, fashion tips, and lifestyle content.

Fashion Innovation Hackathon

A fashion innovation hackathon is an event or competition that brings together fashion designers, entrepreneurs, technologists, and industry experts to collaborate and innovate in the field of fashion design. It typically involves a set timeframe, usually ranging from a few hours to a couple of days, during which participants work in teams to develop creative solutions and prototypes that address challenges or explore opportunities within the fashion industry. At a fashion innovation hackathon, participants are encouraged to think outside the box and challenge traditional norms and practices in fashion design. They can leverage cutting-edge technologies, such as augmented reality, virtual reality, wearable tech, and 3D printing, to explore new possibilities for garment design, production, sustainability, retail experiences, and more. The hackathon format fosters a collaborative environment where participants with diverse backgrounds and skill sets can exchange ideas, share knowledge, and combine their expertise to create innovative solutions. Designers can work hand in hand with engineers, software developers, data analysts, and business strategists to develop transformative concepts that push the boundaries of fashion. Throughout the event, participants are guided by mentors and industry professionals who provide insights, feedback, and guidance to help them refine their ideas and projects. These mentors share their expertise and offer industry-specific knowledge to ensure the concepts developed during the hackathon meet the requirements and demands of the fashion industry. A fashion innovation hackathon is not only a competition but also a platform for networking and building meaningful connections within the fashion and technology community. It provides an opportunity for participants to showcase their skills, gain exposure, and even secure potential collaborations or investment for their innovative fashion projects. In summary, a fashion innovation hackathon is a collaborative event where fashion designers, technologists, and industry experts come together to explore and develop groundbreaking solutions for the fashion industry. By leveraging technology and embracing creative thinking, participants aim to disrupt and transform traditional fashion practices, ultimately shaping the future of the industry.

Fashion Innovation

Fashion innovation refers to the creative and forward-thinking processes and techniques employed in fashion design to push the boundaries of traditional fashion concepts and develop novel ideas. It involves the development and implementation of unique and original designs, fabrics, patterns, materials, and technologies that revolutionize the fashion industry. Fashion innovation is driven by artistic creativity, technological advancements, cultural influences, and consumer demand for novel and cutting-edge fashion.At its core, fashion innovation challenges traditional norms and perceptions of fashion, breaking away from conventional styles and practices. It encompasses various aspects of design, including clothing, accessories, footwear, and textiles. Fashion innovators strive to create aesthetically pleasing and functional garments that reflect the zeitgeist of a particular era while creating something entirely new and exceptional.

Fashion Insider

Fashion Insider refers to an individual who possesses extensive knowledge, experience, and influence in the field of fashion design. This individual is a key player within the fashion industry, typically working behind the scenes to shape and direct the direction of fashion trends. A Fashion Insider is someone who is highly knowledgeable about fashion and is well-connected within the industry. They have a keen understanding of current fashion trends, historical influences, and upcoming styles. Their expertise allows them to forecast and predict the future direction of fashion, making them invaluable resources for fashion designers, brands, and retailers.

Fashion Institute

A fashion institute is an educational institution that offers programs and courses in the field of fashion design. It provides students with the necessary knowledge and skills to pursue a career in the fashion industry. The primary focus of a fashion institute is to train individuals in the creative and technical aspects of fashion design. Students learn about various elements of fashion such as fabric selection, garment construction, pattern making, and fashion illustration. They are also taught about fashion history, trends, and the business side of the industry.

Fashion Internship

A fashion internship refers to a structured program or work experience in the field of fashion design, typically offered to students or recent graduates. It provides an opportunity to gain practical knowledge, hands-on experience, and industry exposure in the fashion industry. During a fashion internship, individuals work under the guidance and supervision of experienced professionals in fashion design or related areas. They may be assigned various tasks and responsibilities, such as assisting in designing and creating garments, conducting research, participating in fashion shows or events, organizing materials, or contributing to the overall design process. The primary objective of a fashion internship is to provide individuals with a real-life experience of working in the fashion industry. This includes understanding the different aspects of fashion design, production, marketing, and distribution. Interns often get the chance to work closely with designers, pattern makers, stylists, and other fashion professionals, allowing them to learn from their expertise and build a professional network. Furthermore, a fashion internship allows individuals to develop and enhance key skills required in the fashion industry. These skills may include but are not limited to, creative thinking, problem-solving, attention to detail, time management, teamwork, communication, and adaptability. It also helps individuals understand the importance of meeting deadlines, managing resources, and working effectively in a fast-paced and dynamic environment. Fashion internships are valuable opportunities for aspiring fashion designers to apply and improve their technical skills, such as sewing, patternmaking, draping, sketching, and fabric selection. Interns may get the chance to work with various types of fabrics, tools, and equipment, allowing them to gain firsthand experience in the practical aspects of fashion design. Moreover, fashion internships provide individuals with a platform to showcase their talent, creativity, and commitment to the fashion industry. It can help them build a portfolio of their work, which is essential for securing future employment in the field of fashion design. In conclusion, a fashion internship is a structured program that offers individuals the opportunity to gain practical experience, industry exposure, and develop key skills in the field of fashion design. It serves as a stepping stone for individuals who aspire to pursue a career in the fashion industry and provides a platform to learn, grow, and showcase their talent.

Fashion Jewelry

Fashion jewelry, also known as costume jewelry or imitation jewelry, refers to accessories made from non-precious materials that are designed to complement and enhance an individual's outfit. Unlike fine jewelry, which is made from precious metals and gemstones, fashion jewelry is created using more affordable materials such as brass, copper, acrylic, glass, or plastic. With its focus on style, affordability, and versatility, fashion jewelry has become increasingly popular in the world of fashion design. It allows individuals to express their personal style without the need for expensive investments, as it offers a wide range of options at accessible price points.

Fashion Journalism

Fashion journalism is a form of journalism that focuses on reporting and analyzing the latest trends, events, and developments in the fashion industry. It involves the creation and dissemination of written content, such as articles and reviews, as well as visual content, including photographs and videos, that capture and convey the essence of fashion. As a specialized area of journalism, fashion journalism encompasses a wide range of topics and areas of interest within the field of fashion design. It involves providing coverage and commentary on fashion shows, fashion weeks, and other industry events, as well as profiling and interviewing designers, models, and other influential figures in the fashion world. Fashion journalists not only report on the latest trends and fashion news but also interpret and critique them. They provide analysis and opinions on collections presented by designers, offering insights into the creative process and the significance of the designs. This includes examining the use of fabrics, colors, and silhouettes, as well as assessing the overall impact and relevance of the collections in the context of contemporary fashion. In addition to reporting on fashion shows and events, fashion journalists also cover a variety of other aspects of the industry, including retail and marketing strategies, sustainability and ethical practices, and cultural and social influences on fashion. They explore the intersection between fashion and other fields, such as art, music, and popular culture, and examine how fashion reflects and shapes societal trends and values. Overall, fashion journalism plays a crucial role in informing and inspiring both industry professionals and fashion enthusiasts. By providing a platform for discussion and analysis, it contributes to the ongoing dialogue and evolution of fashion as a form of expression and an industry. Through the written word and visual storytelling, fashion journalists capture and convey the ever-changing landscape of fashion design, offering insights, perspectives, and an appreciation for the artistry and innovation that define this dynamic realm.

Fashion Journalist

A fashion journalist is a professional who specializes in reporting, analyzing, and critiquing fashion trends, events, and designers. Their primary role is to provide objective and informative coverage of the fashion industry, including runway shows, fashion weeks, retail trends, and style icons. As experts in the field, fashion journalists possess a deep understanding of fashion design, fabrics, colors, and silhouettes. They are knowledgeable about the historical context and cultural influences that shape fashion movements. Using their expertise, they write articles, reviews, and features for newspapers, magazines, online publications, and television programs.

Fashion Knitwear

Fashion knitwear refers to clothing items created using the knitting technique, in which yarn or thread is interlooped to form fabric. Knitwear is known for its softness, flexibility, and comfort, making it a popular choice in the fashion industry. Knitwear can be created using various types of knitting machines or by hand using knitting needles. It encompasses a wide range of garments, including sweaters, cardigans, scarves, hats, and socks. These pieces can be made using different weights and types of yarn, resulting in various textures and thicknesses. The design possibilities with knitwear are vast. It can be shaped, patterned, and textured in numerous ways to create unique and fashionable garments. Knitting techniques like ribbing, cabling, and lacework can add visual interest and dimension to the fabric. Additionally, different types of stitches, such as garter stitch, stockinette stitch, and seed stitch, can achieve different surface textures. Fashion knitwear offers versatility in terms of styling and functionality. It can be worn as a standalone piece or layered with other clothing items to create stylish and cozy outfits. Knitwear is commonly used for winter and fall collections due to its ability to provide insulation and warmth. Knitwear has a long history and has evolved significantly over time. Traditionally, it was handcrafted by skilled artisans using natural fibers like wool and cotton. However, with advancements in technology and the availability of synthetic fibers, knitwear can now be mass-produced and offers a wider range of material options. In contemporary fashion, knitwear continues to be a staple in designer collections. It caters to various consumer preferences, from classic and timeless designs to avant-garde and experimental pieces. The combination of functionality, comfort, and style makes fashion knitwear a sought-after choice for both everyday wear and special occasions.

Fashion Label

A fashion label refers to a distinctive brand or name associated with a particular fashion designer or fashion house. It represents the designer's unique identity and style, and is used to market and promote their fashion creations. A fashion label serves as a means of communication between the designer and their target audience, conveying the designer's vision and aesthetic through various fashion products. The creation of a fashion label involves the development of a brand identity, which includes a name, logo, and visual elements that reflect the designer's signature style. The fashion label acts as a symbol of quality, craftsmanship, and innovation, distinguishing the designer's creations from others in the industry. It encapsulates the designer's values, inspiration, and artistic vision, which are translated into their fashion collections. A fashion label plays a crucial role in the fashion industry as it helps consumers identify and connect with a specific designer or brand. It allows consumers to associate themselves with the designer's values and lifestyle, creating a sense of identity and belonging. Fashion labels also serve as a reference point for consumers to explore and appreciate the designer's previous and future collections, enabling them to develop a loyal following of customers. The establishment and success of a fashion label requires a combination of creative talent, business acumen, and effective marketing strategies. Fashion designers must constantly innovate and adapt to changing fashion trends, while also maintaining a strong brand identity that resonates with their target audience. They need to create compelling and desirable collections that attract attention and generate demand in the market. A fashion label is not limited to clothing and accessories but can extend to other lifestyle products and services associated with the designer's brand. It can include fragrance lines, home decor, beauty products, and collaborations with other brands or artists. The versatility of a fashion label allows designers to expand their creative expression and reach new markets, further enhancing their brand's reputation and success.

Fashion Lace

Fashion lace refers to a delicate and decorative fabric that is woven or knitted in an openwork pattern. It is commonly used in fashion design to add a touch of elegance and femininity to garments, accessories, and even shoes. Lace can be made from a variety of materials, including silk, cotton, synthetic fibers, or a combination of these. Lace has a long history in fashion and has been used for centuries to create intricate designs and embellishments. It is often associated with vintage and romantic aesthetics, but can also be incorporated into contemporary and edgy fashion styles. The unique texture and look of lace make it a versatile material that can be used in a wide range of designs, from delicate and ethereal to bold and avant-garde.

Fashion Launch Party

A Fashion Launch Party is a highly anticipated event in the fashion industry, where a fashion designer or brand unveils their latest collection to the public. It is a glamorous occasion that combines elements of fashion, entertainment, and networking, and serves as a platform for designers to showcase their creative vision and generate buzz for their brand. The primary purpose of a Fashion Launch Party is to generate excitement and build anticipation for a new fashion collection. This event typically takes place before the collection is available for purchase, allowing industry professionals, celebrities, influencers, and other key stakeholders to preview the designs and provide feedback. By creating a sense of exclusivity and prestige, the designer aims to cultivate interest and desire among potential buyers, media representatives, and fashion enthusiasts.

Fashion Law

Fashion Law is a specialized area of law that focuses on the legal aspects of the fashion industry, specifically pertaining to fashion design. It encompasses a range of legal issues and regulations that affect fashion designers, brands, and retailers. One of the key areas of Fashion Law is intellectual property, which includes copyright, trademark, and design protection. Copyright protects original creative expressions, such as fashion designs, from unauthorized copying or reproduction. Trademark protects brand names, logos, and symbols associated with fashion brands, ensuring their exclusive use and preventing consumer confusion. Design protection safeguards the unique and new visual appearance of a fashion design from being copied.

Fashion Leather

Fashion Leather is a term used in the fashion design industry to refer to leather materials that are specifically utilized for creating stylish and trendy garments, accessories, and footwear. Leather, which is derived from the hides of various animals such as cows, pigs, goats, and sheep, is known for its durability, flexibility, and unique texture. Its use in fashion dates back centuries, and it continues to be valued for its luxurious and timeless appeal.

Fashion Lecture

A fashion lecture refers to a formal presentation or discourse in the context of fashion design. It is a structured talk delivered by an expert or industry professional in order to educate, inform, and inspire individuals interested in the field of fashion. These lectures are typically delivered in academic settings, such as universities or design schools, or in industry events, seminars, or conferences. Fashion lectures aim to provide a comprehensive understanding of various aspects of fashion design, including history, theory, technical aspects, trends, and industry practices. They serve as a platform for sharing knowledge, exchanging ideas, and fostering critical thinking within the fashion community.

Fashion Licensing Agreement

A fashion licensing agreement is a formal legal contract between a fashion designer (licensor) and a manufacturer or distributor (licensee), granting the licensee the rights to produce and distribute products under the designer's brand name or trademark.This agreement outlines the specific terms and conditions under which the licensee can use the licensor's brand, designs, patterns, trademarks, and other intellectual property rights.

Fashion Licensing

Fashion licensing, in the context of fashion design, refers to the legal agreement between a fashion designer or brand and another party (licensee) that grants the licensee the rights to use and produce the designer's or brand's intellectual property, such as logo, name, designs, trademark, or even entire collections, for commercial purposes. Through fashion licensing, the licensee gains the legal permission to manufacture, distribute, and sell fashion products under the designer's or brand's name, allowing them to tap into the established reputation, style, and brand equity of the designer.

Fashion Line Development

A fashion line development refers to the process of creating and establishing a collection of garments or accessories that embodies a specific brand or designer's vision and style. It involves various stages of designing, planning, and producing a range of products that align with the brand's aesthetic and target market. The first stage of fashion line development is the conceptualization and research phase. This involves identifying the target market, studying current trends, and conducting market research to gather insights and inspiration. Designers then create mood boards, sketches, and prototypes to develop a cohesive concept for the collection. Once the concept is finalized, the next stage is the design and technical development process. Designers create detailed technical drawings and patterns for each garment, specifying materials, colors, and trims. They also consider factors like fit, comfort, and functionality to ensure the garments are not only aesthetically pleasing but also well-constructed and wearable. After the designs are finalized, the production planning phase begins. This involves sourcing and ordering materials, coordinating with manufacturers or production teams, and creating a detailed production timeline. Designers and production teams work closely together to ensure that the garments are produced to the desired quality standards and within the designated timeframe. Additionally, fashion line development also includes branding and marketing strategies. Designers and brand managers collaborate to create a brand identity, logo, and visual assets that effectively communicate the essence and values of the fashion line. They also develop marketing materials, such as lookbooks, catalogs, and promotional campaigns, to showcase the collection to potential buyers and consumers. In conclusion, fashion line development encompasses the entire process of creating and bringing to life a collection of garments or accessories. It involves a combination of creative, technical, and strategic elements to create a cohesive and marketable line that reflects the brand's unique vision and style.

Fashion Line Merchandising

A fashion line merchandising is a strategic and creative process within the fashion design industry that involves the planning, development, and marketing of a specific line of clothing or accessories. It encompasses the activities and decisions made by fashion designers, buyers, and merchandisers to bring a cohesive and visually appealing collection to market.At its core, fashion line merchandising aims to create a desirable and marketable range of products that aligns with current fashion trends, target audience preferences, and brand image. This process involves various stages, including trend research, product design and development, sourcing and production, and retail planning and marketing.Firstly, trend research and analysis play a crucial role in fashion line merchandising. Designers and merchandisers constantly monitor fashion trends, cultural influences, and consumer behavior to identify the direction and themes for their collections. They gather inspiration from various sources, such as runway shows, fashion magazines, street style, and social media, to ensure their designs are relevant and in demand.Secondly, the product design and development phase involves translating the chosen trend or theme into tangible garments or accessories. Fashion designers work on sketching, draping, and creating prototypes to bring their creative vision to life. They collaborate with patternmakers, tailors, and sample makers to refine the designs and ensure the quality and fit of the final products.The sourcing and production stage is vital for fashion line merchandising as it involves finding reliable manufacturers and suppliers to produce the garments or accessories in bulk. Merchandisers negotiate prices, quantities, and delivery schedules to ensure both profitability and timely availability of the products. They also oversee the sampling, fitting, and quality control processes to maintain the desired standards.In the retail planning and marketing phase, fashion line merchandisers strategize the distribution and promotion of the collection to maximize sales and brand exposure. They work closely with buyers and retailers to plan assortments, pricing, and merchandising displays. They also collaborate with marketing and advertising teams to develop effective campaigns, communicate brand messages, and create visual merchandising materials to attract customers to the collection.Overall, fashion line merchandising is a multifaceted process that requires a combination of creativity, business acumen, and market knowledge to successfully bring a fashion collection to the consumer market. It involves continuous inspiration, coordination, and collaboration between designers, merchandisers, manufacturers, and retailers to meet the evolving demands of the fashion industry.

Fashion Line Sheet

A fashion line sheet is a document used in the fashion industry to present a collection of clothing or accessories designed by a fashion designer or brand. It serves as a comprehensive visual and informational guide for retailers, buyers, and other industry professionals who are interested in carrying or purchasing the products. The fashion line sheet typically includes the following key elements: The first element is the brand or designer's logo, which is usually placed at the top of the sheet for branding purposes. This helps to establish brand identity and build recognition among buyers and retailers. The second element is the product images, usually displayed in a grid format. These images showcase the different styles, colors, and details of each product in the collection. High-quality and visually appealing images are crucial to attract attention and engage potential buyers. The third element is the product information, which provides essential details about each item. This includes the product name, style number, color options, sizes available, and materials used. It may also include additional information such as care instructions or any special features or details that make the product unique. The fourth element is the pricing information, which can be displayed alongside each product or in a separate section of the line sheet. This includes the suggested retail price (SRP) and any applicable discounts or promotions. Clear and transparent pricing information is crucial for buyers to make informed decisions and compare prices across different brands or collections. The fifth element is the order information, which includes details on how buyers can place orders or inquire about the products. This may include contact information such as phone numbers, email addresses, or website links. It is important to make this information easily accessible and visible to buyers to facilitate the ordering process. In addition to these key elements, a fashion line sheet may also include other supplementary information such as a brief brand or designer introduction, a lookbook or campaign images, or any other relevant information that helps communicate the brand's aesthetic and story. In summary, a fashion line sheet is a crucial tool for fashion designers and brands to showcase their collections to potential buyers and retailers. It provides a visually appealing and informative overview of the products, helping to attract attention, generate interest, and facilitate the ordering process.

Fashion Linen

Fashion Linen is a natural fabric derived from the stalks of the flax plant, known as Linum Usitatissimum. It is a versatile and breathable material widely used in fashion design due to its numerous beneficial properties. One of the most notable features of Fashion Linen is its exceptional strength and durability. Despite being a lightweight fabric, it possesses high tensile strength, making it resistant to tear and wear. This attribute makes it an ideal choice for garments that need to withstand frequent use and laundering without compromising quality.

Fashion Lingerie

Fashion lingerie refers to intricately designed undergarments that are specifically produced for aesthetic appeal and fashion purposes rather than purely functional ones. This branch of lingerie design focuses on creating pieces that are visually appealing, trendy, and fashionable, while still providing some degree of support and comfort. The concept of fashion lingerie emerged as a response to the increasing demand for undergarments that are not only functional but also stylish. Unlike traditional lingerie, which is mainly designed for basic support and coverage, fashion lingerie is crafted with an emphasis on style, design, and visual appeal. It often incorporates delicate fabrics, intricate lacework, decorative embroidery, and various embellishments to create visually striking and alluring pieces.

Fashion Logistics

Fashion Logistics refers to the management and coordination of the complex process of delivering fashion products from the point of creation to the point of sale in an efficient and timely manner. It involves various activities such as sourcing, production, distribution, and retailing, which are essential in ensuring that fashion products are available to customers when and where they want them. In the context of fashion design, fashion logistics encompasses the entire supply chain of the fashion industry. It starts with the sourcing of raw materials, which can include fabrics, trims, and other components needed for garment production. These materials are often sourced from different suppliers, both locally and internationally, and need to be carefully selected based on factors such as quality, cost, and sustainability. Once the materials are acquired, the production process begins. This involves the transformation of the raw materials into finished fashion products through various stages such as pattern-making, cutting, sewing, and finishing. Fashion logistics ensures that production is carried out efficiently, with consideration given to factors such as productivity, quality control, and lead times. After production, the next stage of fashion logistics involves the distribution of the fashion products to retailers or directly to customers. This can be done through various channels such as wholesale distribution, brick-and-mortar stores, e-commerce platforms, or a combination of these. Effective logistics management is crucial in ensuring that the right products are available in the right quantities at the right locations, taking into account factors such as demand forecasting, inventory management, and order fulfillment. Finally, fashion logistics also plays a role in the retailing phase of the fashion industry. This includes activities such as visual merchandising, store layout, and customer service, all of which contribute to the overall shopping experience and customer satisfaction. Fashion logistics ensures that the retail operations are well-coordinated and optimized to attract customers and drive sales. In summary, fashion logistics is the coordinated management of the entire supply chain in the fashion industry, from sourcing raw materials to delivering finished products to customers. It involves various activities and considerations, all aimed at ensuring that fashion products are available to customers in a timely and efficient manner.

Fashion Look Of The Day

A fashion look of the day refers to a specific outfit or ensemble that is chosen and styled by an individual or a fashion designer to showcase their personal style or the current fashion trends. It is a snapshot of an individual's fashion choices on a particular day and can be seen as a form of self-expression or a representation of their fashion identity. The concept of a fashion look of the day has gained popularity with the rise of social media platforms like Instagram, where individuals share their outfit choices and fashion inspirations with their followers. Fashion bloggers and influencers often create daily fashion looks to provide inspiration to their audience and showcase their fashion expertise.

Fashion Lookbook

A fashion lookbook is a compilation of images or photographs that showcase a collection of clothing or accessories designed by a fashion designer or brand. It serves as a visual representation of the overall style, aesthetic, and theme of the collection, allowing viewers to get a sense of the designer's creative vision and the intended look and feel of the pieces. The lookbook is typically used as a marketing tool, often distributed to media outlets, buyers, and potential customers. It offers an opportunity for the designer or brand to communicate their brand identity, demonstrate their design skills, and generate interest and excitement around their latest collection.

Fashion Loungewear

Fashion Loungewear Fashion loungewear refers to a clothing category that combines elements of comfort and style, specifically designed for leisure and relaxation. It is a versatile and modern approach to casual attire, blurring the lines between traditional loungewear and fashionable streetwear. Loungewear typically includes pieces such as sweatpants, hoodies, sweatshirts, joggers, pajama sets, robes, and oversized t-shirts. Unlike traditional loungewear, fashion loungewear explores unique silhouettes, materials, and design details that elevate the overall aesthetic. It focuses on creating a stylish yet relaxed look that can be worn both indoors and outdoors. The key principles of fashion loungewear lie in its emphasis on comfort, functionality, and effortless style. Fabrics used are often soft, breathable, and stretchy, such as cotton, jersey, fleece, and knits. These materials allow for ease of movement and provide a cozy feel against the skin. Additionally, the incorporation of functional features like drawstrings, elastic waistbands, and pockets enhance the practicality of the garments. Design-wise, fashion loungewear often showcases minimalist aesthetics and clean lines, embracing neutral colors and subtle patterns. The focus is on achieving a sleek and refined look while maintaining a relaxed vibe. However, fashion loungewear also allows for playful elements, such as color-blocking, graphic prints, and logo placements, which add a distinctive touch to the overall design. The versatility of fashion loungewear extends beyond its comfort and style. It offers individuals the flexibility to transition from home to casual outings effortlessly. By accessorizing and incorporating complementary pieces, such as sneakers, statement jackets, or statement jewelry, fashion loungewear can effortlessly be elevated for various occasions. In summary, fashion loungewear is a stylish reinterpretation of traditional loungewear, designed to offer comfort, functionality, and a modern aesthetic. It presents an opportunity to blend relaxation and fashion, allowing individuals to express their personal style while embracing comfort.

Fashion Made-To-Measure

Fashion Made-to-Measure refers to the process of creating custom clothing that is tailored to a specific individual's measurements and preferences. It involves taking precise body measurements and using them as the basis for creating a unique garment that fits the individual perfectly. This approach to fashion design allows for a high level of customization, as every aspect of the garment can be tailored – from the style, silhouette, and fabric choice to the details such as buttons, pockets, and trimmings. Made-to-measure garments are created with meticulous attention to detail, ensuring a superior fit and quality compared to ready-to-wear clothing.

Fashion Magazine

A fashion magazine is a publication that focuses on the latest trends, styles, and designs within the fashion industry. It serves as a platform for designers, photographers, stylists, and models to showcase their work and inspire readers to stay up-to-date with the ever-changing world of fashion. A fashion magazine typically contains a wide range of content, including editorials, features, and interviews with industry insiders. These articles highlight the work of talented designers, discuss emerging fashion trends, and provide insights into the creative process behind fashion collections. In addition to written content, a fashion magazine is also known for its visually appealing layout and high-quality photography. Fashion editorials often showcase models wearing the latest designer clothes, accessories, and beauty looks in a variety of editorial spreads and fashion shoots. Alongside the editorial content, fashion magazines also include advertisements from various brands and designers. These ads not only provide financial support for the magazine but also help readers discover new products and designers in the market. Furthermore, fashion magazines play a significant role in shaping and influencing the fashion industry. They act as a source of inspiration for both consumers and professionals, acting as a guide for what is considered stylish and fashionable at any given time. Overall, fashion magazines serve as a valuable resource for anyone interested in fashion design, providing a glimpse into the world of high fashion and allowing readers to explore and appreciate the creative work of designers and other fashion industry professionals.

Fashion Makeup

Fashion makeup refers to the application of cosmetics to enhance and alter a person's appearance in the context of fashion design. It plays a vital role in bringing a particular fashion concept or vision to life, emphasizing and complementing the overall aesthetic of a fashion ensemble or style. Fashion makeup is an art form that involves creativity, skill, and an understanding of current fashion trends. Artists specializing in fashion makeup work closely with fashion designers, photographers, models, and stylists to create visually captivating looks that align with the desired fashion direction. They use various cosmetic products, tools, and techniques to achieve the desired effects. Fashion makeup is not solely limited to enhancing facial features but can also involve body painting and other forms of artistic expression on the body.

Fashion Marketing Campaigns

A fashion marketing campaign refers to a coordinated series of promotional activities and strategies that aim to create awareness, generate interest, and drive sales for a particular fashion design or collection. It involves the implementation of various marketing techniques, both online and offline, to effectively communicate the brand's message, enhance its image, and captivate the target audience. The primary goal of a fashion marketing campaign is to create a buzz around a brand or specific fashion product, enticing consumers to purchase and become loyal customers. It requires a deep understanding of the target market, including their demographics, preferences, and lifestyle, in order to develop compelling messages and visuals that resonate with them. A successful fashion marketing campaign typically consists of several key elements. Firstly, market research and analysis are conducted to identify consumer trends, competitors, and potential market opportunities. This information serves as the foundation for developing a comprehensive marketing strategy and campaign plan. Next, branding and positioning strategies are employed to differentiate the fashion design from its competitors and establish a unique identity in the market. This involves creating a strong brand image, including a distinctive logo, tagline, and brand story that can evoke emotions and connect with consumers on a deeper level. Furthermore, a fashion marketing campaign utilizes a wide range of communication channels and mediums to reach the target audience effectively. This may include traditional advertising methods such as print ads, billboards, and television commercials, as well as digital marketing techniques like social media marketing, influencer collaborations, and content creation. To maximize the impact of a fashion marketing campaign, strategic partnerships and collaborations with industry influencers, celebrities, or other relevant stakeholders are often pursued. This helps to leverage their existing fan base and credibility, thereby increasing the brand's reach and exposure to a wider audience. Throughout the campaign, careful tracking and analysis of key performance indicators (KPIs) such as website traffic, social media engagement, and sales conversions are essential to measure the effectiveness of the campaign and make necessary adjustments if needed. In conclusion, a fashion marketing campaign plays a vital role in promoting and selling fashion designs by utilizing various marketing strategies to capture the attention and interest of the target audience. It aims to establish a strong brand identity, increase brand awareness, and ultimately drive sales for the fashion design or collection.

Fashion Marketing Seminar

A fashion marketing seminar is a formal event or gathering in the context of fashion design, where industry professionals and enthusiasts come together to discuss and exchange ideas, strategies, and best practices for promoting and selling fashion products. It is typically organized by fashion schools, industry associations, or marketing agencies, and can be attended by fashion designers, marketers, retailers, and other key stakeholders in the fashion industry. The main purpose of a fashion marketing seminar is to provide a platform for learning, networking, and professional development in the field of fashion marketing. Participants have the opportunity to engage with industry experts, gain valuable insights into the latest trends and innovations in fashion marketing, and enhance their knowledge and skills in this specialized area. The topics covered in a fashion marketing seminar may include branding and positioning, consumer behavior and market research, digital marketing and social media strategies, retail merchandising and visual presentation, public relations and fashion events, as well as ethical and sustainable fashion practices. Through presentations, panel discussions, workshops, and case studies, participants can learn about successful marketing campaigns, industry trends, and the latest technologies and tools used in fashion marketing. Attending a fashion marketing seminar can offer several benefits for professionals in the fashion industry. Firstly, it provides a platform to network and connect with like-minded individuals and industry leaders, fostering collaborations, partnerships, and potential business opportunities. Secondly, it serves as a platform for personal growth and professional development, allowing attendees to expand their knowledge, skills, and expertise in the field of fashion marketing. Lastly, it offers a forum to gain inspiration, fresh ideas, and insights into emerging trends, enabling marketers to stay ahead in a highly competitive industry. In conclusion, a fashion marketing seminar provides a valuable learning and networking opportunity for professionals and enthusiasts in the fashion industry. It serves as a platform to exchange ideas, strategies, and best practices in fashion marketing, aimed at promoting and selling fashion products effectively. By attending such seminars, participants can enhance their knowledge, skills, and professional network, ultimately contributing to their success in the dynamic world of fashion marketing.

Fashion Marketing

Fashion Marketing is a strategic approach focused on the promotion and sale of fashion products or services in a way that creates value for both the brand and the target audience. It involves the application of marketing principles and techniques to the fashion industry, with the aim of understanding and satisfying the needs and desires of consumers. At its core, fashion marketing encompasses various activities that contribute to the overall success of a fashion brand. These activities include market research, trend forecasting, product development, branding, advertising, and retailing. By conducting market research, fashion marketers gain valuable insights into consumer preferences, behavior, and trends, which inform the development and promotion of fashion products. Trend forecasting is a crucial aspect of fashion marketing as it helps brands anticipate and adapt to changing consumer tastes and preferences. This involves analyzing fashion shows, street styles, social media, and other cultural influences to identify upcoming trends. By understanding future trends, fashion marketers can align their product offerings and marketing strategies accordingly, enhancing their brand's relevance and appeal. Product development is another key component of fashion marketing. It involves creating and designing fashion products that align with the brand's identity and target market. Fashion marketers collaborate with designers, merchandisers, and suppliers to ensure that the products meet quality, aesthetic, and functional standards. Additionally, they consider factors such as pricing, distribution channels, and packaging to maximize the product's appeal and accessibility to consumers. Branding plays a crucial role in fashion marketing, as it helps differentiate a brand from its competitors and creates a distinct identity in the minds of consumers. Fashion marketers develop brand strategies that encompass visual elements, messaging, and values, evoking emotions and aspirations that resonate with the target audience. These strategies are implemented through various channels, including advertising campaigns, social media, and influencer partnerships, to enhance brand awareness and create an emotional connection with consumers. Finally, retailing is an integral part of fashion marketing, encompassing both physical and virtual channels. Fashion marketers collaborate with retailers to create engaging in-store experiences that reflect the brand's identity and values. They also leverage e-commerce platforms and digital marketing strategies to reach a wider audience and facilitate online sales.

Fashion Marketplace

A fashion marketplace is an online platform that connects fashion designers and brands with consumers, providing a virtual space for buying and selling fashion products. It serves as a digital marketplace where users can discover, browse, and purchase a wide range of fashion items, including clothing, accessories, and footwear. In a fashion marketplace, designers and brands can showcase their collections, promoting their unique styles and designs to a global audience. This platform allows them to reach a larger customer base without the limitations of physical stores. It offers them the opportunity to establish their brand presence and gain exposure in the highly competitive fashion industry. For consumers, a fashion marketplace provides a convenient and accessible way to explore and shop for the latest fashion trends. It offers a variety of options to suit different preferences, styles, and budgets. Users can easily search for specific items or categories, filter their search results, and compare prices and product details. The platform often includes features such as customer reviews and ratings, helping buyers make informed purchasing decisions. In addition to facilitating transactions, a fashion marketplace may also offer additional services such as style inspiration, trend forecasts, and personalized recommendations. This creates a holistic shopping experience and enhances customer satisfaction. Some fashion marketplaces operate on a commission-based model, where designers or brands pay a percentage of each sale to the platform. Others may charge a subscription fee or offer a freemium model, providing basic features for free and additional benefits for a premium membership. The revenue generated from these sources helps support the maintenance and development of the platform. Overall, a fashion marketplace plays a crucial role in the fashion industry by bridging the gap between designers and consumers. It serves as a dynamic and inclusive online space where fashion enthusiasts can indulge in their passion for style, discover new brands, and stay up-to-date with the latest fashion trends.

Fashion Masterclass

Fashion Masterclass is a comprehensive and interactive educational program designed to provide in-depth knowledge and practical skills in the field of fashion design. It is an advanced learning initiative that aims to enhance the expertise of aspiring fashion designers and individuals passionate about the fashion industry. Throughout the Fashion Masterclass, students are exposed to a wide range of topics and techniques, including trend forecasting, sketching, pattern making, garment construction, and fashion illustration. The program covers both theoretical concepts and hands-on exercises, allowing participants to develop a strong foundation and gain valuable insights into the world of fashion. By enrolling in a Fashion Masterclass, aspiring designers have the opportunity to refine their creative abilities and refine their artistic vision. They are encouraged to explore various design aesthetics, experiment with different materials and textures, and harness their unique perspectives to create innovative and boundary-pushing fashion collections. In addition to technical skills, Fashion Masterclass also emphasizes the importance of understanding the business side of fashion. Participants learn about fashion marketing, brand development, retail strategies, and industry trends, equipping them with the knowledge and tools to succeed in the highly competitive fashion industry. Moreover, Fashion Masterclass provides a platform for students to network and collaborate with industry professionals, fashion experts, and fellow designers. Through workshops, seminars, and mentorship programs, participants can receive valuable guidance and feedback, enabling them to further refine their skills and enhance their professional growth. Upon completion of a Fashion Masterclass, graduates have an enhanced understanding of various aspects of fashion design, from conceptualization to execution. They are equipped with a diverse set of skills that can be applied in different areas of the industry, such as fashion styling, design consultancy, fashion journalism, or establishing their own fashion label. In summary, Fashion Masterclass is a comprehensive educational program that offers aspiring fashion designers the opportunity to acquire in-depth knowledge, develop practical skills, and gain valuable industry insights. It prepares individuals to excel in the dynamic and ever-evolving world of fashion, fostering creativity, innovation, and professionalism.

Fashion Material Swatches

Fashion material swatches are small samples or pieces of various fabrics and materials used in fashion design. These swatches are essential tools for designers, allowing them to visually and tactually evaluate and select materials for their creations. Material swatches provide a tangible representation of the fabric's quality, texture, color, pattern, weight, and other characteristics, enabling designers to assess how the fabric behaves, drapes, stretches, and moves. By examining and comparing different swatches, designers can make informed decisions about which materials best suit their designs and objectives.

Fashion Media Planning

Fashion media planning refers to the strategic process of creating and implementing an effective media campaign to promote and showcase fashion designs. It involves the analysis of target audience, selection of appropriate media channels, creation of engaging content, and the execution of the campaign to ensure maximum visibility and impact. In the context of fashion design, media planning plays a crucial role in bringing the designer's vision to a wider audience. It involves understanding the target market, their preferences, and the most effective ways to reach them through various media platforms. The first step in fashion media planning is conducting research to identify the target audience. This involves studying demographics such as age, gender, location, and lifestyle preferences. By understanding the audience's characteristics, fashion designers can tailor their campaigns to appeal to their specific interests and needs. Once the target audience is identified, the next step is selecting the most suitable media channels to reach them. This may include traditional channels such as television, print magazines, and newspapers, as well as digital platforms such as social media, websites, and online publications. Fashion designers must carefully evaluate the reach, cost, and effectiveness of each channel to determine the best mix for their campaign. Creating engaging content is a key aspect of fashion media planning. This involves developing captivating visuals, impactful messages, and compelling stories that resonate with the target audience. Fashion designers often collaborate with photographers, models, stylists, and writers to create content that showcases their designs in the most appealing and aspirational manner. Execution is the final step in the fashion media planning process. This involves implementing the campaign across selected media channels, monitoring its performance, and making adjustments as needed. By closely tracking audience engagement, fashion designers can gauge the effectiveness of their campaign and make informed decisions for future media planning efforts.

Fashion Mentorship Program

A Fashion Mentorship Program is a formal arrangement in the field of fashion design where an experienced and knowledgeable professional, known as a mentor, provides guidance, support, and advice to a less experienced individual, known as a mentee, to help them develop their skills, knowledge, and career in the fashion industry. The objective of a Fashion Mentorship Program is to create a structured relationship between the mentor and the mentee, fostering an environment of mutual trust, respect, and openness. The mentor, based on their expertise and experience, assists the mentee in identifying and setting professional goals, providing feedback, and offering constructive criticism to enhance the mentee's growth and development in the field of fashion design. The mentor in a Fashion Mentorship Program acts as a role model and source of inspiration for the mentee. They share their industry insights, knowledge of current trends, and practical advice on various aspects of fashion design, such as garment construction, textile selection, sketching techniques, color theory, and styling. Additionally, the mentor may guide the mentee in developing a unique design aesthetic, honing their creativity, and refining their technical skills. The mentee, on the other hand, benefits from the mentor's experience and expertise by gaining valuable exposure to real-world fashion scenarios, professional networks, and potential career opportunities. The mentorship relationship also offers the mentee a platform to seek guidance and seek solutions to challenges they may encounter in their fashion design journey. A Fashion Mentorship Program typically involves regular meetings or interactions between the mentor and the mentee, which can be conducted in person, online, or through a combination of both. These engagements may include portfolio reviews, design critiques, industry event attendance, and networking opportunities. The duration of the program can vary, ranging from a few months to a year or longer, depending on the agreed-upon arrangement between the mentor and mentee.

Fashion Mentorship

A fashion mentorship is a specialized professional relationship in the field of fashion design, where an experienced and successful fashion designer guides and advises a less experienced individual, known as the mentee, in their journey to develop their skills, knowledge, and career in fashion design. The mentorship relationship is based on mutual trust, respect, and shared goals. The fashion mentor, with their in-depth knowledge and experience in the industry, provides guidance, support, and constructive feedback to the mentee, helping them navigate the complexities of the fashion design world and effectively grow their creative abilities.

Fashion Merchandiser

A Fashion Merchandiser can be defined as an individual within the fashion industry who is responsible for the planning and execution of the product assortment for a fashion brand or retailer. They play a crucial role in the fashion design process by analyzing sales data, market trends, and customer preferences to determine the best assortment of products to be offered to consumers. The primary goal of a Fashion Merchandiser is to ensure that the right products are available at the right time, in the right quantities, and at the right price. They collaborate closely with designers, buyers, and suppliers to develop and implement strategies that will maximize sales and profitability. By effectively managing the product assortment, a Fashion Merchandiser helps to attract and retain customers, enhance brand image, and drive overall business success.

To achieve these goals, a Fashion Merchandiser must possess a diverse set of skills and knowledge. They need to have a strong understanding of fashion trends, consumer behavior, and market dynamics. This allows them to identify and capitalize on emerging trends, while also ensuring the brand's products align with the preferences and needs of its target customers. Additionally, a Fashion Merchandiser must have excellent analytical and forecasting skills. They use sales and inventory data to evaluate the performance of different product categories and make informed decisions about future assortments. This requires the ability to analyze complex data sets, identify patterns and trends, and make accurate projections about future demand. Communication and collaboration are also essential skills for a Fashion Merchandiser. They need to effectively communicate their merchandising strategies and objectives to various stakeholders, including designers, buyers, suppliers, and retail teams. This requires strong interpersonal skills and the ability to build and maintain relationships across different functions. Overall, a Fashion Merchandiser plays a critical role in translating the creative vision of a fashion brand into a commercially successful product assortment. They combine their knowledge of fashion, market trends, and consumer behavior with strong analytical and communication skills to optimize sales and drive business growth. In conclusion, a Fashion Merchandiser is responsible for the strategic planning and implementation of the product assortment for a fashion brand or retailer. They use their knowledge of fashion trends, consumer behavior, and market dynamics to ensure the right products are available at the right time, in the right quantities, and at the right price. By effectively managing the product assortment, a Fashion Merchandiser contributes to the overall success and profitability of a fashion brand.

Fashion Merchandising

Fashion merchandising is the strategic process of planning, developing, and executing marketing and sales strategies for fashion products within the retail industry. It involves analyzing market trends, selecting and procuring merchandise, and creating compelling visual displays to attract and engage customers. Fashion merchandisers play a crucial role in bridging the gap between fashion designers and consumers. They are responsible for ensuring that the right products are available at the right time, in the right quantities, and at the right prices to meet consumer demands and maximize sales. One of the key tasks of a fashion merchandiser is to conduct thorough market research to identify emerging fashion trends, consumer preferences, and buying habits. This information is then used to create a merchandising plan, which includes deciding on the assortment of products to be offered, setting price points, and determining the quantity of each item to be stocked. Once the products have been selected, fashion merchandisers work closely with designers and manufacturers to ensure that they are produced according to the desired specifications and quality standards. They negotiate and finalize purchasing contracts, monitor production timelines, and coordinate the delivery of goods to retail stores. In addition to product selection and procurement, fashion merchandisers are also responsible for visual merchandising. They collaborate with store designers to create attractive and engaging displays that effectively showcase the products and inspire customers to make purchases. This involves arranging clothing, accessories, and other fashion items in visually appealing ways, selecting appropriate props and lighting, and regularly refreshing displays to maintain customer interest. Another important aspect of fashion merchandising is sales analysis. Merchandisers monitor sales data, identify patterns and trends, and use this information to make informed decisions about inventory replenishment, pricing adjustments, and promotional strategies. They work closely with store managers and sales associates to ensure that sales goals are met and profits are maximized. Overall, fashion merchandising requires a combination of creativity, analytical skills, and business acumen. It involves staying up-to-date with the latest fashion trends, understanding consumer behavior, and effectively communicating and collaborating with various stakeholders within the fashion industry. Successful fashion merchandisers are able to anticipate and respond to market demands, resulting in increased sales and profitability for retail establishments.

Fashion Minimalist Style

Minimalist style in fashion design refers to a simplistic and understated approach that focuses on essential elements and clean lines. This style emphasizes functionality, practicality, and simplicity, as opposed to excessive ornamentation or embellishments. Minimalist fashion often features neutral colors such as black, white, gray, and earth tones, which create a timeless and elegant look. The emphasis is on creating a harmonious and balanced ensemble, with a minimal use of patterns or prints. The clothing and accessories are typically made from high-quality materials with a focus on craftsmanship and durability.

Fashion Mixer

A fashion mixer is a term commonly used in the fashion design industry to describe an event or platform where designers, creatives, industry professionals, and influencers come together to network, collaborate, and showcase their work. It is a space where different individuals with diverse backgrounds and talents in the fashion industry can connect and explore opportunities for collaboration and growth. The main purpose of a fashion mixer is to foster connections and promote collaboration among professionals in the fashion industry. It allows designers to showcase their latest collections or designs, and provides them with a platform to gain exposure and recognition. Additionally, fashion mixers often provide an opportunity for emerging designers to gain valuable feedback and advice from more experienced professionals in the industry.

Fashion Model Agency

A fashion model agency is a specialized organization that manages the careers of fashion models. It serves as the intermediary between fashion designers, brands, and clients who require models for various purposes such as runway shows, magazine editorials, advertising campaigns, or product launches. These agencies are responsible for scouting new faces and discovering potential talent for the fashion industry. They actively seek out individuals who possess the desired look, height, body proportions, and unique features that align with the current fashion trends and the specific requirements of their clients. Once models are signed with an agency, the agency takes on the vital role of promoting and representing them. This includes organizing castings, go-sees (meetings with potential clients), and photo shoots to build the models' portfolios. The agency also negotiates contracts and sets the models' rates for their work. Furthermore, a fashion model agency provides guidance and support to its models. This involves offering professional advice on body care, nutrition, fitness, and grooming to help models maintain their physical appearance and meet the industry's standards. The agency may also provide training and development opportunities to enhance the models' skills and increase their overall marketability. These agencies work with a wide range of clients, including renowned fashion designers, magazines, commercial brands, and advertising agencies. They aim to match the right model with the right project, taking into account the specific requirements and desired aesthetic of the client. By building relationships with both models and clients, a fashion model agency acts as a crucial link in the fashion industry, facilitating collaborations and ensuring the successful execution of projects.

Fashion Model Casting

A fashion model casting is a formal process conducted by fashion designers to select models for their upcoming fashion shows or campaigns. This casting brings together a group of potential models to showcase their suitability for the designer's collection or project. During a fashion model casting, designers evaluate various aspects of the models, including their physical appearance, runway skills, ability to pose for photographs, and overall presence. The casting process enables designers to choose models that align with their brand image and enhance the visual presentation of their designs.

Fashion Model

A fashion model is a person who poses or displays clothing, accessories, or other fashion products to promote them and showcase their design. They serve as a live mannequin, exhibiting garments in various settings such as fashion shows, photo shoots, or promotional events. The role of a fashion model is to convey the desired image and aesthetic of a fashion brand or designer. They are selected based on specific physical attributes that match the brand's vision and target audience. These attributes include height, body proportions, facial features, and overall body shape. Fashion models are often expected to have a slim and toned physique, although there is a growing demand for diversity in body sizes and shapes to reflect an inclusive and realistic representation of customers. Once selected, fashion models work closely with designers, photographers, stylists, and casting directors to bring a collection or fashion concept to life. They undergo fittings and rehearsals to ensure that the garments fit properly and are presented in the most flattering way. During fashion shows, models walk the runway, showcasing designs with confidence and elegance, while photographers capture their movements and poses. Photographic modeling is another important aspect of a fashion model's work. They collaborate with photographers to create visually captivating images that highlight the clothing or accessories being showcased. These photographs are then used in advertising campaigns, editorial spreads, and online promotions. Being a fashion model requires more than just looking good in clothes. They must possess strong interpersonal and communication skills, as they often interact with designers, stylists, photographers, and other team members. Professionalism, adaptability, and the ability to take direction are also essential qualities for a successful fashion model. In recent years, the fashion industry has made efforts to embrace diversity and inclusivity. There is now a greater demand for models of all ethnicities, ages, sizes, and genders, reflecting the diverse range of consumers and challenging traditional beauty standards.

Fashion Mood Boards

A fashion mood board is a visual tool used by fashion designers to communicate and explore their ideas and inspirations for a particular collection or project. It is a collage of images, textures, colors, and materials that help designers visually represent their vision and concept for a fashion line. Mood boards act as a visual reference point and serve as a starting point for the design process. They help designers capture and convey the overall mood, theme, and aesthetic they want to achieve. By gathering and arranging various visual elements, designers can create a cohesive and cohesive visual story that guides them throughout the design process.

Fashion Museum

A fashion museum is a dedicated institution or exhibition space that showcases and preserves the history, craftsmanship, and evolution of fashion design. It serves as a cultural and educational hub for the fashion industry and provides a platform for the public to engage with and appreciate fashion as an art form. At its core, a fashion museum is a repository of fashion artifacts, garments, accessories, textiles, and other related objects that have historical, cultural, artistic, or societal significance. These collections are carefully curated and displayed in a way that highlights their aesthetic and conceptual value, as well as their historical and cultural context. A fashion museum plays a vital role in documenting and interpreting fashion history. It preserves and conserves garments and textiles, ensuring their longevity and protecting them as valuable cultural artifacts. Through exhibitions, the museum presents a chronological narrative of fashion, showcasing iconic designs, designers, and movements from different eras. In addition to its physical collections, a fashion museum often hosts temporary exhibitions that explore specific themes, concepts, or designers. These exhibitions can be retrospective, highlighting the work of a particular designer or fashion house, or they can focus on a specific era, region, or cultural influence. They provide opportunities for in-depth exploration and analysis of specific aspects of fashion design. A fashion museum also serves as an educational resource, offering opportunities for research, study, and public programs. It may house a library or archive dedicated to fashion, providing access to a wide range of resources for students, researchers, and fashion enthusiasts. Workshops, lectures, and symposiums are often organized to foster dialogue and knowledge exchange among industry professionals, scholars, and the public. Overall, a fashion museum celebrates and promotes the significance of fashion design as a form of artistic expression and cultural heritage. It seeks to inspire and inform visitors about the creativity, innovation, and craftsmanship behind fashion, fostering a deeper understanding and appreciation of this dynamic industry.

Fashion Museums

A fashion museum is a physical institution that preserves and exhibits artifacts related to the history, development, and evolution of fashion design. These museums play a crucial role in showcasing the artistic and cultural significance of fashion, serving as educational resources for designers, students, researchers, and the general public. Fashion museums curate and display a wide range of garments, accessories, textiles, and other items that have played a significant role in the fashion industry. These items can include historical pieces from various time periods, iconic designs from renowned fashion houses, avant-garde creations from cutting-edge designers, and culturally significant garments from different regions of the world. One of the primary functions of fashion museums is to preserve and conserve these artifacts, ensuring their long-term viability and accessibility. Museums employ trained professionals, such as conservators and archivists, who handle these items with utmost care, utilizing specialized techniques and technologies to prevent damage and decay. By doing so, these museums contribute to the preservation of fashion history and heritage. In addition to preservation, fashion museums serve as platforms for exhibition and education. They organize curated displays and temporary exhibitions that showcase specific themes or eras, highlighting the cultural, social, and artistic contexts in which fashion has evolved. Through these exhibitions, visitors can gain a deeper understanding of fashion as an art form and its interconnectedness with history and society. Fashion museums also offer educational programs, workshops, and seminars that cater to designers, students, and enthusiasts. These programs provide valuable insights into various aspects of fashion design, including garment construction, textile development, historical fashion movements, and fashion theory. By offering these educational opportunities, museums contribute to the growth and development of the fashion industry. Last but not least, fashion museums often house extensive archives, libraries, and research facilities. These resources support scholarly research and facilitate academic discourse on fashion design. Researchers can access rare publications, fashion journals, photographs, and manuscripts, providing a comprehensive understanding of fashion's evolution and its impact on society. In summary, fashion museums are physical institutions that preserve, exhibit, and educate on the history and development of fashion design. By preserving artifacts, organizing exhibitions, offering educational programs, and providing research resources, these museums play a vital role in celebrating and furthering the understanding of fashion as an art form.

Fashion Networking Event

A fashion networking event is a gathering or event specifically designed for professionals in the fashion industry to meet, connect, and collaborate with one another. It provides a platform for fashion designers, artists, stylists, influencers, manufacturers, retailers, and other industry individuals to build relationships, share ideas, and explore potential collaborations. The primary goal of a fashion networking event is to create an environment that fosters professional growth and opportunities within the fashion industry. Participants are able to showcase their work, learn from industry experts, and gain insights into current trends and practices. It also allows attendees to establish connections with potential clients, mentors, and business partners.

Fashion Networking

Fashion networking refers to the process of connecting and building relationships within the fashion industry for professional purposes. It involves creating and maintaining connections with individuals and organizations involved in various aspects of the fashion design industry, including designers, manufacturers, suppliers, retailers, fashion influencers, and other industry professionals. The primary goal of fashion networking is to develop a strong and diverse network of contacts that can facilitate collaboration, growth, and success in the fashion design industry. It provides opportunities for designers to showcase their work, seek advice, gain exposure, and expand their business or career opportunities.

Fashion Outlet

A fashion outlet is a physical or online store that sells discounted or clearance clothing, accessories, and other fashion items. It is often associated with designer brands or high-end fashion labels. A fashion outlet differs from a regular retail store in that it offers products at a lower price point. This is achieved through various means, such as sourcing overstocked or last season's items, products with slight imperfections, or merchandise that is being phased out of the regular retail line. These items are then sold at a reduced price to attract value-conscious customers.

Fashion PR Workshop

Fashion PR Workshop is a comprehensive training program that focuses on the intersection of public relations and fashion design. It is designed to equip individuals with the essential knowledge and skills needed to effectively manage and enhance the public image of fashion brands and designers. This workshop covers various aspects of fashion PR, including media relations, brand messaging, event planning, social media management, and crisis communication. Participants will learn how to create compelling press releases, pitch stories to journalists, cultivate relationships with fashion influencers, and execute successful publicity campaigns. Through a combination of theoretical teachings and practical exercises, participants will gain a deep understanding of the fashion industry and the role of PR in shaping its narrative. They will learn how to develop and implement strategic PR plans that align with the brand's vision and objectives, promote new collections or fashion shows, and generate positive media coverage. The workshop also delves into the power of social media in fashion PR, providing insights into how to leverage platforms such as Instagram, Facebook, and Twitter to engage with the target audience, build brand awareness, and foster a loyal community of followers. Participants will explore strategies for content creation, influencer partnerships, and measuring the impact of social media efforts. Furthermore, the Fashion PR Workshop addresses crisis communication within the fashion industry. Participants will learn how to effectively handle and respond to negative publicity, manage reputation crises, and maintain brand authenticity and integrity. The workshop emphasizes the importance of transparency, accountability, and ethical practices in fashion PR. By the end of the workshop, participants will have acquired the necessary skills and knowledge to navigate the dynamic world of fashion PR and effectively promote fashion brands and designers. They will be equipped with a comprehensive toolkit of PR strategies and techniques that can be applied to enhance the visibility and reputation of fashion brands in an increasingly competitive industry.

Fashion PR

Fashion PR, or fashion public relations, is a specialized area within the field of public relations that focuses on promoting and generating positive publicity for fashion brands, designers, and industry professionals. It involves managing the public image and reputation of fashion brands, creating buzz and excitement around new collections, and building and maintaining relationships with key stakeholders such as journalists, influencers, and celebrities. The primary goal of fashion PR is to create a positive perception of a fashion brand or designer in the eyes of the public, media, and potential consumers. This is achieved through various strategies and tactics, including media relations, event planning and execution, brand partnerships, and social media management. One of the key responsibilities of a fashion PR professional is to secure press coverage for their clients. This may involve pitching story ideas and press releases to journalists, arranging interviews and photo shoots, and coordinating press events such as fashion shows and product launches. By generating positive media coverage, fashion PR helps to increase brand awareness and visibility, and ultimately drive sales and growth for the fashion brand. In addition to media relations, fashion PR also involves managing relationships with influencers and celebrities. These individuals have a strong impact on consumer buying decisions and can greatly influence the success of a fashion brand. Fashion PR professionals often collaborate with influencers and celebrities by gifting them products, inviting them to fashion events, and seeking their endorsement and support. By associating a brand with well-known and respected individuals, fashion PR helps to enhance the brand's image and credibility. Furthermore, fashion PR plays a crucial role in crisis management and damage control. In the fast-paced and highly competitive fashion industry, issues and controversies can arise that may negatively impact a brand's reputation. Fashion PR professionals are responsible for mitigating potential damage by developing strategic communications plans, addressing negative press, and effectively managing public perception during challenging times. In conclusion, fashion PR is a specialized branch of public relations that focuses on building and maintaining the positive image and reputation of fashion brands and designers. Through media relations, event planning, influencer partnerships, and crisis management, fashion PR professionals work to create buzz, generate positive publicity, and ultimately drive growth for their clients in the dynamic world of fashion design.

Fashion Panel

A fashion panel in the context of fashion design refers to a group of industry experts who come together to discuss and evaluate various aspects of fashion, including trends, designs, and techniques. The main purpose of a fashion panel is to provide insight, guidance, and critique to both established and emerging fashion designers. The fashion panel typically consists of individuals with extensive knowledge and experience in different areas of the fashion industry, such as designers, stylists, fashion editors, buyers, and influencers. These experts have a deep understanding of current and upcoming fashion trends, as well as a keen eye for evaluating the quality, creativity, and marketability of fashion designs. The role of the fashion panel is to offer constructive feedback and advice to fashion designers, which helps them refine and improve their work. Through a collaborative and critical discussion, the panel members provide valuable insights on design aesthetics, fabrication choices, color combinations, and overall presentation. They also consider factors like target audience, market demand, and cultural influences when evaluating the potential success of a fashion collection or individual garments. Fashion panels are often featured in fashion shows, design competitions, and industry events. Designers present their collections or individual garments to the panel, who then assess and provide feedback on various aspects of the designs. This feedback helps designers make informed decisions during the design process and enhances their chances of creating desirable and commercially viable fashion products. In addition to critiquing designs, fashion panels also discuss broader industry topics, such as sustainability, inclusivity, and innovation. They contribute to the advancement of the fashion industry by sharing their insights and expertise, thereby shaping the direction and future of fashion design.

Fashion Pattern Making

Fashion pattern making is an essential process in the field of fashion design that involves creating precise templates or pattern pieces as a foundation for creating garments. These patterns serve as a blueprint, guiding fashion designers in the construction of clothing items with the desired fit, structure, and aesthetic appeal. The process of pattern making starts with a fashion designer conceptualizing a design and translating it into a tangible form. They typically begin by sketching the garment on paper, providing a visual representation of the desired style and silhouette. From this initial sketch, the designer then creates a pattern by using basic geometric shapes and measurements to draft individual pattern pieces for different sections of the garment. Once the initial pattern is created, it serves as a starting point for further refinement and adjustment. Fashion pattern makers meticulously measure and analyze the pattern's dimensions, making necessary alterations to ensure an accurate fit and aesthetic outcome. They consider factors such as the body's shape, proportions, and movements, as well as specific design elements such as darts, pleats, and seams. Pattern making involves technical skills and knowledge, including understanding fabric properties, garment construction techniques, and body measurements. It requires a keen eye for detail and precision, as small errors in pattern creation can result in ill-fitting garments. Pattern makers often work closely with fashion designers, using their expertise to transform design concepts into practical patterns that can be replicated and produced in various sizes. The significance of pattern making extends beyond the design process. Accurate and well-drafted patterns are crucial for efficient and cost-effective garment production. They serve as a guide for garment factories and manufacturers, enabling them to reproduce the designer's vision at a larger scale and across different sizes. In summary, fashion pattern making plays a vital role in fashion design by creating precise templates that serve as foundations for garment construction. It involves the technical skill of transforming design concepts into tangible patterns, ensuring accurate fit and aesthetic outcomes. With its significance in both design and production processes, pattern making is an integral part of the fashion industry.

Fashion Philanthropy

Fashion philanthropy is a concept in the field of fashion design that involves the use of fashion as a means of giving back to society. It encompasses various initiatives and activities undertaken by fashion designers, brands, and individuals to make a positive impact on social, humanitarian, and environmental issues. In the context of fashion design, fashion philanthropy means using one's creative skills, influence, and resources to support charitable causes and contribute to the betterment of society. It goes beyond creating aesthetically pleasing garments and focuses on using fashion as a medium for social change.

Fashion Photographer

A fashion photographer is a professional who specializes in capturing photographs that showcase clothing, accessories, and fashion designs. They have a keen eye for detail and are skilled at using lighting, composition, and posing techniques to create visually striking images.

Fashion photographers play a crucial role in the fashion industry as they bring clothing and designs to life through their photographs. They work closely with designers, stylists, and models to ensure that the images effectively communicate the desired message and aesthetic. One of the key responsibilities of a fashion photographer is to accurately depict the clothing and accessories being showcased. They must showcase the cut, fit, and texture of the garments to highlight their unique features. The photographer also needs to capture the overall mood and concept that the designer wants to convey, whether it's glamorous, edgy, or romantic. To achieve this, fashion photographers must have a good understanding of fashion trends and styles. They need to stay up-to-date with the latest collections, designers, and industry influencers. This knowledge allows them to provide valuable input and creative direction during photoshoots. Another important aspect of a fashion photographer's role is to work with models and direct them to create the desired poses and expressions. They need to have strong communication skills and the ability to make the models feel comfortable and confident. This helps in capturing natural and authentic moments that reflect the essence of the fashion design. In addition to technical skills and industry knowledge, fashion photographers need to be highly creative and artistic. They must be able to envision the final result and bring their artistic vision to life through their photographs. This involves making decisions about the location, background, props, and styling, which contribute to the overall aesthetic of the image. Post-production is also a significant part of a fashion photographer's work. They edit and retouch the images to enhance the colors, composition, and overall visual impact. This ensures that the photographs align with the client's brand image and vision. In conclusion, a fashion photographer is a professional who uses their technical skills, industry knowledge, creativity, and artistic vision to capture visually stunning photographs that showcase clothing, accessories, and fashion designs. They play a crucial role in the fashion industry, collaborating with designers, stylists, and models to bring fashion concepts to life through their images.

Fashion Photography Studio

A fashion photography studio is a dedicated space where professional photographers and their team capture images of clothing, accessories, and models for fashion publications, advertisements, and branding purposes. These studios are equipped with specialized lighting equipment, backdrops, and props to create a visually appealing and high-quality imagery that showcases the aesthetic of fashion brands and designers. Fashion photography studios are usually located in urban areas, often in close proximity to the fashion and design industry hubs. The main objective of a fashion photography studio is to create striking visuals that effectively communicate the essence and personality of a fashion brand or designer. The photographers work closely with stylists, makeup artists, and hair stylists to ensure that the overall concept of the shoot aligns with the brand's identity and vision. During a photoshoot in a fashion photography studio, multiple photographs are taken of different outfits and accessories. The models are carefully posed and directed by the photographer to capture the desired look and mood. The studio is equipped with various props and set designs to create different scenes and backdrops that complement the clothing being photographed. After the photoshoot, the selected images are carefully edited and retouched to enhance their visual impact. This editing process may involve adjusting the colors, lighting, and overall composition of the photographs. The final images are then delivered to the fashion brand or designer for use in marketing materials, social media campaigns, and other promotional channels. In addition to clothing and accessories, fashion photography studios may also specialize in other areas of fashion photography, such as beauty, editorial, and runway photography. Some studios offer additional services such as model casting, art direction, and post-production editing to provide a comprehensive solution for fashion brands and designers.

Fashion Photography Workshop

A Fashion Photography Workshop is an educational event in the field of fashion design that provides participants with the opportunity to learn and develop photography skills specifically focused on fashion. It is a formal gathering where aspiring fashion photographers, both beginners and intermediate level, come together to enhance their knowledge and technical expertise in capturing fashion images. The main objective of a Fashion Photography Workshop is to equip participants with the necessary skills and techniques required to create visually captivating and aesthetically pleasing photographs that emphasize the beauty and uniqueness of fashion garments, accessories, and models. By attending such workshops, aspiring fashion photographers gain insight into the best practices and strategies employed in the fashion industry, enabling them to produce professional-grade images that meet industry standards. During the workshop, participants are immersed in a hands-on learning environment that includes practical sessions featuring live models, professional fashion stylists, and hair and makeup artists. Through these practical sessions, participants have the opportunity to apply their newly acquired skills in real-world scenarios, addressing challenges such as lighting, composition, and directing models. They learn to work collaboratively with a team to create cohesive fashion imagery that communicates the desired message and evokes the intended visual impact. In addition to the technical aspect, Fashion Photography Workshops also emphasize the conceptual and artistic elements of fashion photography. Participants learn about the importance of storytelling through imagery, understanding how to convey a brand's identity or a designer's vision through visual narratives. They explore various styles and genres within fashion photography, such as editorial, commercial, and street fashion, to broaden their creative repertoire and develop their unique artistic voice. Fashion Photography Workshops often feature industry professionals, such as established fashion photographers, experienced fashion editors, or renowned fashion designers, who share their insights and expertise with the participants. Through interactive sessions, participants gain valuable knowledge about the business side of fashion photography, including portfolio development, client management, and marketing strategies. By attending a Fashion Photography Workshop, aspiring fashion photographers acquire the necessary skills, knowledge, and industry connections to kickstart their career in the competitive world of fashion photography. It serves as a platform for personal growth and fosters a sense of community among like-minded individuals who share a passion for fashion and photography, inspiring collaboration and creative exchange. In conclusion, a Fashion Photography Workshop is a formal educational event that provides aspiring fashion photographers with an immersive learning experience, enabling them to develop technical proficiency, artistic vision, and valuable industry insights required to pursue a successful career in the field of fashion photography.

Fashion Photography

Fashion Photography is a specialized genre of photography that focuses on capturing images of fashion and clothing for promotional and artistic purposes. It plays a crucial role in the fashion industry by showcasing garments and accessories in a visually captivating and aesthetically pleasing manner. The primary objective of fashion photography is to capture the essence and mood of a fashion collection or a specific clothing item. Through composition, lighting, and styling, fashion photographers create visually stunning images that not only showcase the design and craftsmanship of the garments but also evoke emotions and tell stories. Fashion photographers work closely with fashion designers, stylists, makeup artists, and models to bring their creative visions to life. They collaborate with a team of professionals to create a narrative that aligns with the brand's identity and the designer's aesthetic. The photographers need to have a deep understanding of fashion trends, as well as the ability to interpret and translate them into compelling visual narratives. Aside from capturing the garments, fashion photographers also play a significant role in creating a mood or atmosphere around the fashion brand or item being photographed. They use various techniques, such as lighting, composition, and post-production editing, to create an atmosphere that enhances the clothing's appeal and brings it to life. The choice of location, props, and even models' poses all contribute to building a cohesive narrative that resonates with the target audience. In addition to editorial fashion photography, fashion photographers also work on advertising campaigns, lookbooks, catalogues, and runway shows. Each of these platforms requires a different approach, but the goal remains the same: to showcase the fashion in a way that is visually compelling and aligned with the brand's image. Overall, fashion photography is a critical element in the fashion industry, playing an integral role in showcasing designs, promoting brands, and enticing consumers. It combines artistic vision, technical skills, and a deep understanding of fashion to create visually captivating images that capture attention and inspire consumers' desires.

Fashion Pleats

Fashion Pleats: Fashion pleats refer to a design technique utilized in clothing and textile products that involves folding or creasing fabric to create elegant and structured effects. Pleats can be seen in various garments such as skirts, dresses, trousers, and even accessories like scarves and handbags. Pleats are created by folding fabric in a controlled manner, which adds volume, texture, and visual interest to the garment. This technique is achieved by manipulating the fabric through folding, then securing it in place by stitching or pressing. The resulting folds can be arranged in different ways, such as accordion pleats, box pleats, knife pleats, or inverted pleats, each producing a distinct aesthetic appeal. The use of pleats in fashion design dates back centuries, with evidence of its presence in ancient Egyptian and Greek clothing. Throughout history, pleats have been employed not only for their aesthetic qualities but also for their functional benefits. Pleated garments often exhibit increased flexibility and movement due to the added fabric volume, making them suitable for activewear and dance costumes. Pleats can create various visual effects depending on their placement, width, and direction. For example, vertical pleats can elongate the body, creating a slimming effect, while horizontal pleats can add volume and fullness. Pleats can also be strategically positioned to accentuate certain features or disguise areas of the body. In addition to their visual appeal, pleats can also enhance the drape and flow of a garment. Designers often experiment with pleats to create innovative and unique looks. They may incorporate pleats as a primary design element or use them as subtle accents. Pleats can be combined with other design elements such as color, pattern, texture, and shape to create visually striking and dynamic garments. In conclusion, fashion pleats are a design technique involving controlled folding or creasing of fabric to create distinctive aesthetic effects. Whether used to add volume, texture, or visual interest, pleats have a long history in fashion and continue to be a versatile and beloved design element.

Fashion Podcast

A fashion podcast is a digital audio or video series that provides informative and engaging content related to fashion design. It is usually hosted by industry professionals, designers, or fashion enthusiasts, who share their knowledge, insights, and experiences in the field. The main aim of a fashion podcast is to educate, inspire, and entertain its audience by covering various topics within the realm of fashion design. These topics may include trends, styles, fashion history, industry news, interviews with designers, and tips for aspiring fashion designers. By utilizing the audio or video format, podcasts allow for a more dynamic and immersive learning experience, enabling listeners to hear the voices, opinions, and stories behind the fashion world.

Fashion Police

Fashion Police is a term used in the fashion industry to refer to individuals or groups who critique and evaluate fashion designs, trends, and styles. They act as a form of authority, enforcing and upholding certain standards and norms within the fashion world. The Fashion Police's role is to assess and judge the visual aesthetics, creativity, and overall appeal of fashion designs. They evaluate various elements such as clothing silhouettes, fabrics, colors, patterns, and accessories to determine their quality, uniqueness, cohesiveness, and relevance to current trends or specific events. In their evaluation, the Fashion Police often consider factors like fit, proportion, balance, and technical craftsmanship. They may also take into account historical references, cultural influences, and socio-political contexts. Their goal is to determine whether a fashion design is successful in conveying a particular message or evoking a desired response from the audience. Fashion Police can be individuals, such as fashion critics, journalists, bloggers, or influencers, who express their opinions through various media platforms such as magazines, newspapers, websites, or social media. They provide commentary, reviews, and analyses on fashion collections, runway shows, red carpet events, and celebrity outfits. Their assessments can influence public opinions and trends by highlighting what is considered fashionable or stylish. Additionally, Fashion Police can also refer to panels of experts who judge fashion design competitions or participate in fashion-related TV shows. These panels use their expertise and industry knowledge to assess the designs and skills of aspiring fashion designers, providing constructive criticism and feedback. While the role of the Fashion Police is to critique and offer opinions, it is essential to acknowledge that fashion is subjective and inherently personal. One's taste and perception of fashion may differ from others, emphasizing the importance of diversity and individual expression within the industry. Overall, the Fashion Police play a significant role in shaping and influencing fashion trends, providing guidance and standards within the fashion industry. Their assessments and critiques contribute to the ongoing evolution and development of fashion design, pushing boundaries, and challenging conventions.

Fashion Polyester

Fashion Polyester is a versatile synthetic fabric commonly used in the fashion industry. It is made from polyester fibers, which are a type of plastic that is created through a chemical process known as polymerization. This process involves combining chemicals such as ethylene glycol and dimethyl terephthalate to create long chains of repeating units. The properties of fashion polyester make it an attractive choice for designers. It is known for its durability, wrinkle resistance, and ability to hold its shape, making it ideal for clothing items such as dresses, shirts, and skirts. It is also lightweight and breathable, allowing for comfortable wear. Fashion polyester is a popular choice for its affordability as well. It is a cost-effective fabric compared to natural fibers like cotton or silk, making it accessible to a wide range of consumers. Its synthetic nature also allows for a wide variety of colors and patterns, as it can be easily dyed and printed on, offering endless design possibilities. In addition to its practical qualities, fashion polyester is also known for its versatility. It can be blended with other fibers such as cotton or rayon to enhance specific characteristics, such as adding softness and moisture-wicking properties. This blend allows for the creation of fabrics that combine the best qualities of both fibers. However, it is important to note that fashion polyester does have some drawbacks. It is not as breathable as natural fibers, which can make it less comfortable in hot and humid climates. It is also not biodegradable, contributing to environmental concerns. Nonetheless, efforts are being made to develop more sustainable and eco-friendly alternatives.

Fashion Pop-Up Event

A fashion pop-up event is a short-term retail experience that aims to create a unique and immersive environment for fashion designers and brands to showcase their products to the public. It is a temporary event typically lasting from a few hours to a few days, often set up in unconventional and non-traditional locations such as empty warehouses, industrial spaces, or outdoor venues. The purpose of a fashion pop-up event is to generate buzz and excitement around a particular brand or collection, while also creating a sense of urgency and exclusivity for consumers. By creating a limited-time shopping experience, fashion pop-up events attract a sense of scarcity and desirability, encouraging consumers to make a purchase on the spot. This format also allows designers to test new markets, engage with customers directly, and gauge the demand for their products before committing to a long-term retail space. At a fashion pop-up event, the venue is transformed into a visually captivating space that reflects the brand's aesthetic and values. The layout and design of the space are carefully curated to provide an immersive experience for visitors, often including customized fixtures, creative lighting, and engaging displays. The goal is to create an environment that not only showcases the products but also evokes emotion and tells a story. In addition to shopping opportunities, fashion pop-up events often feature a range of experiential elements such as live performances, art installations, workshops, or panel discussions. These activities help to create a multi-sensory experience that goes beyond traditional retail and fosters a deeper connection between the brand and the consumer. Overall, a fashion pop-up event serves as a strategic marketing tool for fashion designers and brands to create brand awareness, drive sales, and connect with their target audience in a unique and memorable way. It offers an opportunity for designers to experiment with innovative retail concepts, build relationships with customers, and leave a lasting impression that extends beyond the duration of the event.

Fashion Pop-Up Shop

A fashion pop-up shop is a temporary retail space that showcases and sells fashion products for a limited time. It is typically set up in an unconventional, non-permanent location, such as a vacant storefront or an event space, and is designed to create a sense of exclusivity and urgency among potential customers. The concept of a pop-up shop is rooted in the idea of creating a unique and immersive shopping experience. By offering a limited-time opportunity to discover and purchase fashion items, pop-up shops generate excitement and drive consumer engagement. These temporary spaces often feature eye-catching displays, interactive installations, and curated assortments of merchandise, all of which are designed to capture the attention and interest of fashion-forward consumers. One of the key benefits of a fashion pop-up shop is its ability to create a sense of novelty and surprise. As the shop appears for a limited period, customers are enticed to visit and explore the unique fashion offerings, knowing that once the shop is gone, so are the opportunities to purchase those specific items. This limited-time aspect fosters a sense of urgency and exclusivity, encouraging customers to act quickly and make purchases. Moreover, fashion pop-up shops serve as a platform for emerging designers and brands to gain exposure and build brand awareness. By offering a temporary space to showcase their collections, these designers can reach a wider audience and connect with potential customers who may not have otherwise discovered their brand. This temporary nature also allows designers to experiment with new concepts, test market demand, and gather valuable customer feedback. In recent years, fashion pop-up shops have become increasingly popular due to their ability to create buzz and generate social media engagement. The unique and visually appealing nature of these spaces often leads to sharing on platforms such as Instagram, allowing the brands to maximize their exposure and reach wider audiences. In conclusion, a fashion pop-up shop is a temporary retail space that provides a unique and immersive shopping experience, featuring limited-time fashion collections and creating a sense of urgency and exclusivity. By showcasing emerging designers and brands, pop-up shops serve as a platform for building brand awareness and engaging with potential customers.

Fashion Portfolio

A fashion portfolio is a collection of a fashion designer's work that showcases their creativity, technical skills, and design aesthetic. It serves as a visual representation of their talent and serves as a tool to present their work to potential employers, clients, or fashion schools. The purpose of a fashion portfolio is to demonstrate the designer's ability to create innovative and well-executed designs. It includes a range of design projects, such as sketches, illustrations, photographs of finished garments, and technical drawings. These projects can showcase the designer's ability to create unique garment shapes, experiment with different fabric textures, incorporate various colors and patterns, and develop cohesive collections.

Fashion Preppy Style

Fashion Preppy Style is a fashion trend characterized by clean and polished looks inspired by the clothing styles traditionally associated with Ivy League universities in the United States. This style emerged in the 1950s and has remained popular ever since, particularly among young adults and college students. The key elements of Preppy Style include a focus on classic and timeless clothing pieces, such as button-down shirts, polo shirts, blazers, chinos, and knee-length skirts. Neat and well-fitted silhouettes are favored, with a preference for tailored and structured garments. Typical colors of Preppy Style include pastels, nautical elements, and vibrant combinations. Stripes, plaids, and checks are commonly seen in Preppy fashion, often mixed and matched to create an effortless yet put-together look. Accessories play an important role in completing the Preppy Style. Here, we see items like loafers, boat shoes, Mary Jane pumps, pearl necklaces, and headbands. Handbags tend to be medium-sized and structured, often made of materials like leather or canvas. The fashion Preppy Style is known for its attention to detail and the use of high-quality materials. Fabrics like cotton, linen, silk, and cashmere are often chosen for their timeless appeal and luxurious feel. The Preppy Style can be worn in various settings, from casual outings to formal events. During the colder months, layering is common, with sweaters, cardigans, and blazers being paired with collared shirts or dresses. Although the Preppy Style has its roots in the Ivy League culture of the past, it continues to evolve and adapt to modern fashion trends. This style is favored by those who appreciate a classic and polished look, yet want to incorporate their personal style into it.

Fashion Production Coordinator

A Fashion Production Coordinator is an essential role within the fashion design industry. They are responsible for managing and coordinating the production process of fashion garments and accessories, ensuring that each step is executed smoothly and efficiently.The primary role of a Fashion Production Coordinator is to oversee the entire production process, from the initial design concept to the final delivery of the products. They work closely with the design team, suppliers, manufacturers, and other stakeholders to ensure that all aspects of production are carried out with the utmost attention to detail.One of the main responsibilities of a Fashion Production Coordinator is to create production schedules and timelines. They must carefully plan the production process, taking into consideration factors such as the availability of materials, production capacity, and delivery deadlines. This requires excellent organizational skills and the ability to multitask effectively.In addition to creating schedules, Fashion Production Coordinators also play a vital role in sourcing and managing the supply chain. They work closely with suppliers and manufacturers to source the required materials and negotiate favorable prices. They also monitor the production progress and quality, ensuring that all products meet the desired standards.Another important aspect of the role is ensuring effective communication and coordination between different departments and stakeholders involved in the production process. Fashion Production Coordinators act as a liaison between the design team, production team, suppliers, and manufacturers, ensuring that all parties are aligned and working towards the common goal of delivering high-quality fashion products.Overall, a Fashion Production Coordinator is a crucial link in the fashion industry, ensuring that the production process runs smoothly and efficiently. With their attention to detail, organizational skills, and ability to coordinate multiple tasks, they play a crucial role in bringing fashion designs to life.

Fashion Production Manager

A Fashion Production Manager is a professional responsible for overseeing the entire production process in the fashion industry. They play a crucial role in ensuring that designs are brought to life, from the initial concept to the final product. The primary responsibilities of a Fashion Production Manager include coordinating with designers to understand the vision and requirements of each collection, developing production plans, and managing the production schedule. They are involved in every step of the process, from sourcing raw materials to coordinating with manufacturers, ensuring that all aspects of production are executed efficiently and within budget. One of the key tasks of a Fashion Production Manager is to oversee the sourcing and procurement of materials, including fabric, trims, and accessories. They work closely with suppliers to ensure that materials meet quality standards and are delivered on time. Additionally, they negotiate pricing and quantities to ensure cost-efficient production. Once the materials are ready, the Fashion Production Manager collaborates with patternmakers and sample machinists to create prototypes. They ensure that the prototypes meet the designer's specifications and make any necessary adjustments. During the production phase, the Fashion Production Manager is responsible for coordinating with manufacturers and factories. They oversee the production processes to ensure that quality standards are maintained, and production timelines are met. They also manage any issues or delays that may arise, finding solutions to minimize disruptions. To ensure smooth operations, a Fashion Production Manager communicates regularly with the design team and other stakeholders involved in the production process. They provide status updates, address concerns, and make any adjustments necessary to meet deadlines. Overall, a Fashion Production Manager plays a critical role in bringing fashion designs to life. They are responsible for coordinating all aspects of production, from sourcing materials to overseeing manufacturing. They ensure that the production process runs smoothly and efficiently, resulting in high-quality fashion products that align with the designer's vision. In conclusion, a Fashion Production Manager is an integral part of the fashion industry, ensuring that designs are transformed into tangible products through efficient and effective production processes.

Fashion Prototyping

Fashion prototyping is a method used in the field of fashion design to test and visualize ideas before producing a final garment or collection. It involves creating a sample or prototype that represents the intended design and allows designers to assess its fit, look, and functionality. The process of fashion prototyping typically starts with sketching or creating a digital design that captures the designer's vision. This initial concept is then translated into a three-dimensional prototype using various materials and techniques. The prototype can be a simplified version of the final design, made with inexpensive materials or even created digitally using software or 3D modeling. The purpose of fashion prototyping is to refine and perfect the design by identifying any potential issues or improvements. Designers can use the prototype as a tool for experimentation and exploration, making adjustments to the shape, cut, or fabric choice to achieve the desired outcome. By physically experiencing the design, they can evaluate its aesthetics, functionality, and overall appeal. During the fashion prototyping process, designers may also involve other professionals such as pattern makers, sewers, and sample makers who can provide valuable input and expertise. Their collaboration helps ensure that the prototype reflects the intended design accurately and meets the requirements for production. The feedback gained from the fashion prototype informs the designer's decision-making process. It helps them refine and iterate on the design, making necessary changes or improvements to achieve the desired result. By testing the prototype on a fit model or through fittings, designers can also gather insights on the garment's comfort, drape, and wearability, allowing them to make necessary adjustments for optimal functionality and fit. In summary, fashion prototyping is a critical step in the fashion design process that allows designers to test, refine, and evaluate their ideas before committing to the final production. It enables them to visualize their design in three dimensions, explore different materials and techniques, and gather feedback to improve the overall quality and functionality of their creations.

Fashion Prêt-À-Porter

Fashion Prêt-à-Porter refers to ready-to-wear clothing that is mass-produced and available for purchase in standard sizes from retail stores. Derived from French, the term Prêt-à-Porter translates to "ready-to-wear" in English. This concept emerged in the mid-20th century as a response to the increasing demand for more accessible and affordable fashion. The advent of Fashion Prêt-à-Porter revolutionized the fashion industry by democratizing style and making high-fashion aesthetics accessible to a broader audience. Instead of exclusively targeting elite clientele, designers began producing garments in bulk quantities, allowing customers to enjoy the latest trends without the need for custom tailoring. The production process of Prêt-à-Porter garments involves creating patterns and prototypes based on standard body measurements. These patterns are then replicated multiple times to achieve economies of scale, resulting in a lower cost per unit. The use of standardized sizes allows customers to easily find garments that fit them well without the need for extensive alterations. Fashion Prêt-à-Porter caters to a wide range of consumers, offering clothing options for various occasions and style preferences. Collections typically include everyday essentials, formal attire, casual wear, and seasonal trends. Designers and brands showcase their creations through runway shows and presentations, allowing retailers and buyers to select pieces for their stores based on market trends and customer demands. While Fashion Prêt-à-Porter prioritizes accessibility and availability, it does not compromise on design quality or creativity. Designers still focus on creating aesthetically pleasing and innovative garments that reflect current fashion movements. Materials, techniques, and craftsmanship play essential roles in ensuring that Prêt-à-Porter clothing maintains a level of sophistication and style. In conclusion, Fashion Prêt-à-Porter represents ready-to-wear clothing that is produced in large quantities and available to the general public through retail stores. It aims to make fashion more accessible, affordable, and convenient for a broader customer base. Despite its mass production nature, Prêt-à-Porter garments uphold design excellence and reflect the current trends of the fashion industry.

Fashion Public Relations

Fashion Public Relations is a strategic communication practice within the fashion industry that aims to create and maintain a positive public image for fashion designers, brands, and products. It involves managing the relationships between fashion brands and the media, influencers, celebrities, and other stakeholders in order to generate publicity and enhance brand awareness. The primary objective of Fashion Public Relations is to promote and elevate a fashion brand's visibility, reputation, and credibility to its target audience and key stakeholders. This is achieved through various PR tactics such as media relations, press releases, fashion shows, celebrity collaborations, social media campaigns, and event sponsorships. One key aspect of Fashion Public Relations is media relations, which involves building and maintaining relationships with journalists, editors, and influencers within the fashion industry. Fashion PR professionals aim to secure press coverage in fashion magazines, newspapers, blogs, and social media platforms to create buzz and increase brand exposure. Another important role of Fashion Public Relations is managing fashion shows and events. Fashion PR professionals work closely with fashion designers to organize and promote their runway shows, presentations, and store openings. They invite influential people from the fashion industry, media, celebrities, and stylists to attend these events, generating publicity and fostering brand engagement. Additionally, Fashion Public Relations professionals often collaborate with celebrities and influential individuals to endorse fashion brands and products. By dressing celebrities for red carpet events or securing brand partnerships with influential figures, fashion PR professionals aim to create positive associations and enhance brand desirability. Furthermore, Fashion Public Relations plays a crucial role in crisis management. In the event of negative publicity or controversies, PR professionals work to mitigate potential damage to the brand's reputation by addressing the issue promptly and strategically communicating the brand's response. In summary, Fashion Public Relations is the practice of strategically managing communication and relationships between fashion designers, brands, and their target audience, media, influencers, and key stakeholders. Through various

PR tactics, Fashion PR professionals aim to generate positive publicity, enhance brand visibility, and foster brand engagement, ultimately contributing to the success and growth of fashion brands within the competitive fashion industry.

Fashion Publicist

A fashion publicist is a professional in the fashion industry who is responsible for managing the public image and publicity of a fashion brand or designer. They work closely with fashion designers, retailers, and brands to create and implement strategic public relations campaigns and initiatives. One of the main duties of a fashion publicist is to generate media coverage and create buzz around a fashion brand or designer. This can include securing press coverage in magazines, newspapers, and on websites, as well as organizing and managing fashion shows, events, and product launches. They also act as the main point of contact for media inquiries and requests, and are responsible for managing relationships with the press. In addition to generating publicity, a fashion publicist also plays a crucial role in creating and maintaining the public image of a fashion brand or designer. They work closely with the creative team to develop messaging and branding strategies, as well as to create and distribute press releases, lookbooks, and other marketing materials. They also assist with the production of photo shoots and fashion campaigns, and may be involved in selecting models, stylists, and photographers. Furthermore, a fashion publicist is responsible for managing and promoting collaborations and partnerships between fashion brands and other industry stakeholders. This may include working with celebrities and influencers to dress them in the brand's designs, as well as organizing and promoting events and activations that align with the brand's image and target audience. In summary, a fashion publicist is a critical member of a fashion brand or designer's team, responsible for managing the public image and publicity of the brand. They generate media coverage, create buzz, and maintain the brand's image through strategic public relations campaigns and initiatives.

Fashion Quality Control

Fashion Quality Control is a critical process in the field of fashion design that ensures the consistency and excellence of products throughout their production cycle. It involves a series of measures taken to assess and maintain the desired quality standards in terms of materials, construction, and overall design of fashion items. The primary objective of Fashion Quality Control is to detect and eliminate any defects or imperfections in the products before they reach the market. This helps in upholding the brand's reputation, meeting customer expectations, and maximizing customer satisfaction. Fashion brands strive to provide high-quality products that are visually appealing, comfortable, and durable. During Fashion Quality Control, various aspects of the garments or accessories are checked and evaluated. This includes the selection and inspection of fabrics, trims, and other components used in the production. The quality control team scrutinizes the materials for any flaws, such as color fading, uneven textures, or inadequate strength. In addition, the construction and workmanship of the fashion items are closely examined. This involves checking the accuracy of stitching, seam strength, and overall structural integrity. The goal is to ensure that the garments fit well, have proper finishing, and are free from any manufacturing defects. Another important aspect of Fashion Quality Control is assessing the design and aesthetics of the products. The team looks for consistency in design elements, such as prints, patterns, and embellishments, to maintain the brand's signature style. They also evaluate the visual appeal, proportions, and overall appearance of the fashion items. Furthermore, functionality and comfort are key considerations in Fashion Quality Control. The garments and accessories must be practical to wear and should meet the requirements of the intended use. Factors like ease of movement, proper sizing, and comfort on the body are carefully assessed during the quality control process. Fashion Quality Control plays a vital role in maintaining high standards and ensuring that the final products align with the brand's vision and customer expectations. By carefully monitoring and addressing any quality issues, fashion brands can establish reliability and trust among their target consumers, ultimately contributing to their success in the competitive fashion industry.

Fashion Rayon

Fashion Rayon is a synthetic fabric widely used in the field of fashion design. It is derived from the natural fiber cellulose, often sourced from wood pulp or bamboo. Rayon is known for its soft and silky texture, which makes it a popular choice for creating comfortable and flowy garments. Rayon is valued in fashion design for its versatility. It can be manufactured to mimic various textures such as cotton, silk, wool, or linen, allowing designers to achieve different looks and aesthetics. This fabric can be easily dyed and printed, enabling an array of vibrant and intricate designs to be applied.

Fashion Red Carpet

The fashion red carpet is a significant aspect of the fashion industry, specifically in relation to fashion design. It refers to the area or space where celebrities, models, and notable individuals walk during events such as film premieres, award ceremonies, and fashion shows. The red carpet symbolizes glamour, sophistication, and exclusivity. During a red carpet event, fashion designers have the opportunity to showcase their latest creations and gain exposure for their fashion labels. These designs are usually meticulously crafted and tailored to suit the specific occasion and the individual wearing them. The fashion red carpet serves as a platform for designers to display their aesthetic vision, creativity, and technical skills to a global audience.

Fashion Research Symposium

A Fashion Research Symposium is an academic event, typically held in the field of fashion design, that brings together scholars, industry professionals, and students to explore and discuss contemporary issues and developments in fashion research. It provides a platform for sharing innovative ideas, theories, and methodologies related to fashion design, fashion history, textile technology, sustainability, cultural studies, and critical analysis of fashion. Participants of a Fashion Research Symposium engage in a range of activities, such as presenting their research papers, delivering keynote speeches, participating in panel discussions, and showcasing their creative work through exhibitions or fashion shows. The symposium offers a unique opportunity for researchers to present their findings, exchange insights, and receive constructive feedback from their peers and experts in the field. By gathering researchers and professionals from various disciplines within fashion design, such as fashion marketing, visual merchandising, pattern making, and fashion journalism, the symposium encourages interdisciplinary collaborations and fosters a holistic understanding of the multifaceted nature of the fashion industry. The primary objectives of a Fashion Research Symposium are to promote dialogue and critical thinking within the fashion community, pushing boundaries and challenging conventional notions of fashion. It aims to inspire new perspectives and approaches in fashion research, contributing to the advancement of the field and its sustainable development. Overall, a Fashion Research Symposium serves as a platform for intellectual discourse, knowledge sharing, and networking in the realm of fashion design. It supports the growth of the fashion industry by encouraging research-driven practices and fostering collaborations that lead to innovative and sustainable fashion solutions.

Fashion Research

Fashion research in the context of fashion design refers to the systematic investigation and analysis of various elements and concepts that influence the development and direction of the fashion industry. It involves gathering and interpreting data and information to enhance the understanding of trends, consumer behavior, cultural influences, historical references, and technological advancements. The primary objective of fashion research is to create a comprehensive understanding of current and future fashion trends, as well as their potential impact on design, production, and marketing strategies. It helps designers and fashion professionals make informed decisions by providing valuable insights into consumer preferences, market demands, and industry challenges. Fashion research encompasses both qualitative and quantitative methods. Qualitative research involves techniques such as interviews, focus groups, and observations, which aim to gain a deeper understanding of consumers' perceptions, preferences, and motivations. This type of research explores subjective experiences, emotions, and cultural influences to identify emerging trends and design directions. Quantitative research, on the other hand, relies on numerical data and statistical analysis to identify patterns, correlations, and trends on a larger scale. This includes analyzing sales figures, market reports, and consumer surveys to quantify consumer behavior, market size, and market segmentation. These findings help fashion designers and companies develop products and services that meet the needs and desires of their target audience. Furthermore, fashion research also involves the study of historical and cultural contexts, examining past fashion movements and their impact on contemporary design. It helps designers gain insight into the evolution of fashion and tradition, enabling them to create innovative designs that bridge the gap between the past and present. Overall, fashion research plays a critical role in the creative and strategic decision-making processes within the fashion industry. By understanding consumer behavior, market trends, and historical influences, fashion designers and professionals can develop unique and relevant designs that cater to the ever-changing demands of the fashion market.

Fashion Retail Analytics

Fashion Retail Analytics refers to the use of data analysis techniques to understand and optimize various aspects of the fashion retail industry. It involves the collection, interpretation, and application of data to make informed and strategic decisions related to fashion design and retail operations. With the rise of digital technology and e-commerce, fashion retail has become highly competitive, making it crucial for fashion designers and retailers to gain a deeper understanding of their customers, market trends, and business performance. Fashion Retail Analytics helps in achieving this by providing actionable insights derived from data. One aspect of Fashion Retail Analytics is customer analytics. This involves analyzing data on customer preferences, shopping behavior, and demographics to better understand their needs and preferences. By understanding the customer's likes and dislikes, fashion designers can create targeted designs that are more likely to resonate with their target audience. This can lead to increased customer satisfaction and sales growth. Another aspect of Fashion Retail Analytics is inventory analytics. This involves analyzing data on inventory levels, sales performance, and demand forecasting to optimize inventory management. By understanding which fashion items are selling well and which are not, fashion retailers can make more informed decisions on their product selection, pricing, and promotions. This can help reduce overstocking and minimize the risk of stockouts, leading to improved profitability. Pricing analytics are also an important part of Fashion Retail Analytics. By analyzing data on pricing trends, competitor prices, and customer price sensitivity, fashion retailers can optimize their pricing strategy. This involves determining the optimal price points that maximize both customer demand and profit margins. Finally, Fashion Retail Analytics includes sales and marketing analytics. This involves analyzing data on sales performance, marketing campaigns, and customer acquisition to measure the effectiveness of marketing initiatives and identify areas for improvement. By understanding which marketing efforts are most successful, fashion retailers can allocate their resources more effectively and improve their return on investment. In conclusion, Fashion Retail Analytics is the use of data analysis techniques to gain insights into various aspects of the fashion retail industry. By leveraging data, fashion designers and retailers can make more informed decisions related to customer preferences, inventory management, pricing strategy, and sales and marketing efforts. This can ultimately lead to improved business performance and competitiveness in the fashion retail market.

Fashion Retail Conference

A Fashion Retail Conference is an event specifically designed for professionals in the fashion industry to gather and share knowledge, ideas, and insights about the latest trends, strategies, and challenges in the retail sector. This conference focuses on the intersection of fashion and retail, providing a platform for designers, retailers, marketers, and other industry experts to network, collaborate, and learn from each other. During a Fashion Retail Conference, participants engage in panel discussions, workshops, keynote speeches, and presentations, led by distinguished individuals who have extensive experience and expertise in the fashion and retail industries. The topics covered at these conferences often include retail innovation, consumer behavior, omnichannel marketing, sustainability, technology advancements, and global market trends. Through these sessions, attendees gain valuable insights into the ever-evolving fashion landscape, helping them stay ahead of the curve and make informed decisions for their businesses. One of the main objectives of a Fashion Retail Conference is to provide a platform for networking and establishing meaningful connections within the industry. Participants have the opportunity to meet and interact with fashion influencers, industry leaders, and potential collaborators, fostering mutually beneficial relationships that can contribute to the growth and success of their respective organizations. In addition to knowledge sharing and networking, a Fashion Retail Conference often showcases the latest fashion collections and product innovations through exhibitions and fashion shows. These showcase events offer attendees a firsthand look at the latest designs and trends, allowing them to stay up-to-date and acquire inspiration for their own creations or business strategies. Overall, a Fashion Retail Conference is a vital event in the fashion industry, providing professionals with a unique opportunity to gain insights, connect with peers, and explore new possibilities for growth and innovation. By participating in such conferences, individuals and organizations can stay informed about the ever-changing dynamics of the fashion retail world, enabling them to adapt and thrive in an increasingly competitive marketplace.

Fashion Retail Management

Fashion Retail Management is a professional field within the fashion industry that focuses on the strategic planning, coordination, and execution of various activities involved in the buying, merchandising, and selling of fashion products to consumers. It encompasses the management of retail businesses, such as clothing stores, boutiques, department stores, and online fashion platforms. The main objective of Fashion Retail Management is to optimize sales and profitability by effectively managing the entire retail process, from the selection of products to their display and promotion, while keeping in mind the ever-changing trends and demands of the fashion market. This requires a combination of business acumen, creativity, and an understanding of consumer behavior.

Fashion Retail Store

A fashion retail store is a physical or online establishment that sells clothing, footwear, accessories, and other fashion-related products to consumers. It serves as a platform for designers, brands, and manufacturers to showcase their latest collections and styles to the target audience. In a fashion retail store, customers can explore a wide range of fashion products, including apparel for men, women, and children, shoes, bags, jewelry, cosmetics, and more. These stores often feature displays, mannequins, and organized sections to make the shopping experience visually appealing and convenient for customers. One of the primary functions of a fashion retail store is to provide customers with the opportunity to stay up-to-date with the latest fashion trends. They curate and stock items that reflect the current and upcoming styles preferred by consumers. By partnering with various designers and brands, these stores ensure they offer a diverse selection of products that cater to different fashion preferences and budgets. Additionally, fashion retail stores often employ knowledgeable sales associates who can assist customers in finding the right sizes, styles, and outfits based on individual preferences and requirements. These associates are trained to provide fashion advice, coordinate outfits, and suggest accessories that complement a customer's desired look. In recent times, fashion retail stores have started incorporating online platforms to reach a wider customer base and offer convenience through online shopping. These online stores provide customers with the flexibility to browse and shop from the comfort of their homes, making it easier to explore and purchase fashion products from anywhere at any time. In conclusion, a fashion retail store encompasses both physical and online establishments where customers can access a wide range of fashionable products. These stores play a crucial role in presenting the latest trends, providing diverse options, and assisting customers in finding their desired fashion items.

Fashion Retail

Fashion retail refers to the business of selling clothes, accessories, and other fashion-related products to customers through physical stores or online platforms. It involves various processes such as buying, merchandising, marketing, and selling fashion products to consumers. Fashion retail encompasses a wide range of players in the industry, including fashion designers, manufacturers, distributors, and retailers.

Fashion Retailer

A fashion retailer is a company or individual who sells clothing, accessories, and other fashion items to consumers. The role of a fashion retailer is to curate a collection of merchandise that appeals to their target market and create an inviting shopping experience for customers. Fashion retailers can sell their products through various channels, including physical brick-and-mortar stores, online platforms, or a combination of both. They may operate as standalone boutiques or as part of a larger retail chain. Regardless of the platform or business model, the primary objective of a fashion retailer is to meet the fashion needs and desires of their customers.

Fashion Retreat

A fashion retreat is a specialized program or event that offers fashion designers, industry professionals, and enthusiasts an immersive and transformative experience in the world of fashion design. During a fashion retreat, participants are provided with a unique opportunity to engage in a variety of activities that foster creativity, skill development, and networking within the fashion industry. The retreat typically takes place in a serene and inspiring environment, away from the hustle and bustle of everyday life, allowing attendees to fully focus on their artistic pursuits and personal growth. One of the key components of a fashion retreat is the workshops and masterclasses conducted by renowned fashion designers and industry experts. These sessions cover a wide range of topics, such as fashion illustration techniques, garment construction, draping, textile manipulation, and trend forecasting. Participants have the chance to learn directly from established professionals, gaining insights into the latest industry practices and honing their skills. Another important aspect of a fashion retreat is the opportunity to collaborate and network with fellow designers, stylists, photographers, and other industry professionals. Through group projects, discussions, and social activities, participants can exchange ideas, gain feedback on their work, and build valuable connections that may lead to future collaborations or job opportunities. Immersing oneself in a fashion retreat also allows attendees to find inspiration in new surroundings and cultural experiences. Exploring different landscapes, visiting local markets and museums, and engaging with local artisans can broaden perspectives and stimulate fresh ideas in design. These diverse experiences often lead to the development of unique and authentic fashion concepts. Overall, a fashion retreat serves as a platform for personal and professional growth within the fashion industry. It offers a nurturing and supportive environment for designers to enhance their skills, expand their creative vision, and establish meaningful connections. By taking part in a fashion retreat, individuals can unlock their potential and gain the tools and inspiration needed to excel in the competitive world of fashion design.

Fashion Retro Fashion

Fashion Retro Fashion refers to a design style that takes inspiration from the fashion trends, styles, and aesthetics of a previous era, typically from the 20th century. It involves incorporating elements from the past in a modern context, creating a nostalgic and vintage-inspired look. This design approach emphasizes the revival and reinterpretation of iconic fashion trends, clothing silhouettes, fabrics, prints, colors, and accessories that were popular during a specific period. The chosen era may vary, but often includes the 1920s to the 1990s, encompassing iconic decades such as the Roaring Twenties, the swinging sixties, and the grunge-filled nineties.

Fashion Ruffles

Fashion ruffles refer to decorative and ornamental details designed to add volume, texture, and movement to garments. They are created by gathering or pleating fabric in a deliberate and controlled manner, resulting in a series of fluted or frilly edges that cascade or fall in a graceful manner. Ruffles have a long history in fashion, dating back to the Renaissance period when their extravagant use was associated with wealth and status. Over time, ruffles have evolved and found their way into various styles and trends, ranging from romantic and feminine to edgy and avant-garde. In contemporary fashion design, ruffles are often incorporated into garments such as blouses, dresses, skirts, and sleeves. They can be positioned strategically to accentuate specific body parts or to create a dramatic effect. Ruffles may be added along the neckline to draw attention to the wearer's face or cascading down the front of a dress to enhance the overall silhouette. Designers implement ruffles using different techniques, depending on the desired effect. Ruffles can be made by gathering and stitching a strip of fabric, creating a pleated or wavy appearance. They can also be achieved by using layers of fabric or adding trim along the edges. The size, shape, and placement of ruffles can vary to achieve a specific aesthetic or to complement the overall design of a garment. Ruffles offer designers a versatile tool to express their creativity and add depth to their designs. They can be used to create soft and romantic looks or to add a touch of whimsy and playfulness. Additionally, ruffles can be used strategically to balance proportions or to draw attention to certain areas of the body. When working with ruffles, designers consider factors such as fabric choice, color, and silhouette to ensure the overall harmony of the garment. While ruffles can be visually striking, an excessive or poorly executed use of ruffles can overwhelm the wearer and disrupt the intended aesthetic.

Fashion Ruler Sets

A fashion ruler set, in the context of fashion design, refers to a collection of specialized rulers that are used to create accurate and precise patterns and designs in the fashion industry. These ruler sets typically consist of a range of rulers, each with specific shapes and measurements that cater to different aspects of garment design. The rulers are made from durable materials such as clear plastic or metal, ensuring longevity and accuracy in their usage.

Fashion Runway Collection

A fashion runway collection refers to a cohesive and curated set of garments or designs that a fashion designer presents on the runway during a fashion show. It is a carefully planned and executed showcase of a designer's creative vision, often displaying their aesthetic, style, and innovative techniques. The fashion runway collection is typically created by a designer or fashion house for a specific season or occasion. This collection serves as a representation of the designer's interpretation of current fashion trends and influences. It is a visual and artistic expression that aims to captivate and inspire the audience, while showcasing the designer's skill and craftsmanship.

Fashion Runway Lighting

Fashion runway lighting refers to the art and technique of illuminating a fashion runway or stage to enhance the presentation of fashion designs during a fashion show. It plays a crucial role in creating a captivating and immersive atmosphere that showcases the garments in the best possible light. The lighting design for fashion runways is a collaborative effort between fashion designers, lighting designers, and production teams. The primary goal is to create a visually striking and dynamic lighting scheme that complements the designs, captures the attention of the audience, and conveys the desired mood and ambiance. One of the key considerations in fashion runway lighting is achieving the right balance between the overall brightness and the accentuation of specific elements on the runway. This is typically done by combining different types of lighting fixtures, such as spotlights, floodlights, and LED strips, strategically placed around the runway to direct the focus on the models and their outfits. Color temperature also plays a significant role in fashion runway lighting. The choice of warm or cool lighting can dramatically alter the perception and mood of the fashion show. Warm tones can create a cozy and intimate atmosphere, while cool tones can impart a sense of sophistication and modernity. Lighting designers carefully select the color temperature for each fashion show, taking into account the theme, aesthetics, and intended message of the designs. In addition to color temperature, lighting designers also consider the angle and direction of the light to create visual interest and add depth to the runway. This can be achieved by using techniques such as backlighting, side lighting, and cross lighting. These techniques add dimensionality to the garments, highlight textures, and create captivating shadows, enhancing the overall visual impact. Furthermore, timing and sequencing of the lighting cues are crucial in fashion runway lighting. The lighting changes need to be synchronized with the pace and choreography of the models to ensure a cohesive and harmonious presentation. Transitioning from one lighting setup to another can enhance the dramatic effect, emphasize specific moments, or guide the audience's attention. Overall, fashion runway lighting is an art form that combines technical expertise, creative expression, and aesthetic sensibility to create an immersive visual experience that elevates the fashion show. It enhances the presentation of the designs, highlights their unique features, and sets the mood and atmosphere, allowing the audience to truly appreciate and connect with the fashion creations.

Fashion Runway Photography

Fashion Runway Photography is a specialized field of photography that focuses on capturing fashion designs as they are presented on the runway during fashion shows. It is a creative and dynamic form of photography that requires a keen eye for detail, an understanding of fashion trends, and the ability to capture the essence and movement of the garments. During fashion shows, models walk down a long runway while showcasing the latest fashion designs created by fashion designers. Fashion runway photographers strategically position themselves along the runway, often in a designated pit or area to ensure good angles and clear shots of the models and their outfits. One of the primary goals of fashion runway photography is to capture the essence and details of the fashion designs. The photographers aim to highlight the fabrics, silhouettes, colors, and intricate details of the garments, ensuring that the viewers can appreciate and understand the designer's vision. They utilize various techniques such as close-ups, full-body shots, and movement shots to capture the overall look and feel of the designs. Timing plays a crucial role in fashion runway photography. The photographers need to anticipate the movements of the models and capture shots at the right moment to showcase the garments in the best possible way. They often use high-speed continuous shooting mode to capture a series of images, ensuring that they have options to choose from and select the most captivating shots. As fashion designers invest significant time, effort, and resources into creating their collections and presenting them on the runway, fashion runway photography serves as a critical documentation and promotional tool. High-quality runway photographs are used for press releases, editorial features, advertising campaigns, and online promotions. They provide a visual record of the designer's work, helping to generate interest and excitement about the collection among fashion enthusiasts, buyers, and industry professionals. In conclusion, fashion runway photography is a specialized form of photography that focuses on capturing fashion designs as they are presented on the runway during fashion shows. It requires technical skills, creativity, and a deep understanding of fashion to effectively showcase the essence and details of the garments. Fashion runway photographers play a crucial role in documenting and promoting the work of fashion designers.

Fashion Runway Soundtrack

A fashion runway soundtrack refers to the collection of music that is played during a fashion show as models walk down the runway to showcase the latest clothing designs. It is an essential element in creating an immersive and impactful experience for the audience and enhancing the overall atmosphere of the event. The choice of music for a fashion runway soundtrack is crucial as it sets the tone and mood of the show, complementing the aesthetics and artistic vision of the designer. The soundtrack is carefully curated to create a harmonious blend between the fashion pieces being presented and the accompanying music. It serves as a backdrop to the visual spectacle, amplifying the emotions and narratives conveyed through the clothing.

Fashion Runway

A fashion runway is a platform or a stage where fashion designers present their latest collections to an audience, typically composed of industry professionals, journalists, celebrities, and potential buyers. It serves as a crucial element in the fashion industry, providing a showcase for designers to display their creativity and expertise in clothing design. The fashion runway is meticulously designed to create an immersive and visually captivating experience that enhances the presentation of the garments. It serves as a backdrop for models to walk and showcase the new collection in a manner that highlights the designer's vision. Runways are often constructed with specific themes or concepts in mind to further enhance the overall aesthetic and narrative of the collection being presented.

Fashion Sales Representative

A fashion sales representative is an individual who is responsible for promoting and selling fashion products on behalf of a fashion brand or retailer. They act as a liaison between the company and the customers, ensuring that the latest trends and designs are presented and sold to the target audience. The primary role of a fashion sales representative is to establish and maintain strong relationships with existing and potential customers. They do this by attending fashion events, trade shows, and exhibitions to showcase the brand's products and engage with potential buyers. They also reach out to potential clients through cold calls, emails, and social media platforms to generate leads and increase sales. Once they have established contact with customers, the sales representative uses their knowledge of fashion trends, product features, and customer preferences to provide personalized recommendations and assistance. They help customers make informed purchasing decisions by suggesting suitable fashion items based on their individual style, body type, and occasion. In addition to sales, a fashion representative also plays a critical role in marketing and brand promotion. They work closely with marketing teams to develop promotional strategies, campaigns, and initiatives to increase brand visibility and attract new customers. They may collaborate with fashion influencers, bloggers, and celebrities to endorse and showcase the brand's products. To excel in this role, a fashion sales representative must possess excellent communication and interpersonal skills. They should be able to confidently engage with customers, convey product information, answer queries, and address concerns. They should also have a strong understanding of the fashion industry, including its latest trends and emerging styles. Overall, a fashion sales representative is crucial in driving sales, expanding customer base, and promoting a fashion brand's image. Their ability to build relationships, provide personalized recommendations, and stay up-to-date with industry trends makes them an integral part of the fashion sales process.

Fashion Scarf

A fashion scarf is a versatile accessory and a must-have item in the world of fashion design. It is a long, narrow piece of fabric that can be worn around the neck, tied in various ways to add style and flair to an outfit. Fashion scarves come in a variety of fabrics, colors, patterns, and sizes, allowing individuals to express their personal style and enhance their overall look. They can be made from lightweight materials such as silk, chiffon, or cotton for a more delicate and feminine appearance, or from heavier fabrics like wool or cashmere for warmth and coziness during colder seasons.

Fashion Scholarship

A fashion scholarship refers to a monetary award or program given to individuals pursuing a career in the field of fashion design. It is typically offered by educational institutions, fashion organizations, or companies within the fashion industry. The purpose of a fashion scholarship is to provide financial support and recognition to talented individuals who show promise and potential in the field of fashion design. These scholarships aim to encourage and promote the development of creative and innovative fashion designers who can contribute to the growth and progress of the industry.

Fashion Season

A fashion season refers to a specific time period during which fashion designers showcase their new collections to potential buyers, the media, and the public. It is a crucial concept in the fashion industry and plays a significant role in determining the trends and styles that will be popular in the upcoming months. Each fashion season typically lasts for about six months and is divided into two main categories: the spring/summer season and the fall/winter season. The spring/summer season, also known as the "warm" season, usually takes place from September to February, while the fall/winter season, or the "cold" season, occurs from March to August. During a fashion season, designers present their new collections in fashion shows, events, and presentations that are attended by fashion industry professionals, including buyers, stylists, journalists, and influencers. These showcases often take place in major fashion capitals such as New York, Paris, London, and Milan. Designers use fashion seasons as a way to introduce their latest creations, set trends, and establish their brand identity. They draw inspiration from a variety of sources, such as art, culture, history, and current events, to create innovative and unique designs. The collections are typically composed of various garments, including clothing, accessories, and footwear, which are presented through runway shows or lookbooks. After the fashion shows, buyers from retail stores and boutiques attend trade events, such as market weeks or showroom appointments, to make their selections and place orders for the upcoming season. This buying process allows designers to generate revenue and establish partnerships with retailers. Furthermore, the media and fashion influencers play a crucial role in promoting the new collections to the wider public. They attend the fashion shows, write reviews, and feature the designs in magazines, online publications, and social media platforms. This exposure helps create awareness and generates interest among consumers, driving sales and influencing fashion trends. In conclusion, a fashion season refers to a specific time period during which designers present their new collections to buyers, the media, and the public. It serves as a platform for designers to showcase their creativity, set trends, and establish their brand identity, while also providing opportunities for retailers to make purchasing decisions and for the media to promote the latest fashion offerings.

Fashion Seminar

A fashion seminar is an organized event or gathering where industry professionals, designers, students, and fashion enthusiasts come together to discuss various aspects of the fashion world and share knowledge, ideas, and insights related to fashion design. During a fashion seminar, participants engage in discussions, debates, presentations, workshops, and demonstrations focused on different areas of fashion design, such as trends, techniques, sustainability, innovation, branding, marketing, and more. The aim is to foster learning, creativity, and collaboration within the fashion industry.

Fashion Sequins

Fashion sequins are small, shiny, flat discs that are used as embellishments in fashion design. They are typically made of metal or plastic and are often sewn or glued onto garments to add texture, depth, and visual interest. Sequins can be applied in various patterns and arrangements, including as all-over embellishments, scattered accents, or intricate designs. The use of sequins in fashion design dates back many centuries, with ancient civilizations such as the Egyptians, Greeks, and Romans adorning their clothing and accessories with small, reflective disks. However, it wasn't until the early 20th century that sequins became popularized in the world of fashion. Film stars and performers in the 1920s and 1930s, such as flappers and showgirls, often wore sequined outfits to enhance their stage presence and create a glamorous, eye-catching look.

Fashion Sewing Techniques

Fashion Sewing Techniques refer to the specific methods and skills used in the construction of clothing and accessories within the realm of fashion design. These techniques are essential for creating garments that are not only stylish but also well-structured and durable. One of the key aspects of fashion sewing techniques is pattern making. This involves creating a blueprint or template for the garment using measurements and specific design details. By drafting and manipulating the pattern, designers can achieve the desired fit and silhouette for the garment. Once the pattern is created, it is transferred onto the fabric, which is then cut according to the pattern pieces. This requires precision and accuracy to ensure that the fabric pieces align perfectly and match the intended design. Seam allowances are typically included in the pattern, allowing for the stitching or joining of the fabric pieces together. Sewing techniques also encompass a wide range of stitching methods. These include basic stitches such as the straight stitch, which is used for joining seams, and the backstitch, which reinforces seams and prevents them from unraveling. Other stitches, such as the blind hem stitch and the slip stitch, are used for more specialized purposes, such as hemming and attaching trims or closures. In addition to stitching, fashion sewing techniques involve various techniques for finishing the raw edges of fabric. This can be done through methods such as pinking, serging, or binding, which help prevent fraying and give the garment a clean and polished look. Details such as pleats, darts, gathers, and tucks are also part of fashion sewing techniques. These techniques add depth, shape, and visual interest to the garment, enhancing its overall design. They require careful folding, stitching, and pressing to achieve the desired effect. Furthermore, fashion sewing techniques may encompass the application of closures and fastenings. This includes sewing zippers, buttons, snaps, hooks, and other types of closures onto garments. Proper application of these closures ensures that the garment can be easily worn and securely fastened. Overall, fashion sewing techniques are crucial for fashion designers in creating well-constructed, aesthetically pleasing garments. Through the mastery of these techniques, designers can bring their creative visions to life and produce high-quality pieces that embody both style and functionality.

Fashion Shoot

A fashion shoot is a creative process in fashion design that involves capturing and showcasing clothing and accessories through photography or videography. It is an essential part of the fashion industry as it helps promote and market the designer's creations. During a fashion shoot, a team of professionals work together to bring the designer's vision to life. This team typically consists of a fashion photographer, stylist, makeup artist, hair stylist, and models. Each member plays a crucial role in creating a visually appealing and captivating final result. The fashion photographer is responsible for capturing the essence of the clothing and accessories in the most flattering and visually appealing way possible. They use their expertise in lighting, composition, and post-processing techniques to create stunning images that highlight the unique features and details of the designs. The stylist plays a vital role in choosing the clothing, accessories, and props for the shoot. They work closely with the designer to ensure that the overall aesthetic is cohesive and on-brand. The stylist also collaborates with the photographer to create visually pleasing outfits and looks that complement the setting and theme of the shoot. The makeup artist and hair stylist work together to create the perfect look for the models. They use their skills and creativity to enhance the models' features and bring out the best in the designs. The makeup artist carefully chooses the makeup products and techniques that will enhance the overall look, while the hair stylist creates hairstyles that complement the clothing and accessories. Models are an essential component of the fashion shoot. They bring the designs to life by wearing them with confidence and grace. Models need to have a good understanding of the designer's vision and be able to convey the intended message through their poses and expressions. Overall, a fashion shoot is a collaborative effort that brings together various professionals to showcase and promote fashion designs. It is a creative process that requires meticulous planning, attention to detail, and an understanding of the designer's vision. Through the art of photography or videography, a fashion shoot captures the beauty and essence of the designs, allowing them to be shared with a broader audience.

Fashion Show Afterparty

A fashion show afterparty is a social event that takes place immediately after a fashion show, typically held to celebrate and commemorate the completion of the show. It serves as an opportunity for designers, models, industry professionals, and other attendees to come together and unwind, fostering a sense of camaraderie and celebration within the fashion community. The afterparty is usually hosted by the fashion show organizer or the designer themselves and is held in a separate venue or a designated area within the event space. The venue for the afterparty is carefully chosen to create a vibrant and lively atmosphere that complements the energy and excitement of the fashion show. It may range from exclusive clubs and lounges to trendy bars or even outdoor locations, depending on the desired vibe and theme. During the afterparty, attendees can indulge in various activities such as dancing, mingling, enjoying music performances, and partaking in refreshments. The purpose of these activities is to provide a platform for networking and socializing, allowing individuals to connect and build relationships within the fashion industry. It is common to find renowned fashion icons, celebrities, and influencers in attendance, adding to the allure and prestige of the event. Additionally, the afterparty often includes elements of fashion-centric entertainment, such as live showcases of clothing collections, runway presentations, or pop-up shops. This serves as an excellent opportunity for designers to showcase their work in a more intimate and interactive setting, allowing guests to experience their creations up close and personal. Overall, a fashion show afterparty acts as an extension of the fashion show itself, providing a platform for celebration, networking, and continued fashion immersion. It serves as a essential component of the overall fashion event experience, fostering an environment where connections are forged, inspirations are shared, and the love for fashion is celebrated.

Fashion Show Art Installations

Fashion show art installations are creative and visually stunning installations that are designed and showcased during fashion shows to enhance the overall aesthetic and theme of the event. These installations serve as a means to create a memorable and immersive experience for the audience, while also serving as a backdrop to the fashion designs being presented. These art installations can take various forms and can incorporate different artistic mediums such as sculpture, painting, photography, lighting, and technology. They are not simply decorative elements but are carefully curated to complement and amplify the fashion designs being presented on the runway. These installations often convey a specific concept, narrative, or message that aligns with the designer's vision and the overall theme of the fashion show.

Fashion Show Augmented Reality

Fashion Show Augmented Reality is an innovative technology that combines virtual reality and fashion design to create an immersive and interactive experience for both designers and viewers. By superimposing computer-generated images onto the real world, this technology allows fashion designers to showcase their creations in a virtual environment. With Fashion Show Augmented Reality, designers can create virtual models by using 3D modeling software and incorporating their designs onto these virtual representations. This enables them to experiment with various styles, fabrics, and colors without the need for physical prototypes. It also provides them with the opportunity to explore unconventional or avant-garde concepts that may not be feasible in traditional fashion shows.

Fashion Show Backdrops

Fashion Show Backdrops are the visual elements placed behind the models and clothing on the runway during a fashion show, serving as a backdrop to enhance the overall aesthetic and theme of the event. These backdrops are an important component of fashion design as they provide a visual context and create an atmosphere that complements the clothes being showcased. Backdrops are carefully selected based on the designer's vision for the collection, the overall theme of the show, and the desired mood and ambiance. They can range from simple and minimalistic to elaborate and extravagant designs, depending on the creative direction and concept of the fashion show. The purpose of the backdrop is to create a visually appealing and cohesive environment that allows the audience to focus on the garments and accessories being presented.

Fashion Show Backstage Management

A fashion show backstage management refers to the organization and coordination of various aspects behind the scenes of a fashion show. It involves ensuring that all necessary preparations are made to create a successful and seamless runway presentation. Backstage management typically begins with the creation of a detailed schedule and timeline. This includes coordinating the arrival times and order of appearance for models, makeup artists, hairstylists, and dressers. The backstage manager is responsible for maintaining an efficient flow of activities, ensuring that each individual involved knows their role and responsibilities. In addition to managing the schedule, backstage management involves overseeing the setup and organization of the backstage area. This includes arranging the dressing area, ensuring all garments are properly organized and labeled, and providing a comfortable and well-equipped space for hair and makeup artists. During the show, the backstage manager plays a crucial role in maintaining order and resolving any issues that may arise. They must be able to handle high-pressure situations, such as last-minute changes or wardrobe malfunctions, while keeping the show running smoothly. Effective communication and problem-solving skills are essential in this role. Furthermore, the backstage manager works closely with the show producer and director to ensure that the overall vision and theme of the show are met. They may assist in coordinating the music, lighting, and special effects, as well as ensuring that all models are styled appropriately according to the designer's vision. Overall, fashion show backstage management is the behind-the-scenes coordination and organization necessary to execute a successful runway presentation. It involves managing schedules, preparing the backstage area, resolving issues, and ensuring that the overall vision of the show is realized. A skilled and efficient backstage manager is crucial in creating a memorable and seamless fashion show experience.

Fashion Show Casting Calls

A fashion show casting call is a formal process conducted by fashion designers or fashion show organizers to select models to showcase their clothing and accessories in a fashion runway show or presentation. It is an essential step in the fashion show preparation as it determines the lineup of models that will wear the designer's creations and represent their brand. During a fashion show casting call, models are introduced to the designer or casting director and given the opportunity to showcase their modeling skills, physical appearance, and versatility. The casting calls are usually held before the fashion show and may take place at the designer's studio, a casting agency, or a specific location designated for the purpose.

Fashion Show Choreography

Fashion Show Choreography refers to the art and technique of planning, organizing, and executing the runway walk and presentation of garments and accessories in a fashion show. It involves the strategic placement, movement, and coordination of models, as well as the selection of music, lighting, and stage design to enhance the overall aesthetic and impact of the show. The choreography of a fashion show plays a crucial role in showcasing the designer's vision and creating a memorable experience for the audience. It helps to communicate the narrative, theme, or concept behind the collection and ensures that each look is presented in its best light. This choreography is often a collaboration between the designer and a professional choreographer or fashion show director who understands how to translate the designer's vision into a fluid and visually captivating runway presentation.

Fashion Show Community Building

A fashion show community building refers to the process of organizing and presenting a fashion show event that aims to bring together individuals interested in fashion design and promote a sense of unity and collaboration within the fashion industry. This community building activity involves various elements such as selecting a theme or concept for the fashion show, curating a diverse range of fashion designs, and creating an inclusive and supportive environment for participants and attendees. The first step in the fashion show community building process is choosing a theme or concept that will guide the overall aesthetic and message of the event. This theme can be inspired by a particular era, culture, or social cause, and sets the tone for the designs that will be showcased on the runway. Once the theme is established, the organizers of the fashion show reach out to fashion designers, both established and emerging, who are interested in participating. This inclusivity helps to foster a sense of community within the fashion industry, as it allows for collaboration and cross-promotion between designers with different styles and backgrounds. In addition to the designers, models, hair stylists, makeup artists, and photographers also contribute to the fashion show community building. By involving professionals from various sectors of the fashion industry, the event becomes a platform for networking, learning, and sharing ideas. During the fashion show itself, the community building aspect is further emphasized through the supportive and inclusive atmosphere created for both participants and attendees. Fashion shows often provide an opportunity for emerging designers to gain exposure and build connections, and the event organizers strive to create an environment that encourages professional growth and networking. In conclusion, a fashion show community building is an event that promotes collaboration, inclusivity, and professional growth within the fashion industry. By bringing together designers, models, and various other professionals, these events contribute to the development of a strong and connected fashion community.

Fashion Show Dressers

Fashion Show Dressers Fashion show dressers are professionals responsible for assisting models in changing their outfits and ensuring that they are dressed correctly during a fashion show. They play a crucial role in the smooth running of the event, as they help to maintain the overall aesthetic and ensure that each model looks their best on the runway. The primary duty of a fashion show dresser is to help models change quickly between outfits. They work backstage to ensure that the transition between looks is seamless and efficient, minimizing any delays during the show. Dressers must have a keen eye for detail and a thorough knowledge of the designer's collection, as they need to know how each garment should be worn and styled to achieve the desired look. Before the show, dressers work closely with the designer, stylist, and other members of the production team to understand the vision and concept of the show. They receive detailed instructions on how each outfit should be presented, including the order of the looks and any specific styling requirements. They also familiarize themselves with the garments, accessories, and footwear to be worn by the models. During the fashion show, dressers are responsible for helping models change quickly and efficiently. They assist with unbuttoning or unzipping garments, adjusting fit, and fastening any closures. They also ensure that accessories such as jewelry, belts, and hats are correctly positioned and secure. Dressers must be skilled in handling delicate and expensive garments, as they need to maintain the quality and integrity of the designer's creations. In addition to their dressing duties, fashion show dressers may also assist with other backstage tasks. They may help with organizing and steaming garments, preparing outfits for each model, and keeping the backstage area clean and organized. They must be able to work well under pressure, as fashion shows often have tight schedules and require quick changes and last-minute adjustments. In conclusion, fashion show dressers are essential members of the fashion show production team. They ensure that models are dressed and styled correctly, contributing to the overall success of the event. With their attention to detail, quick-thinking abilities, and expertise in fashion, dressers play a crucial role in bringing the designer's vision to life on the runway.

Fashion Show Event Accessibility

Fashion Show Event Accessibility refers to creating a fashion show environment that is inclusive and accessible to all individuals, regardless of their physical or cognitive abilities. It involves implementing design strategies, accommodations, and considerations that ensure everyone can fully participate and enjoy the fashion show experience. This includes several key aspects: 1. Physical Accessibility: Fashion show venues should be designed and organized in a way that allows individuals with mobility challenges to navigate easily. This may include providing wheelchair ramps, stair lifts, or elevators for easy access to different areas of the venue. Adequate seating arrangements should be available, with options for individuals with different needs, such as accessible seating spaces or areas for guide dogs. 2. Visual Accessibility: Fashion shows should consider the visual needs of attendees, including individuals with low vision or blindness. This can be achieved by ensuring that lighting is appropriate, with contrasting colors and well-lit areas to aid visibility. Clear signage, including braille or tactile signs, can assist individuals in finding their way around the venue. 3. Audio Accessibility: Hearing-impaired individuals should be able to fully enjoy the fashion show experience. This can be achieved by providing assistive listening devices, such as hearing loop systems or wireless headphones, to amplify the sound. Captioning or sign language interpreters can also be made available for individuals who are deaf or hard of hearing. 4. Sensory Accessibility: Fashion shows can be overwhelming for individuals with sensory sensitivities or autism spectrum disorders. Design considerations should be made to create a comfortable and less stimulating environment. This may include providing quiet spaces, minimizing excessive noise or bright lights, and offering sensory-friendly options for attendees. Overall, fashion show event accessibility aims to create an inclusive and enjoyable experience for people of all abilities. By implementing these accessibility measures, fashion designers and event organizers can ensure that everyone has the opportunity to engage with and appreciate the artistic expressions of fashion.

Fashion Show Event Advocacy

A fashion show event advocacy in the context of fashion design refers to the promotion and support of a fashion show as a means to showcase new collections, emerging trends, and talented designers. It involves organizing and executing an event that provides a platform for designers to present their work to a wide audience, including industry professionals, media, buyers, and fashion enthusiasts. The primary objective of a fashion show event advocacy is to create a captivating and memorable experience that effectively communicates the designer's vision and brand identity. It involves meticulous planning and coordination to ensure that every element, from the venue and set design to the lighting, music, and choreography, aligns with the desired atmosphere and narrative of the collection being showcased. Through a fashion show event advocacy, designers aim to generate buzz and excitement around their brand, creating brand awareness and increasing its visibility in the industry. It provides an opportunity for designers to form connections with industry experts, influential figures, and potential buyers, potentially leading to collaborations, partnerships, and business opportunities. In addition to promoting individual designers and brands, a fashion show event advocacy also contributes to the overall growth and development of the fashion industry. By bringing together designers, models, stylists, hair and makeup artists, photographers, and various other professionals, it fosters a sense of community and collaboration, nurturing talent and encouraging innovation. Furthermore, a fashion show event advocacy serves as a platform for designers to address social and cultural issues, using fashion as a form of expression and activism. By incorporating diverse models, themes, and narratives in their shows, designers can advocate for inclusivity, sustainability, gender equality, and other important causes.

Fashion Show Event Animal Welfare

A fashion show event animal welfare refers to the incorporation of ethical and sustainable practices in the fashion industry to promote the well-being and protection of animals. It involves the design, production, and showcasing of fashion collections that are cruelty-free, environmentally responsible, and socially conscious. In the context of fashion design, animal welfare encompasses various aspects. Firstly, it focuses on eliminating the use of materials derived from animals such as fur, leather, and exotic skins. Designers opt for alternative materials that are synthetic or plant-based, working towards a more compassionate and environmentally friendly approach. By doing so, they aim to prevent the harm and suffering inflicted on animals in the name of fashion. Animal welfare in fashion design also promotes responsible sourcing of materials. Designers strive to ensure that any animal-derived materials used in their collections are obtained from ethical and sustainable sources. This includes partnering with suppliers who adhere to strict animal welfare standards and avoid engaging in practices like factory farming or animal testing. In addition to material choices, animal welfare in fashion design extends to the treatment of animals during the production process. Designers and fashion houses employ ethical manufacturing practices, ensuring that animals involved in processes like shearing or silk production are treated with respect and care. This may involve supporting initiatives that promote fair trade and fair wages for farmers and workers involved in the production of animal-derived materials. Furthermore, fashion show event animal welfare also takes into account the conservation and preservation of wildlife. Designers may collaborate with organizations dedicated to protecting endangered species and their habitats, raising awareness and funds through their fashion shows. By using their platform to promote animal welfare, designers can inspire change and encourage consumers to make more informed and compassionate choices when it comes to fashion.

Fashion Show Event Artistic Exploration

A Fashion Show Event Artistic Exploration refers to a curated showcase of innovative and avant-garde fashion designs, where designers have the opportunity to express their creativity and artistic vision through the presentation of their collections. It is a platform that allows designers to push the boundaries of traditional fashion and experiment with unconventional materials, silhouettes, and concepts. The purpose of a Fashion Show Event Artistic Exploration is to challenge conventional ideas of beauty and fashion, and to inspire both industry professionals and the general public with fresh and thought-provoking designs. It serves as a platform for emerging talents to gain recognition and exposure in the fashion industry, and also provides established designers with a platform to showcase their latest works.

Fashion Show Event Attendee Engagement

A fashion show event attendee engagement refers to the level of interaction, participation, and emotional connection that attendees experience during a fashion show event. It encompasses the various activities and elements that are designed to captivate and involve the audience, leaving a lasting impact on their perception of the fashion show and the showcased designs. Attendee engagement can be achieved through multiple means, such as captivating runway presentations, interactive exhibits, multimedia displays, and immersive sensory experiences. These elements are strategically incorporated to stimulate attendees' senses, evoke emotions, and foster a deep connection with the showcased designs.

Fashion Show Event Biodiversity Conservation

Biodiversity conservation in the context of a fashion show event refers to the efforts made to protect and preserve the variety of plant and animal species that inhabit our planet, ensuring their survival for future generations. In the realm of fashion design, biodiversity conservation encompasses a range of sustainable practices that promote the responsible use of natural resources, reduce environmental impacts, and prioritize ethical production. It involves creating fashion collections and runway shows that celebrate and respect the unique and diverse ecosystems that provide us with raw materials and inspiration.

Fashion Show Event Body Positivity

Fashion Show Event Body Positivity refers to a runway presentation or exhibition of clothing and accessories aimed at promoting inclusivity and diversity in the fashion industry, specifically with regard to body image and size. It is an event designed to challenge traditional beauty standards and celebrate the uniqueness and individuality of all body types. The Fashion Show Event Body Positivity encompasses a variety of features and elements that contribute to its overall message of acceptance and self-love. One of the key aspects is the showcasing of clothing designs that are specifically tailored to flatter and accentuate a diverse range of body shapes and sizes. This may include offerings such as designs with adjustable or flexible features, innovative cuts and patterns, and fabrics that provide both comfort and style. The event also emphasizes the representation of models who are representative of the diverse population, with a focus on showcasing individuals who may not fit into traditional fashion industry standards. This can include models of various ethnicities, ages, genders, and sizes. By featuring a broad range of models, the fashion show aims to promote inclusivity and challenge societal norms surrounding beauty and body image. In addition to the runway presentation, a Fashion Show Event Body Positivity typically includes educational components and discussions centered on body positivity. This may involve workshops, talks, or panel discussions that explore topics such as self-acceptance, mental health, and the importance of embracing individuality. By providing a platform for dialogue, the event encourages participants to reflect on their own attitudes towards body image and promotes a more inclusive and compassionate fashion industry.

Fashion Show Event Budgeting

A fashion show event budgeting refers to the process of estimating and allocating financial resources for organizing a fashion show. It involves determining the costs associated with various aspects of the event, such as venue rental, runway construction, lighting, sound equipment, models' fees, makeup artists, hairstylists, and other necessary expenses. The budgeting process starts with identifying the key elements required for the fashion show, such as the number of outfits to be showcased, the duration of the event, and the target audience. Once these elements are determined, the event organizer can start allocating funds accordingly. One crucial aspect of fashion show budgeting is determining the venue and its associated costs. The venue should be chosen based on factors like its capacity, location, and aesthetic appeal. The rental charges, including any additional costs for customization or decoration, should be taken into account. Another significant component of the budget is the cost of production, including runway construction, lighting, and sound equipment. The runway should be designed in a way that complements the fashion collection and provides an engaging experience for the audience. The lighting setup needs to be well-planned to showcase the garments effectively, and the sound equipment should ensure clear playback of music and announcements. The models' fees and their accommodations, if required, form a significant part of the budget. The number of models needed will depend on the number of outfits to be showcased, and their fees should be negotiated based on their experience and popularity. Accommodation expenses, such as lodging and meals, should also be considered if models are from out of town. Additionally, budgeting for makeup artists, hairstylists, and other backstage staff is essential. Their expertise is crucial in bringing the fashion collection to life and ensuring that the models look their best. Considering their fees and any necessary supplies is crucial in creating a comprehensive budget. Overall, fashion show event budgeting involves meticulously estimating the costs of various elements required for a successful show. By carefully considering all the expenses from venue rental to models' fees, event organizers can ensure that the show is executed within the allocated budget while still maintaining a high level of creativity and professionalism.

Fashion Show Event Carbon Footprint

Fashion Show Event Carbon Footprint refers to the total amount of greenhouse gas emissions produced directly and indirectly throughout the lifecycle of a fashion show event, including pre-production, production, event management, and post-event activities. This carbon footprint encompasses various sources of emissions, including but not limited to energy consumption, transportation, waste management, and the production of materials used in the event. Energy consumption includes the electricity used for lighting, heating, and air conditioning, as well as the energy required for sound systems, backstage equipment, and other technical aspects. Transportation emissions result from the transportation of models, designers, staff, and attendees to and from the event venue, as well as the transportation of event materials and equipment. Waste management emissions include the disposal of event waste, such as packaging materials, food waste, and promotional materials. The production of materials used in the event, such as clothing, runway sets, and promotional materials, also contributes to the fashion show event carbon footprint through the emission of greenhouse gases during manufacturing and distribution processes.

Fashion Show Event Catering

A fashion show event catering refers to the provision of food and beverages for guests attending a fashion show. It plays a crucial role in enhancing the overall experience and ambiance of the event. The catering aspect of a fashion show is not only about serving food; it is an opportunity to create a unique and immersive experience that aligns with the theme and atmosphere of the event. The food and beverages served should complement the style, elegance, and creativity associated with fashion design. The menu for a fashion show event catering should be thoughtfully curated to suit the tastes and preferences of the attendees. It should incorporate a diverse range of options to cater to different dietary restrictions and preferences. The presentation of the food should also be visually appealing, reflecting the artistry and aesthetics of fashion design. This can be achieved through creative plating, use of vibrant colors, and the incorporation of elements that evoke the essence of fashion. In addition to the food and beverages, the service provided by the catering staff is crucial in ensuring a seamless experience. The staff should be well-trained, professional, and attentive, ensuring that guests are well taken care of throughout the event. This can include efficient and discreet serving, clearing of plates, and addressing any special requests or dietary requirements promptly and courteously. Fashion show event catering is an opportunity to showcase innovation and creativity in the culinary sphere. Collaborations between fashion designers and renowned chefs can create a fusion of art forms and elevate the overall experience. The menu can be tailored to reflect the designer's style, incorporating unique flavors, textures, and presentation techniques that mirror the creativity and craftsmanship showcased on the runway. In conclusion, fashion show event catering is an integral part of creating a memorable and immersive fashion event. It goes beyond simply providing sustenance and nourishment; it is an opportunity to enchant and captivate guests through a culinary experience that resonates with the artistry and elegance of fashion design.

Fashion Show Event Celebration

A fashion show event celebration is a highly anticipated gathering in the fashion industry that showcases the latest trends and designs of clothing, accessories, and other fashion-related items. It is an occasion where designers, models, industry professionals, media, and fashion enthusiasts come together to witness an extravagant display of creativity and style. During a fashion show event celebration, designers present their collections on a runway or stage, allowing the audience to see and experience their designs firsthand. Models gracefully strut down the catwalk, wearing the clothing and accessories, while music sets the mood and atmosphere of the show. The choreography and lighting enhance the overall impact of the event, creating a captivating and immersive experience for the attendees. Aside from showcasing new collections, a fashion show event celebration serves as a platform for designers to express their unique perspectives and artistic visions. It allows them to push boundaries, explore innovative techniques, and experiment with different fabrics, textures, colors, and styles. Fashion shows often serve as a launchpad for emerging designers to gain recognition and establish their brand in the industry. Beyond the artistic aspect, a fashion show event celebration also plays a significant role in promoting and marketing fashion brands and products. It provides an opportunity for designers to connect with buyers, retailers, and industry professionals who may be interested in stocking their collections or collaborating on future projects. Media coverage and social media exposure further amplify the reach and impact of the event, generating buzz and excitement for the showcased designs. Attending a fashion show event celebration offers fashion enthusiasts a glimpse into the latest trends and upcoming styles, allowing them to stay ahead of the curve. It serves as a source of inspiration and a platform for individuals to express their personal style. Fashion shows also contribute to the conversation around diversity, inclusivity, and body positivity within the industry, as designers continue to embrace models of different backgrounds, sizes, and ethnicities.

Fashion Show Event Charitable Contributions

The Fashion Show Event Charitable Contributions refer to the donations and contributions made by the participants, sponsors, and attendees of a fashion show event for charitable purposes.

These contributions can be in the form of money, designer clothing, accessories, or services, and are aimed at supporting and raising funds for charitable organizations and causes. In the context of fashion design, charitable contributions play a significant role in giving back to society and making a positive impact. Designers, brands, and fashion houses often participate in fashion show events to showcase their latest collections and creations. These events serve as platforms for raising awareness about social issues and garnering support for various charitable causes. The donated funds and designer items collected through the charitable contributions at fashion show events are used to support a wide range of causes. These causes can include but are not limited to, supporting underprivileged communities, providing education and healthcare facilities to those in need, promoting sustainable fashion practices, funding research for diseases, and aiding disaster relief efforts. Fashion show event charitable contributions are not only beneficial for the charities and causes they support, but they also provide a unique opportunity for designers and brands to showcase their commitment to social responsibility. By actively participating in these events and making charitable contributions, fashion designers can demonstrate their dedication to using fashion as a force for good and making a difference in society.

Fashion Show Event Circular Fashion

A fashion show event circular is a formal announcement or invitation to attend a fashion show that promotes the concept of circular fashion. Circular fashion is an innovative approach to the design, production, and consumption of clothing that aims to minimize waste and maximize the lifespan of garments. The fashion industry is notorious for its negative environmental impact, with vast amounts of resources being utilized, and a significant amount of waste being generated. Circular fashion seeks to address these issues by adopting sustainable practices throughout the entire fashion lifecycle. In a circular fashion show event, designers showcase their collections that incorporate principles of circularity. This may include using eco-friendly materials, implementing recycling or upcycling techniques, or promoting garment longevity through classic and timeless designs. The purpose of the fashion show event circular is to create awareness and inspire change within the fashion industry and among consumers. By showcasing the potential of circular fashion, it encourages designers, brands, and consumers to adopt more sustainable practices in their own fashion choices. This type of fashion show event is not only a platform for creativity and artistic expression but also a means of communication and education. Through the visual presentation of sustainable fashion designs, attendees can gain a deeper understanding of circular fashion principles and the benefits of choosing more sustainable clothing options. Furthermore, a fashion show event circular often includes information about the participating designers and brands, giving them exposure and recognition for their commitment to sustainability. It may also feature guest speakers, panel discussions, or workshops to provide further insight into the circular fashion movement. In conclusion, a fashion show event circular serves as an invitation to a fashion show that focuses on circular fashion. It showcases designs that adhere to sustainable practices and aims to inspire change within the fashion industry and among consumers. By raising awareness and promoting alternative approaches to fashion, it encourages a more conscious and responsible approach to clothing consumption.

Fashion Show Event Collaboration

A fashion show event collaboration in the context of fashion design refers to a partnership or joint effort between different entities or individuals to organize and present a fashion show. It involves the coming together of various stakeholders in the fashion industry, such as designers, models, stylists, and event organizers, to showcase their designs and create a memorable fashion experience. Different fashion show event collaborations can take place in various settings, such as runway shows, exhibitions, or even digital platforms. These collaborations aim to merge creative talents, resources, and expertise to curate a fashion spectacle that captures the essence of the designers' vision and brand.

Fashion Show Event Community Building

A fashion show event is a community-building activity that showcases the creativity and talent of fashion designers, models, stylists, and other industry professionals. In the context of fashion design, a fashion show event serves as a platform to present collections of clothing, accessories, and other fashion-related products to a live audience. It is a carefully choreographed presentation that highlights the artistic vision and aesthetic of the designers. The main objective of a fashion show event is to create an immersive experience for the attendees, allowing them to witness the latest trends and designs in a visually captivating way. The event brings together fashion enthusiasts, industry insiders, and potential buyers, fostering a sense of community and collaboration within the fashion industry. During a fashion show event, models walk down a runway, showcasing the designs with grace and precision. The choice of music, lighting, and overall ambiance of the venue adds to the overall atmosphere and enhances the impact of the collections presented. Fashion show events are not only about presenting the latest fashion trends but also serve as a networking opportunity for designers, models, stylists, and other professionals in the industry. The event allows them to connect with potential clients, buyers, and fashion influencers, promoting collaborations and future business opportunities. Moreover, fashion show events often generate buzz and media coverage, providing exposure for both established and emerging designers. This exposure can lead to increased brand recognition, sales, and opportunities to expand their businesses. In conclusion, a fashion show event is an important community-building activity in the fashion industry. It brings together industry professionals, fashion enthusiasts, and potential buyers to showcase and appreciate the creativity and talent of designers. Through captivating presentations and networking opportunities, fashion show events contribute to the growth and success of the fashion industry as a whole.

Fashion Show Event Community Engagement

A fashion show event is a community engagement activity that showcases the creativity, innovation, and trends in fashion design. It serves as a platform for designers, stylist, models, and fashion enthusiasts to come together and celebrate the artistry and craftsmanship of clothing and accessories. The primary objective of a fashion show event is to display the latest collections of established and emerging fashion designers. These collections often reflect the designer's unique style, inspiration, and vision for the season. By presenting their work on the runway, designers are able to express their creativity and showcase their talent to a wider audience. Fashion shows also play a significant role in driving trends and influencing the fashion industry. Through these events, designers have the opportunity to introduce new and experimental designs that can potentially shape the future of fashion. They can inspire other designers and fashion enthusiasts, leading to the adoption and replication of certain styles or trends. Beyond the runway, a fashion show event is a social gathering that brings together members of the fashion community. It serves as a meeting place for industry professionals, fashion lovers, buyers, and media. It allows for networking opportunities, collaboration, and the exchange of ideas and information. Fashion show events are often organized by fashion houses, fashion organizations, or event management companies. They can be held in various venues, such as traditional ballrooms, art galleries, or outdoor spaces. The show may be divided into different segments, each showcasing a different designer or theme. It typically involves models walking down the runway, showcasing the garments and accessories in front of an audience. Furthermore, a fashion show event is not simply a display of clothing, but also an immersive experience. Lighting, music, and stage design are carefully curated to create a specific ambiance that complements the designer's vision. Choreography and model selection also contribute to the overall storytelling and presentation of the garments. In summary, a fashion show event is a community engagement activity that serves as a platform for designers to showcase their collections and for fashion enthusiasts to celebrate and appreciate the artistry of fashion design. It is an important event that influences trends, fosters networking opportunities, and provides a memorable experience for both industry professionals and the fashion community at large.

Fashion Show Event Conscious Consumption

Fashion Show Event Conscious Consumption Fashion show event conscious consumption refers to a principle in fashion design that promotes responsible and sustainable consumption practices. It focuses on creating awareness and encouraging individuals to make mindful choices when it comes to buying and using fashion items. Conscious consumption in the context of fashion shows involves showcasing designs and collections that are produced ethically and sustainably. Fashion designers and brands who prioritize this principle ensure that their products are made using environmentally friendly materials and production processes. They also ensure fair labor practices and support local communities. Through a fashion show event that promotes conscious consumption, designers aim to change the perception of fast fashion and its negative impact on the environment and society. They use the platform to educate consumers about the importance of making informed choices and the power of their purchasing decisions. One of the key elements of conscious consumption is the focus on quality over quantity. Instead of following trends and constantly buying new clothes, conscious consumers invest in pieces that are durable and timeless. They prioritize craftsmanship and value the story behind each garment. Conscious consumption also emphasizes the concept of "slow fashion," which encourages consumers to buy less and buy better. By choosing high-quality garments and taking care of them properly, individuals can reduce waste and contribute to a more sustainable fashion industry. In a fashion show event that promotes conscious consumption, designers may collaborate with sustainable fashion brands, incorporate upcycling and recycling techniques, and highlight the importance of supporting local artisans and craftsmen. They may also use the platform to discuss the social and environmental challenges faced by the fashion industry and propose solutions. In conclusion, fashion show event conscious consumption is a concept in fashion design that promotes responsible and sustainable consumption practices. It encourages individuals to make mindful choices when it comes to buying and using fashion items, focusing on quality, durability, and environmental and social impact.

Fashion Show Event Coordination

A fashion show event coordination refers to the process of organizing and managing a fashion show, a highly anticipated and influential event in the fashion industry. It involves overseeing and coordinating various aspects such as venue selection, model casting, production coordination, and publicity to create a seamless and successful fashion show. The first step in fashion show event coordination is selecting an appropriate venue that aligns with the theme and desired atmosphere of the show. The venue should have adequate space for the runway, backstage areas, dressing rooms, and seating for the audience. Additionally, the venue should offer the necessary lighting and sound equipment to enhance the overall experience of the show. Casting models is a crucial aspect of fashion show event coordination. The coordinator works closely with fashion designers and agencies to select models that fit the aesthetic and vision of the show. Models with different body types, ethnicities, and genders are often chosen to represent diversity and inclusivity in the fashion industry. Production coordination involves managing various backstage activities to ensure a smooth flow of the show. This includes organizing the sequence of outfits, coordinating hair and makeup teams, and managing dress rehearsals. The coordinator is responsible for maintaining a strict timeline to ensure that the show runs punctually and efficiently. Publicity plays a significant role in fashion show event coordination. Coordinators work with public relations teams to generate buzz and attract influential individuals such as fashion editors, celebrities, and buyers. They collaborate with stylists and fashion journalists to secure media coverage and create a positive buzz around the designers and their collections. In conclusion, fashion show event coordination encompasses the organization and management of all aspects of a fashion show, from venue selection to model casting, production coordination, and publicity. It requires careful attention to detail, excellent organizational skills, and a deep understanding of the fashion industry to create a memorable and impactful event that showcases the latest trends and designs.

Fashion Show Event Creative Collaboration

A fashion show event creative collaboration refers to the process of bringing together different individuals and entities in the fashion industry to work together in creating and producing a fashion show. It involves the cooperation and partnership of designers, models, stylists, makeup artists, photographers, event planners, and various other professionals who contribute their skills, expertise, and resources to bring the fashion show to life. The objective of a fashion show event creative collaboration is to present a cohesive and visually captivating showcase of clothing, accessories, and style. It serves as a platform for designers to display their latest collections and for attendees to experience the latest trends and fashion forwardness. The collaboration allows for the exchange of ideas, talents, and inspirations among the participants, resulting in a collaborative and innovative production.

Fashion Show Event Creative Expression

A fashion show event is a creative expression of fashion design that showcases the latest collections of clothing, accessories, and other fashion-related products. It is a highly choreographed event where models walk down a runway or catwalk, presenting the designs to an audience of industry professionals, buyers, media, and fashion enthusiasts. The purpose of a fashion show event is to promote and market the designers' creations, as well as to establish a brand image and identity. It is an opportunity for designers to share their artistic vision, craftsmanship, and innovation with the world. The event allows them to captivate the audience and invoke emotions through their designs, presenting their aesthetic ideas in a visually compelling manner. Fashion show events often follow a theme or concept, which sets the tone and mood for the collection being presented. These themes can be inspired by various sources such as nature, art, culture, or current socio-political issues. They provide a narrative or story that helps to create a cohesive and memorable experience for the audience. The runway itself is a key element of a fashion show event. It acts as a platform for the models to showcase the garments and accessories, allowing the audience to see how they move and fit in motion. The lighting, music, and overall ambience of the runway further enhance the visual impact of the designs, creating a captivating atmosphere. In addition to the garments, fashion show events often incorporate other elements of design, such as hair and makeup, to create a complete look that aligns with the designer's vision. These elements contribute to the overall aesthetic and storytelling of the collection, adding depth and dimension to the presentation. Overall, a fashion show event is a dynamic and immersive experience that celebrates the artistry and craftsmanship of fashion design. It provides a platform for designers to express their creativity, establish their brand, and connect with industry professionals and consumers alike. Through the careful coordination of various design elements, a fashion show event offers a captivating and memorable showcase of the latest fashion trends and innovative designs.

Fashion Show Event Cruelty-Free Fashion

A fashion show event showcasing cruelty-free fashion is an exhibition or presentation of clothing designs that are created without the use of materials derived from animals or any other forms of cruelty towards animals. The event aims to promote and celebrate the emerging trend of fashion that respects the welfare and ethical treatment of animals. Cruelty-free fashion design encompasses various aspects, including the sourcing and production of materials, as well as the design and manufacturing processes. It involves the use of alternative fabrics and materials that mimic the luxurious and high-quality look and feel of animal-derived materials, such as fur, leather, silk, and wool. Designers participating in a cruelty-free fashion show prioritize using innovative synthetic fabrics and organic materials that are environmentally friendly and do not harm animals or exploit their labor. These materials can include recycled fibers, vegan leather, plant-based textiles like bamboo and hemp, and high-quality synthetic alternatives. A cruelty-free fashion show event not only focuses on the materials used but also promotes fashion design that is inspired by and supports ethical and sustainable principles. The designs presented in the show often reflect a fusion of creativity, function, and consciousness, demonstrating that it is possible to create stylish and trendy looks without compromising the well-being of animals or the environment. The models showcasing the cruelty-free designs on the runway also embody the ethos of the event. They are chosen not only for their modeling abilities but also for their commitment to promoting cruelty-free fashion and living a compassionate lifestyle. Their presence serves as a visual representation of the values and message conveyed by the event.

Fashion Show Event Cultural Awareness

A fashion show event cultural awareness in the context of fashion design refers to an event that aims to celebrate and promote diversity and inclusivity in the fashion industry. It highlights different cultural influences, traditions, and aesthetics to foster a deeper understanding and appreciation of the richness and variety of global fashion. Through a fashion show event cultural awareness, designers showcase their collections that are inspired by various cultural elements such as traditional garments, textiles, patterns, colors, and accessories. The event provides a platform for designers from different cultural backgrounds to express their creativity and perspectives, bringing forward unique and authentic voices.

Fashion Show Event Cultural Exchange

A fashion show event cultural exchange is a showcase of clothing designs from different cultures, where designers from various backgrounds come together to celebrate and share their unique fashion aesthetics, traditions, and influences. This event provides a platform for both established and emerging designers to present their designs to a wide audience that includes industry professionals, fashion enthusiasts, and the general public. The aim of a fashion show event cultural exchange is to foster cross-cultural understanding, appreciation, and dialogue through fashion. It promotes diversity and inclusivity in the fashion industry by emphasizing the rich and varied cultural heritage expressed through clothing. This exchange allows designers to learn from one another, exchange ideas, and draw inspiration from different artistic traditions and craftsmanship techniques.

Fashion Show Event Disability Inclusion

p { font-family: Arial, sans-serif; font-size: 14px; } Fashion Show Event Disability Inclusion: The concept of disability inclusion in fashion shows refers to the practice of ensuring equal participation and representation of individuals with disabilities in the fashion industry. It aims to break stereotypes and promote diversity by showcasing the talents, abilities, and unique perspectives of disabled individuals in the world of fashion design. Disability inclusion in fashion shows involves various aspects that designers, event organizers, and industry professionals need to consider. This includes creating accessible and inclusive runway environments, casting models with disabilities, designing adaptive clothing, and promoting awareness and acceptance of disabilities within the broader fashion community.

Fashion Show Event Diversity And Inclusion

A fashion show event that promotes diversity and inclusion in the context of fashion design is a platform where designers showcase their collections that celebrate and represent the rich tapestry of human diversity. It is an inclusive space where models of different races, ethnicities, sizes, ages, and gender identities confidently walk the runway, breaking traditional beauty norms and challenging societal standards. Through diversity and inclusion, fashion designers aim to create a more equitable and representative industry, where every individual is celebrated and empowered. They employ a variety of design techniques and styles to cater to people from diverse backgrounds, ensuring that everyone feels seen and heard.

Fashion Show Event Diversity

A fashion show event diversity refers to a curated showcase of clothing collections, runway presentations, and performances that celebrate and embrace a wide range of cultural, ethnic, and body diversities within the fashion industry. It aims to promote inclusivity, representation, and acceptance by featuring models, designers, and creative talents from different backgrounds, identities, and experiences. By incorporating diversity into fashion show events, designers can break away from outdated beauty standards and traditional norms, creating a platform that reflects and respects the multifaceted nature of society. This allows for a more inclusive and accessible representation of fashion, enabling people from all walks of life to feel seen, valued, and empowered.

Fashion Show Event Eco-Friendly Fashion

An eco-friendly fashion show event refers to a showcase of clothing and accessories that adhere to sustainable practices and materials, promoting environmental consciousness within the fashion industry. It serves as a platform to highlight and celebrate designers who prioritize ethical and eco-friendly approaches in their creations. Eco-friendly fashion emphasizes the use of sustainable materials, such as organic cotton, hemp, or recycled fabrics, which minimize harm to the environment. These materials are sourced in a responsible manner, following fair trade principles and avoiding the use of toxic chemicals or pesticides. Additionally, the production processes involved in creating eco-friendly fashion focus on reducing waste, conserving energy, and minimizing carbon emissions. This includes implementing recycling programs, using renewable energy sources, and adopting innovative technologies that minimize water consumption. The eco-friendly fashion show event aims to raise awareness among fashion consumers and industry professionals about the environmental impact of traditional fashion practices. By showcasing sustainable and ethically produced clothing, it encourages consumers to make informed choices and support brands that prioritize eco-friendly initiatives. The event also promotes collaboration and exchange of knowledge among designers, manufacturers, and consumers, fostering a community dedicated to sustainable fashion. Through the eco-friendly fashion show event, designers have the opportunity to showcase their creativity and talent in sustainable fashion design. It provides a platform for innovative and forward-thinking designers to present their collections, demonstrating that style and sustainability can coexist. By challenging conventional norms and pushing boundaries, eco-friendly fashion designers inspire others to explore and adopt sustainable practices within the industry. In conclusion, an eco-friendly fashion show event educates, inspires, and celebrates the intersection of fashion and sustainability. By highlighting and encouraging sustainable practices in fashion design, it contributes to the larger goal of creating a more environmentally conscious and socially responsible fashion industry.

Fashion Show Event Educational Initiatives

A Fashion Show Event Educational Initiative refers to an event that focuses on educating individuals about the various aspects of fashion design through the medium of a fashion show. This type of initiative seeks to provide participants with insights into the creative process of designing, styling, and showcasing fashion garments. The Fashion Show Event Educational Initiative typically involves the participation of fashion students, industry professionals, and fashion enthusiasts. It serves as a platform for students to apply their theoretical knowledge, gain practical experience, and showcase their creative designs to a wider audience. The event may also feature established designers who can share their expertise and inspire young designers.

Fashion Show Event Empowerment

A fashion show event empowerment is an organized event that showcases the creations of fashion designers, providing them with a platform to express their creativity and talent. It is an occasion where fashion designers, models, and industry professionals come together to celebrate and promote the artistry and innovation in the field of fashion design. During a fashion show event empowerment, fashion designers present their collections through a carefully curated runway show. The event typically includes a diverse range of clothing and accessories, representing various styles, themes, and trends. It serves as a platform for designers to exhibit their unique vision and interpretation of fashion, making a statement about their brand and design philosophy. The main goal of a fashion show event empowerment is to empower fashion designers by giving them exposure and recognition in the industry. It provides a valuable opportunity for designers to showcase their work to a wider audience, including potential buyers, retailers, fashion journalists, and influential figures in the fashion world. Being part of a fashion show event empowerment can significantly elevate a designer's profile and open doors for future collaborations and opportunities. In addition to benefiting designers, a fashion show event empowerment also serves as a source of inspiration and trend forecasting for the industry as a whole. It sets the stage for new ideas, concepts, and aesthetics, influencing the future direction of fashion design. Fashion shows often introduce innovative techniques, materials, and silhouettes that can shape the way clothing is designed and perceived. Overall, a fashion show event empowerment is a dynamic and influential occasion that plays a crucial role in nurturing and promoting creativity in the fashion industry. By providing a platform for designers to showcase their work and inspiring new trends, it contributes to the growth and development of fashion design as an art form.

Fashion Show Event Engagement

A fashion show event engagement refers to the level of interaction and participation between the audience and the fashion designers, models, and overall fashion show experience. It is a measure of how well the fashion show event captivates and engages the attendees, leaving a lasting impression and creating a memorable experience. During a fashion show event, engagement can be achieved through various elements and strategies. One of the key factors is the fashion design itself. The creativity, innovation, and quality of the designs showcased on the runway play a crucial role in captivating the audience's attention and sparking their interest. Unique and visually appealing garments, combined with skilled craftsmanship, can leave a lasting impact on the viewers, making them more engaged with the event. Another aspect of fashion show event engagement is the choreography and presentation of the fashion show. The way models walk, pose, and interact with the audience can significantly enhance the overall experience. Thoughtful choreography that flows seamlessly, combined with well-executed styling and accessorizing, can create a visually stunning and engaging fashion show. The coordination of music, lighting, and stage design also contributes to the immersive experience, further captivating the audience. Interactivity also plays a crucial role in fashion show event engagement. Fashion designers can encourage audience engagement by incorporating interactive elements such as Q&A sessions, social media interactions, or live polling. This allows the attendees to actively participate in the event, share their thoughts, and feel connected to the designers and their creations. Additionally, providing opportunities for attendees to try on or touch the garments further enhances engagement and creates a hands-on experience. In conclusion, a fashion show event engagement refers to the level of interaction and captivation between the audience and the fashion show experience. It is achieved through the creativity and quality of the fashion designs, the choreography and presentation of the show, and the incorporation of interactive elements that allow attendees to actively participate. A successful fashion show event engagement leaves a lasting impression on the audience, ensuring that they are fully engaged and connected to the fashion designs showcased.

Fashion Show Event Entertainment

A fashion show event is a highly anticipated and glamorous affair in the world of fashion design. It serves as a platform for showcasing the latest collections and designs created by fashion designers and brands. During a fashion show, models walk down a runway, also known as a catwalk, to display the clothing and accessories that are a part of the designer's collection. The event not only highlights the creativity and talent of the designer but also creates an atmosphere of excitement and anticipation among fashion enthusiasts and industry professionals.

Fashion Show Event Environmental Impact

A fashion show event refers to a carefully choreographed presentation where designers showcase their latest clothing collections on the runway. This event has a significant environmental impact due to various factors involved in the fashion industry. Firstly, the production of clothing materials contributes to the fashion show event's environmental impact. The majority of fabrics used in fashion are derived from non-renewable resources such as petroleum-based synthetic fibers or resource-intensive materials like cotton. Extraction processes and the use of chemicals during fabric production result in pollution, deforestation, and habitat destruction. Secondly, the manufacturing process of garments also plays a role in the event's environmental impact. The mass production of clothing involves the use of large amounts of water, energy, and chemicals. Water consumption during dyeing and finishing processes contributes to water scarcity, while energy consumption leads to increased carbon emissions. Chemicals used for treatments and finishes often end up in waterways, negatively affecting aquatic ecosystems. Thirdly, the transportation of clothing and accessories for fashion shows adds to the event's environmental impact. Fashion designers and their teams travel from various locations to participate in fashion events. The emissions from these journeys contribute to air pollution and climate change. Moreover, the transportation of garments from manufacturing facilities to the event venue involves the use of fossil fuels and further carbon emissions. Lastly, the waste generated by the fashion industry, including fashion shows, exacerbates its environmental impact. After fashion events, many garments are discarded or go unsold. These unsold items often end up in landfills, contributing to the growing problem of textile waste. The decomposition of textiles in landfills releases greenhouse gases, contributing to climate change.

Fashion Show Event Environmental Stewardship

Fashion Show Event Environmental Stewardship refers to the commitment and practice of implementing sustainable and eco-friendly measures throughout the planning, execution, and aftermath of a fashion show event. This concept aims to minimize the negative environmental impacts of fashion shows, such as excessive waste, energy consumption, water usage, and pollution, while promoting responsible and ethical practices within the fashion industry.

Fashion Show Event Equality

A fashion show event equality refers to the principle of promoting equal opportunity and representation within the context of a fashion show. It encompasses the fair and equitable treatment of all participants, regardless of their gender, race, ethnicity, body size, age, or any other characteristic that may lead to discrimination or disadvantage. Within the fashion industry, there has been a historical lack of diversity and inclusivity, with certain standards of beauty dominating the runway and fashion publications. Fashion show event equality aims to challenge and disrupt these norms by creating an environment that celebrates and showcases a variety of perspectives and experiences.

Fashion Show Event Ethical Fashion

Ethical fashion is a design philosophy that promotes socially and environmentally responsible practices throughout the entire fashion supply chain. It encompasses the principles of sustainability, fair trade, and animal welfare, aiming to address the negative impact of the fashion industry on both people and the planet. In the context of fashion design, ethical fashion focuses on creating garments that are made with materials and processes that minimize harm to the environment and prioritize the well-being of workers involved in the production process. Designers who embrace ethical fashion strive to create collections that are both stylish and sustainable, considering the entire lifecycle of a garment, from its sourcing to its disposal.

Fashion Show Event Ethical Labor Practices

Ethical labor practices in the context of a fashion design fashion show event refer to the responsible and fair treatment of workers involved in the production and organization of the event. It encompasses a range of principles and standards aimed at ensuring that human rights, labor laws, and environmental sustainability are respected and upheld. These practices involve various aspects, starting from the selection and hiring of workers to their working conditions, wages, and overall well-being. The event organizers should prioritize the use of suppliers and contractors who adhere to ethical labor practices, ensuring that no exploitative or unsafe conditions exist in the workplaces.

Fashion Show Event Ethical Production

Event Ethical Production in the context of fashion design refers to the practice of organizing and executing a fashion show event in a socially responsible and sustainable manner. It encompasses all aspects of production, from the selection of materials and manufacturing processes to the treatment of workers and the impact on the environment. When organizing a fashion show event, ethical production involves a careful consideration of the materials used in the garments. Sustainable and environmentally friendly materials, such as organic cotton, recycled fabrics, and ethically sourced animal products, are preferred over materials that contribute to pollution and resource depletion. By utilizing sustainable materials, the fashion industry aims to reduce its carbon footprint and minimize harm to the planet. The manufacturing processes employed in the production of garments for the fashion show event also play a crucial role in ethical production. Garments should be produced under fair and safe working conditions, where workers are treated with respect and paid a fair wage. Sweatshop labor and exploitative practices are strictly avoided in ethical production. Additionally, the fashion industry strives to promote transparency in the supply chain, ensuring that all suppliers and manufacturers adhere to ethical guidelines and standards. Furthermore, event ethical production takes into account the social and cultural impact of the fashion show event. It respects and celebrates diversity, promoting inclusivity and equality. The event should reflect a range of body types, ethnicities, and backgrounds to challenge the narrow beauty standards often perpetuated in the fashion industry. By embracing diversity, the fashion show event fosters a more inclusive and representative environment. In conclusion, event ethical production in fashion design encompasses the consideration of sustainable materials, fair manufacturing processes, and cultural inclusivity. It aims to minimize the negative environmental and social impacts associated with the fashion industry. By promoting ethical production, fashion show events can inspire positive change and contribute to a more sustainable and equitable future.

Fashion Show Event Ethical Sourcing

Ethical sourcing in the context of fashion design refers to the practice of procuring materials, fabrics, and other components for creating fashion products in a manner that is socially responsible and environmentally sustainable. It encompasses various aspects, including fair trade, labor rights, animal welfare, and environmental stewardship.

Fashion Show Event Evaluation

A fashion show event evaluation is a formal assessment or analysis of a fashion show event that has taken place. It involves the examination and evaluation of the various aspects and elements of the fashion show, including the designs, models, production, and overall presentation. The purpose of a fashion show event evaluation is to provide feedback, critique, and recommendations for improvement. It allows the organizers and designers to understand what worked well and what can be improved upon in future events. It also provides an opportunity to recognize and appreciate the creativity, talent, and hard work of the designers, models, and production team.

Fashion Show Event Fair Trade

Fashion Show Event Fair Trade is a concept in fashion design that promotes ethical and sustainable practices throughout the entire fashion industry, including production, sourcing, and selling of fashion products. It emphasizes the principles of fair wages, safe working conditions, and environmental responsibility. It is important to note that Fashion Show Event Fair Trade goes beyond just the final product being showcased at a fashion show. It focuses on the entire supply chain and aims to ensure that the fashion industry operates in a way that is fair to all stakeholders, including the manufacturers, workers, and consumers.

Fashion Show Event Fair Wages

A fashion show event fair wages refer to the appropriate and just remuneration given to individuals involved in the planning, organizing, and execution of a fashion show. These individuals may include designers, models, stylists, hair and makeup artists, event coordinators, production staff, and other professionals who contribute to the overall success of the event. Fair wages in the context of fashion design are determined based on various factors, including the level of expertise, experience, and industry standards. It takes into account the skill set and specialization of each individual, as well as the time and effort invested in executing their respective tasks. For fashion designers, fair wages ensure that their creative talents and efforts are properly compensated. This includes the time spent in designing and creating innovative and original apparel and accessories, as well as the costs of materials and production. Fair wages also acknowledge the designers' experience, reputation, and market value, which may vary depending on their achievements and brand recognition. Models, on the other hand, receive fair wages based on their experience, demand, and the scope of their participation in the fashion show. This includes compensation for their time spent in fittings, rehearsals, and actual runway presentations. Fair wages for models also consider factors such as exclusivity, the number of outfits they showcase, and the level of visibility or exposure they gain from the event. A fair wage for stylists, hair and makeup artists, and other professionals involved in the fashion show is determined by industry standards and their level of expertise. It takes into account their ability to effectively transform models and enhance the overall aesthetic of the fashion show. Fair wages for these individuals also consider the time and resources invested in preparing for the event, including sourcing and maintaining a wide range of beauty products and tools. In summary, a fashion show event fair wages ensure that individuals involved in the fashion industry are compensated appropriately for their contributions. It considers their skill set, experience, and effort, as well as industry standards and market value. Fair wages play a crucial role in promoting professionalism and sustainability within the fashion industry, while also recognizing and valuing the creative talents of all those involved.

Fashion Show Event Fashion Activism

Fashion activism is a concept within the realm of fashion design that combines the elements of style and societal change. It is a movement that seeks to utilize fashion as a means of challenging the norms and addressing important social and political issues. As a form of visual communication, fashion activism aims to bring awareness and create dialogue through the medium of clothing and accessories. Unlike conventional fashion shows that solely focus on showcasing the latest trends and designs, fashion activism events emphasize the power of fashion as a tool for activism. These events serve as platforms for designers and fashion enthusiasts to express their thoughts and opinions on various issues, such as gender inequality, environmental sustainability, body positivity, racial discrimination, and more.

Fashion Show Event Fashion Education

A fashion show event is a highly anticipated gathering in the fashion industry where designers showcase their latest clothing and accessory collections on the runway. It is an organized platform that allows fashion designers to exhibit their creative vision and style to industry professionals, journalists, buyers, and fashion enthusiasts.At a fashion show event, the designers communicate their fashion concepts through the presentation of clothing garments, accessories, and overall styling. The event is typically divided into different segments or shows, each featuring a specific designer or brand. Models walk down the runway, displaying the designer's creations, while a select audience observes and evaluates the collection.Fashion show events serve several purposes. Firstly, they provide a platform for designers to gain recognition, exposure, and potential business opportunities. The event allows fashion industry professionals, such as buyers and retailers, to see the latest trends and products available in the market. Journalists and editors attend these events to report on new collections and showcase them in fashion publications.Furthermore, fashion show events act as a source of inspiration and education for aspiring fashion designers and students. Attending these events can offer valuable insights into current fashion trends, innovative design techniques, and creative approaches to garment construction. Students and emerging designers can observe the unique styles and aesthetics of established designers, helping them develop their own creative vision.In addition to the physical runway shows, fashion show events may also include pre and post-show activities, such as networking opportunities, industry panels, and interviews. These events foster collaboration and exchange of ideas among industry professionals, creating a supportive and dynamic environment for the fashion community. Fashion show events can take place on a regional, national, or international scale, with iconic cities like Paris, Milan, New York, and London hosting renowned fashion weeks.In conclusion, a fashion show event is a vital platform for designers to showcase their collections, gain exposure, and connect with industry professionals. It is an influential event that sets the stage for new trends and creative expressions in the world of fashion.

Fashion Show Event Feedback

A fashion show event is a curated showcase of clothing designs and accessories, typically organized by fashion designers, fashion houses, or fashion organizations. It serves as a platform for designers to present their latest collections to a targeted audience, usually consisting of buyers, industry professionals, press, and fashion enthusiasts.The primary objective of a fashion show event is to display the creativity and unique aesthetic vision of the participating designers. Through carefully choreographed runway presentations, models showcase the garments, allowing the audience to witness their craftsmanship, fit, and overall design. Fashion show events often incorporate music, lighting, and stage props to enhance the visual impact and create an immersive experience that captures the essence of the collection. These events serve multiple purposes within the fashion industry. They provide designers with an opportunity to gain exposure, promote their brand, and attract potential buyers and clients. Fashion show events also act as a market research platform, allowing designers to gauge the audience's reaction to their designs and gather valuable feedback. Furthermore, fashion show events contribute to the overall promotion and advancement of the fashion industry. They help in establishing trends and setting the tone for upcoming seasons. Fashion designers often collaborate with other creative professionals, such as makeup artists, hairstylists, and set designers, to create a cohesive visual story that aligns with the collection's theme or inspiration. Attendees of fashion show events include industry insiders, such as fashion editors, journalists, fashion bloggers, and influencers, who play a crucial role in disseminating information about the showcased designs. This coverage generates publicity and serves as a catalyst for consumer interest and engagement. In conclusion, a fashion show event serves as a platform for fashion designers to showcase their latest collections to industry professionals, buyers, and fashion enthusiasts. It aims to display the creativity, craftsmanship, and unique aesthetic vision of the designers, while also contributing to the promotion and advancement of the fashion industry as a whole.

Fashion Show Event Fundraising

A fashion show event fundraising is a formal gathering that showcases a collection of clothing and accessories created by designers, with the purpose of raising funds for a specific cause or organization. During a fashion show event fundraising, designers present their latest creations on models who walk down a runway or stage in front of an audience. The clothing and accessories showcased usually reflect the designer's unique style and vision. The event may also include live music, dance performances, or other forms of entertainment to enhance the overall experience.

Fashion Show Event Gender Equality

A fashion show event with a focus on gender equality is an innovative platform that promotes equal representation and opportunities for designers, models, and industry professionals of all genders. This event aims to challenge traditional gender norms and stereotypes prevalent in the fashion industry. By hosting a fashion show event that promotes gender equality, the organizers provide a platform for designers to create collections that transcend the boundaries of traditional menswear and womenswear. This encourages creative exploration and pushes the boundaries of fashion design, ultimately leading to a more inclusive and diverse industry.

Fashion Show Event Global Outreach

A fashion show event with global outreach refers to a fashion design exhibition or showcase that aims to reach a worldwide audience. This type of event typically features collections from a variety of designers from different countries or cultures, providing a platform for the global fashion community to come together and celebrate creativity and innovation in fashion. During a fashion show event with global outreach, designers present their latest collections on a runway or stage, using models to showcase their designs. The event may include various elements such as music, lighting, and set design to enhance the overall experience and create a visually stunning presentation.

Fashion Show Event Green Practices

A Fashion Show Event Green Practices is a concept in the fashion industry that focuses on implementing sustainable and environmentally-friendly practices during the planning, execution, and aftermath of a fashion show. It involves adopting strategies and initiatives that minimize the negative impact of the event on the environment, promote sustainability, and raise awareness about eco-friendly fashion practices. Fashion designers and event organizers play a crucial role in incorporating green practices into fashion shows. This can be achieved by: 1. Sustainable Sourcing: Fashion designers can use responsibly sourced materials such as organic cotton, hemp, bamboo, and recycled fabrics. By opting for sustainable materials, designers reduce the carbon footprint in the production and manufacturing stages of their designs. 2. Ethical Production: Green fashion shows promote fair labor practices and prioritize the well-being of workers involved in the production process. Designers can ensure their garments are made in factories that provide safe working conditions, fair wages, and adhere to labor regulations. 3. Energy Efficiency: Fashion show venues can be designed to be energy-efficient by using natural lighting, energy-saving LED bulbs, and smart temperature control systems. This reduces energy consumption and minimizes the use of resources during the event. 4. Waste Management: During fashion shows, proper waste management should be implemented to minimize the amount of waste generated. This can involve recycling bins for paper and plastic, composting stations for organic waste, and donating leftover garments to charities or textile recycling programs. 5. Digital Invitations and Presentations: To reduce paper waste, fashion show organizers can opt for digital invitations and presentations instead of traditional printed materials. This not only saves resources but also allows for creative and interactive digital experiences. By embracing Fashion Show Event Green Practices, the fashion industry can strive towards a more sustainable future, where both the production and consumption of fashion are mindful of the environment and social responsibility.

Fashion Show Event Human Rights

The Fashion Show Event Human Rights is a concept in fashion design that aims to promote and uphold the principles of human rights through the showcase of clothing and accessories. It is an event that utilizes the medium of fashion to raise awareness and advocate for human rights issues such as gender equality, freedom of expression, fair labor practices, and social justice. This fashion event serves as a platform for designers to express their creativity while simultaneously addressing pressing human rights concerns. Through their collections, designers can address and challenge societal norms, stereotypes, and discrimination, promoting a more inclusive and just society.

Fashion Show Event Impact Measurement

A fashion show event impact measurement refers to the evaluation and assessment of the effects and outcomes of a fashion show event. It aims to determine the level of influence, significance, and success of the event in terms of its impact on various aspects related to fashion design. The measurement of fashion show event impact involves analyzing different factors such as audience engagement, media coverage, brand awareness, networking opportunities, and industry recognition. These indicators help determine the effectiveness of the event in achieving its goals and objectives.

Fashion Show Event Inclusivity

In the realm of fashion design, an inclusive fashion show event refers to an exhibition of diverse fashion collections that embraces and celebrates people of all backgrounds, body types, and abilities. It aims to break away from traditional beauty standards and challenges societal norms by promoting inclusivity, representation, and acceptance. The main objective of an inclusive fashion show event is to create an environment where everyone feels welcome and empowered. This is achieved by featuring a wide range of models who represent various ethnicities, genders, ages, and body shapes. By showcasing a diverse group of individuals on the runway, fashion designers can cater to a broader audience, inspire self-confidence, and redefine the notion of beauty to be more inclusive.

Fashion Show Event Industry Collaboration

Fashion Show Event Industry Collaboration refers to the process of cooperation and partnership between the fashion industry and event planners to organize and execute successful fashion shows. This collaboration aims to bring together the creative talents of fashion designers, stylists, models, and event professionals to showcase the latest trends and designs in a visually captivating and engaging manner. In the context of fashion design, collaboration in the fashion show event industry involves various stakeholders working together to create a seamless and memorable fashion show experience. Fashion designers collaborate with event planners to conceptualize and plan the overall theme, aesthetics, and logistics of the fashion show. They work closely with event professionals to determine the ideal location, stage set up, lighting, and sound requirements that will enhance the presentation of their collections. One crucial aspect of collaboration in the fashion show event industry is the partnership between fashion designers and stylists. Stylists collaborate with designers to curate and style the outfits that will be showcased on the runway. They play a vital role in ensuring that the garments are presented in the most visually appealing and impactful way, taking into consideration factors such as styling techniques, accessories, and hair and makeup choices. Collaboration also extends to the selection and casting of models for the fashion show. Designers and event planners work together to choose models who can best embody the essence of their collections and effectively communicate their vision on the runway. The collaboration between designers and models involves fittings, rehearsals, and ongoing communication to create a cohesive and harmonious presentation. Furthermore, collaboration in the fashion show event industry includes partnership with various suppliers and vendors. Event professionals work closely with lighting and sound technicians, stage designers, and AV experts to create a visually stunning and technically flawless runway presentation. Additionally, collaborations with hair and makeup artists, photographers, and videographers contribute to capturing and preserving the overall aesthetics and mood of the fashion show. In summary, fashion show event industry collaboration brings together fashion designers, stylists, models, event planners, and various industry professionals to create a captivating and seamless fashion show experience. This collaboration ensures that the creative vision of designers is effectively translated into a visually stunning and memorable presentation that showcases the latest trends and designs in the fashion industry.

Fashion Show Event Innovation In Fashion

A fashion show event is an innovative platform in the field of fashion design where designers showcase their latest creations and trends on a runway, presenting their collections to an audience of industry professionals, influencers, buyers, and fashion enthusiasts. It is a highly anticipated event that allows designers to establish their brand image, gain exposure, and create buzz around their work. Fashion shows are organized by fashion weeks, fashion organizations, or individual designers, and can take place in various settings such as art galleries, fashion showrooms, or even outdoor locations.

Fashion Show Event Innovation

A fashion show event innovation refers to the introduction of new and creative ideas and concepts in the way fashion shows are organized and presented. It encompasses the integration of novel elements and techniques that enhance the overall experience and impact of the show on the audience. These innovations can include changes in various aspects of fashion show production, such as staging, lighting, music, and choreography, as well as the integration of technology and digital media. Fashion designers and event organizers constantly strive to bring forth fresh and exciting ideas that captivate the audience and create a memorable and immersive fashion experience.

Fashion Show Event Inspiration

A fashion show event inspiration refers to the process of generating ideas and concepts for a runway show that showcases the latest trends and designs in the fashion industry. It involves gathering inspiration from various sources and using creative thinking to curate a visually captivating and unique showcase of clothing, accessories, and styling. The fashion design industry is constantly evolving, and fashion show events play a crucial role in presenting new collections to buyers, the media, and the general public. Fashion show event inspiration begins with research and exploration of different themes, trends, cultures, art movements, and historical eras. The fashion designer or creative team responsible for the event draws inspiration from these sources to create a cohesive concept for the show. This could involve using elements such as color palettes, textures, patterns, or specific references to enhance the overall theme. The goal is to create an immersive experience that captivates the audience and leaves a lasting impression. Once the inspiration is established, the fashion show event planning process begins. This includes selecting models, choosing the appropriate venue, arranging lighting and music, and coordinating hair and makeup styles. The event team works together to ensure that the overall vision is executed flawlessly. The runway itself becomes a platform for the designer's artistic expression. It is carefully choreographed to showcase each garment at its best, taking into consideration the flow, movement, and styling of the models. Attention is paid to the order in which the garments are presented to create a coherent and balanced narrative throughout the show. Throughout the fashion show event, designers and models work together to bring the clothing and accessories to life. The audience experiences the fusion of the designer's inspiration and the individual interpretation of each garment. This collaboration between inspiration, design, and interpretation creates a dynamic and memorable fashion show event.

Fashion Show Event LGBTQ+ Inclusion

A fashion show event with LGBTQ+ inclusion refers to a runway presentation or exhibition that intentionally incorporates and celebrates diverse gender identities and sexual orientations within the fashion industry. It aims to provide a platform where LGBTQ+ individuals can express their authentic selves through fashion, while challenging traditional norms and promoting inclusivity. By including LGBTQ+ representation in fashion shows, designers convey a message of acceptance and support for the community. This can be achieved through various means, such as featuring LGBTQ+ models, showcasing designs that cater to diverse body types and gender expressions, and working with queer designers and stylists. The event also creates an opportunity to address social issues that affect the LGBTQ+ community, such as discrimination and stereotypes, by using fashion as a medium for activism and awareness.

Fashion Show Event Local Engagement

A fashion show event is a local engagement that showcases the latest trends and designs in the world of fashion. It is a platform where fashion designers, models, and industry professionals come together to present their creations and inspire others in the fashion industry. The main objective of a fashion show event is to promote and market the designs of the fashion designers. It serves as a way for them to showcase their talents, craftsmanship, and innovative ideas to a larger audience, including potential clients, buyers, and fashion enthusiasts. Through the fashion show, designers can gain exposure and recognition for their work, which can lead to future collaborations, partnerships, and even opportunities to showcase their designs in retail stores or fashion magazines. During a fashion show event, models walk down a runway or a stage, wearing the latest collections of the designers. The runway serves as the central focal point, where all attention is directed towards the models and their outfits. The models' movements, poses, and expressions are carefully choreographed to effectively highlight the details, uniqueness, and overall aesthetic of the garments. In addition to the runway, a fashion show event may also include other elements such as music, lighting, and stage design, which are used to enhance the overall atmosphere and presentation of the show. These factors contribute to creating a visually appealing and immersive experience for the audience, allowing them to fully appreciate the beauty and creativity behind the designs. Furthermore, fashion show events often attract a diverse range of attendees, including fashion journalists, bloggers, photographers, and celebrities. Their presence adds to the prestige and publicity of the event, as well as provides an opportunity for networking and media coverage. Media outlets often report on fashion show events, generating further exposure and buzz for the designers and their collections.

Fashion Show Event Logistics

A fashion show event logistics refers to the detailed planning and organization of various elements involved in the execution of a fashion show. It encompasses all the behind-the-scenes arrangements required to ensure the smooth running of the event and the successful presentation of the fashion designs. First and foremost, fashion show event logistics involve selecting a suitable venue that can accommodate the runway, seating arrangement for guests, backstage areas for models, and other essential facilities. The logistics team works closely with the venue management to determine the layout and design of the space, considering factors such as the number of expected attendees, lighting requirements, and audiovisual setup. Next, the logistics team is responsible for coordinating the transportation and accommodation of models, designers, and other key personnel involved in the fashion show. They liaise with airlines, hotels, and travel agencies to ensure that everyone arrives on time and is comfortably accommodated throughout the event. Furthermore, fashion show event logistics include the management of the backstage area, which is crucial for the smooth flow of the show. This involves organizing dressing rooms for models, hair and makeup stations, and coordinating the arrival and departure of the models for their respective segments. The logistics team ensures that everything runs according to schedule, managing any last-minute changes or emergencies that may arise. In addition, the logistics team is responsible for handling the technical aspects of the fashion show. This includes coordinating with lighting and sound technicians to create the desired ambiance and mood on the runway. They also collaborate with stage designers to create a visually captivating set that complements the fashion designs being showcased. Lastly, fashion show event logistics involve managing the front-of-house operations, including guest registration, ushering, and seating arrangements. The logistics team ensures that guests are greeted and guided to their assigned seats, taking into consideration any special requirements or preferences they may have. In conclusion, a fashion show event logistics encompasses the various tasks and arrangements required to execute a successful fashion show. From venue selection to backstage management, transportation coordination to technical setup, and front-of-house operations, the logistics team plays a crucial role in ensuring the smooth running and overall success of the event.

Fashion Show Event Marketing

A fashion show event marketing refers to the strategic planning and execution of marketing activities aimed at promoting and creating awareness about a fashion show event. This includes creating buzz, generating excitement, and attracting a target audience to attend the fashion show. The primary objective of fashion show event marketing is to effectively communicate the unique selling points of the fashion show, such as the designers, collections, themes, or collaborations involved, to generate interest and ultimately drive attendance.

Fashion Show Event Mental Health Awareness

A Fashion Show Event Mental Health Awareness is a platform for raising awareness and promoting discussion about mental health within the fashion industry. It is an event where fashion designers, models, and industry professionals come together to use their creative talents to shine a light on mental health issues. Through the art of fashion design, this event aims to break the stigma surrounding mental health and provide a safe space for open conversations. Designers showcase their collections, incorporating elements that reflect different aspects of mental health, such as emotions, struggles, and resilience. The Fashion Show Event Mental Health Awareness encourages designers to use their garments as a means of self-expression and storytelling. Each collection tells a unique narrative, amplifying the experiences of those affected by mental health challenges. Through the use of colors, textures, and silhouettes, designers evoke emotions, capturing the complexity of mental health in a visual medium. Furthermore, this event provides an opportunity for models to share their personal experiences with mental health. By walking the runway, they demonstrate strength and empowerment, challenging societal norms and prejudices. Models become ambassadors, using their platform to start conversations and advocate for positive change. The Fashion Show Event Mental Health Awareness also plays a crucial role in educating the fashion industry and the wider public about mental health. It promotes inclusivity and diversity, celebrating the beauty of individuals regardless of their mental health status. By showcasing diverse models and designers, it challenges the traditional standards of beauty and encourages acceptance and understanding. Overall, a Fashion Show Event Mental Health Awareness is a powerful and impactful gathering that combines the artistry of fashion with the important mission of raising awareness about mental health. It creates a space where creativity and advocacy intersect, striving to promote positive mental health practices and foster a more compassionate industry.

Fashion Show Event Mentorship

A fashion show event mentorship is a program or process in the field of fashion design where established and experienced professionals provide guidance, support, and knowledge to aspiring fashion designers. It involves a mentor who is an experienced individual, usually a successful fashion designer, and a mentee who is an aspiring fashion designer looking to learn and grow in the fashion industry. The main objective of a fashion show event mentorship is to provide guidance and mentorship to the mentee, helping them develop their skills, expand their knowledge, and navigate the complexities of the fashion industry. The mentor acts as a role model and provides valuable insights and advice based on their own experiences and expertise.

Fashion Show Event Networking Opportunities

A fashion show event is an organized platform where fashion designers and industry professionals showcase their latest creations and designs to a targeted audience. It is a significant networking opportunity for individuals working in the fashion industry, including designers, models, journalists, stylists, buyers, and fashion enthusiasts. Networking opportunities in a fashion show event involve establishing connections and relationships with like-minded individuals and professionals in the fashion industry. These events provide a platform for designers and industry professionals to promote their work, seek collaborations, gain exposure, and expand their professional networks.

Fashion Show Event Networking

A fashion show event networking refers to a gathering or event that is specifically organized for fashion designers, fashion industry professionals, models, photographers, and other individuals involved in the fashion industry to come together in one place to showcase their latest designs, creations, and talents. This type of networking event provides a platform for designers to connect with potential clients, buyers, and industry influencers, and also allows participants to expand their professional network by establishing relationships with key figures in the fashion industry. The primary objective of a fashion show event networking is to facilitate the exchange of ideas, knowledge, and resources among fashion professionals. It serves as a space for designers to present their work to a targeted audience, receive feedback and constructive criticism, collaborate with other like-minded individuals, and gain exposure in the fashion industry. Furthermore, fashion show event networking provides an opportunity for designers to stay up-to-date with the latest trends, innovations, and developments in the fashion world.

Fashion Show Event Partnerships

Fashion show event partnerships refer to collaborations and alliances between fashion designers and other entities to organize and execute a fashion show event. These partnerships are crucial in ensuring the success of the event by bringing together different expertise and resources. A fashion show event partnership usually involves the fashion designer or fashion brand collaborating with various stakeholders such as sponsors, event organizers, venues, models, makeup artists, hairstylists, photographers, and media partners. Each partner plays a specific role in contributing to the overall execution and promotion of the fashion show.

Fashion Show Event Philanthropy

A fashion show event philanthropy is a charitable event that combines the elements of fashion design and philanthropic causes. It is a platform where fashion designers showcase their latest collections while raising funds or awareness for a particular charitable organization or cause. In this type of event, fashion designers collaborate with the philanthropic organization to create a runway show that not only displays their artistic creations but also promotes the mission and goals of the charity. The fashion show serves as a means to engage the audience in both the glamour of fashion and the importance of philanthropy. During a fashion show event philanthropy, models walk down the runway wearing the designer's clothing, allowing the audience to appreciate the craftsmanship and aesthetics of the garments. The designs showcased usually align with the theme or purpose of the philanthropic cause, emphasizing its importance and relevance. Besides the fashion presentation, there are often additional activities or elements incorporated into the event to further support the philanthropic cause. These may include speeches from representatives of the charity, video presentations highlighting the organization's work, or interactive experiences that allow attendees to contribute or learn more about the cause. The purpose of a fashion show event philanthropy extends beyond just raising funds. It aims to create a positive impact on society by increasing awareness and promoting a sense of responsibility towards the cause. Through the visual power and influence of fashion, these events have the potential to draw attention to important issues and inspire individuals to take action. Overall, a fashion show event philanthropy combines the glamour and creativity of fashion design with the noble goal of making a difference in the world. It allows fashion designers to use their talent and influence to support and raise awareness for charitable organizations and causes, creating a meaningful and impactful event that brings together both the fashion and philanthropic communities.

Fashion Show Event Planning

A fashion show event planning refers to the process of organizing and executing an event specifically dedicated to showcasing the latest fashion designs and trends. It involves coordinating and managing various aspects of the event, including selecting the venue, recruiting models, arranging for hair and makeup, designing the stage and lighting setup, inviting guests, and ensuring a smooth flow of the entire show. The primary objective of fashion show event planning is to create a platform for fashion designers to exhibit their collections to a targeted audience, which typically consists of industry professionals, buyers, press, celebrities, and fashion enthusiasts. By carefully planning and organizing the event, the aim is to inspire and captivate the attendees, effectively communicate the brand's vision and aesthetic, and generate exposure and buzz around the showcased designs.

Fashion Show Event Positive Change

A fashion show event is a gathering or exhibition that showcases the latest trends, designs, and creations in the world of fashion. It is a platform where fashion designers present their collections to an audience consisting of industry professionals, fashion enthusiasts, and potential buyers. The purpose of a fashion show event is to promote and highlight the creativity, innovation, and skill of fashion designers. It serves as a platform for designers to express their unique artistic vision and communicate their design philosophy to a wider audience. By showcasing their collections on the runway, designers aim to generate interest and excitement around their brand, establish their credibility in the industry, and create a demand for their designs. A fashion show event is not solely about presenting garments; it is a multidimensional experience that combines fashion, music, choreography, and set design to create a captivating and immersive atmosphere. The runway serves as a stage where models strut down, showcasing the garments to their full effect while capturing the attention of the audience. It is a carefully orchestrated production that combines various elements to create a cohesive and impactful presentation. In addition to providing a platform for designers, a fashion show event also plays a significant role in shaping and influencing fashion trends. It sets the tone for what will be considered fashionable and desirable in the upcoming seasons. By bringing together designers, industry professionals, and fashion influencers, a fashion show event fosters collaboration, exchange of ideas, and creative dialogue, leading to the evolution and progression of fashion. Furthermore, a fashion show event has the potential to bring about positive change in the fashion industry. It provides an opportunity for designers to address relevant social, cultural, and environmental issues through their collections. By using fashion as a medium for storytelling and advocacy, designers can raise awareness, provoke thought, and contribute to positive societal change.

Fashion Show Event Positive Impact

A fashion show event is a highly anticipated and glamorous affair in the world of fashion design. It serves as a platform for designers to showcase their latest collections to an influential audience, including fashion industry professionals, celebrities, and the media. The event plays a vital role in promoting and elevating the brand image of designers and fashion houses. One positive impact of a fashion show event is the opportunity it provides for designers to gain exposure and recognition. By presenting their collections on the runway, designers can capture the attention of potential buyers, trendsetters, and fashion enthusiasts. This exposure can lead to increased sales and brand visibility, paving the way for future growth and success.

Fashion Show Event Postmortem

A fashion show event postmortem is an evaluation or analysis of a fashion show event that has already taken place. It involves the examination of various aspects and components of the event to determine its successes and areas for improvement. The purpose of a fashion show event postmortem is to gather feedback and insights that can be used to enhance future events and ensure their overall success. It is an opportunity to assess the effectiveness of different elements, such as the fashion designs, runway setup, lighting, music, models, and overall presentation.

Fashion Show Event Professional Development

A fashion show event is a professional development opportunity in the field of fashion design that showcases the latest trends and designs in clothing, accessories, and styling. It is an organized presentation that allows fashion designers to display their creative work to an audience, which often includes industry professionals, media representatives, and potential clients. The main purpose of a fashion show event is to promote and market the designer's collection, create brand awareness, and generate interest in their designs. It serves as a platform for designers to establish their presence in the fashion industry and gain recognition for their work. Additionally, it provides an opportunity for designers to network and connect with other professionals, such as buyers, stylists, and fashion journalists.

Fashion Show Event Promotion

A fashion show event promotion is a strategic marketing activity designed to create awareness and generate excitement about a fashion show. It involves the use of various communication channels and promotional techniques to reach the target audience and persuade them to attend the event. The aim of a fashion show event promotion is to showcase the latest fashion trends and designs, promote fashion brands and designers, and attract potential buyers, industry professionals, and fashion enthusiasts. The event provides a platform for designers to present their collections, engage with the audience, and create buzz around their brand.

Fashion Show Event Racial Equality

A fashion show event promoting racial equality is an organized display of clothing and accessories designed to celebrate and embrace diversity and inclusivity within the fashion industry. The event aims to challenge and break down racial barriers by showcasing garments that are inspired by different cultural perspectives and traditions, while incorporating a variety of models from different racial and ethnic backgrounds. The fashion designers participating in this event are committed to creating collections that pay homage to various cultures, traditions, and histories, while also promoting social justice and equality. Each designer uses their talent and creativity to blend different styles, fabrics, and aesthetics to create unique and groundbreaking pieces that challenge traditional norms and celebrate the beauty and diversity of all races.

Fashion Show Event Recycling

A fashion show event recycling refers to the practice of incorporating sustainable and eco-friendly elements into a fashion show. It involves reusing, repurposing, and recycling materials and garments in order to reduce waste and promote a more sustainable approach to fashion design. In a fashion show event recycling, designers aim to showcase their creations while also highlighting the importance of sustainable practices and responsible consumption. They incorporate materials that have been recycled or upcycled, such as fabrics made from recycled plastic bottles or reclaimed textiles. They may also use vintage or second-hand garments as a way to promote the concept of longevity and discourage fast fashion. The fashion industry is known for its significant environmental impact, from the production of textiles to the disposal of unwanted clothing. By organizing a fashion show event recycling, designers aim to raise awareness and encourage a shift towards more sustainable fashion practices. During the event, the runway may feature models wearing garments made from recycled materials, demonstrating the potential for creativity and innovation within sustainable fashion. Designers may also showcase the process of repurposing and transforming old garments into new, unique pieces, highlighting the possibilities of upcycling and reducing waste. Additionally, a fashion show event recycling can serve as a platform for educating the audience about the environmental consequences of fast fashion and the benefits of choosing sustainable options. Designers may provide information about the materials used in their collections, as well as the impact of these choices on the planet. Overall, a fashion show event recycling aims to promote sustainability, creativity, and conscious consumption within the fashion industry. It provides an opportunity for designers to showcase their commitment to environmental responsibility and inspire others to reconsider their fashion choices.

Fashion Show Event Representation

A fashion show event representation refers to the process of showcasing a collection of clothing and accessories designed by a fashion designer or fashion brand in a visual and experiential manner. It typically takes place on a runway or stage and is attended by industry professionals, celebrities, influencers, and members of the press. The purpose of a fashion show event representation is to communicate the creative vision and style of the designer or brand to the audience. It allows them to experience the garments and accessories in a dynamic and immersive way, as models walk down the runway wearing the designs. The event representation often incorporates music, lighting, set design, and choreography to enhance the overall presentation. Fashion show event representations are organized by fashion houses, fashion weeks, or individual designers, and are an integral part of the fashion industry. They serve as a platform for designers to showcase their talent, establish their brand identity, and generate buzz and interest among potential buyers, retailers, and consumers. During a fashion show event representation, the garments and accessories are styled and presented in a cohesive and visually appealing manner. The sequence of the runway presentation is carefully curated to create a narrative or tell a story through the designs. The models, chosen for their ability to embody the desired aesthetic and attitude, showcase the clothing and accessories, while also embodying the brand's image and values. Attendees of a fashion show event representation include fashion buyers, who may place orders for the showcased designs to be sold in retail stores or online, as well as members of the press, who will report on the event and the collections presented. Celebrities and influencers are often invited to sit in the front row and create publicity for the designer or brand by wearing their designs and sharing their experience on social media. In conclusion, a fashion show event representation is a highly anticipated and meticulously planned production that serves as a platform for designers and brands to present their collections in a visually captivating and experiential way, with the aim of creating excitement, generating publicity, and driving interest in the fashion industry.

Fashion Show Event Resource Efficiency

The concept of fashion show event resource efficiency in the context of fashion design refers to the effective and sustainable use of resources during a fashion show event. It involves optimizing the use of materials, energy, and other resources to minimize waste, reduce environmental impact, and enhance the overall efficiency of the event. Resource efficiency in a fashion show event encompasses various aspects, including the selection and utilization of fabrics, garments, props, lighting, sound equipment, and other materials. Designers and event organizers strive to make conscious choices that consider the environmental and social impacts of their decisions.

Fashion Show Event Security

Fashion Show Event Security refers to the measures put in place to ensure the safety and smooth execution of a fashion show event. It involves the deployment of skilled security personnel and the implementation of security protocols to protect the event, its participants, and attendees. The primary responsibility of fashion show event security is to maintain order and handle any potential threats or disruptions. This includes managing access control, crowd control, and conducting thorough security checks to prevent unauthorized individuals or items from entering the event premises. Security personnel are trained to identify and respond to any suspicious behavior, trespassing, or other security breaches that may pose a risk to the event or its attendees. In addition to maintaining security, fashion show event security also plays a crucial role in providing a safe and comfortable environment for the participants and guests. They ensure that attendees can enjoy the event without feeling uneasy or threatened. By maintaining a visible presence and offering assistance when needed, security personnel help create a sense of trust and reassurance among the attendees. Furthermore, fashion show event security is responsible for protecting the intellectual property and confidential information associated with the event. This includes safeguarding the designs, collections, and other proprietary assets of the fashion designers and brands participating in the show. Security measures may include restricting unauthorized photography, ensuring the privacy of backstage areas, and closely monitoring the handling of intellectual property throughout the event. In conclusion, fashion show event security encompasses a range of measures aimed at ensuring the safety, order, and protection of the event, its participants, and attendees. It involves the deployment of skilled security personnel, the implementation of security protocols, and the protection of intellectual property. By maintaining security and providing a safe atmosphere, fashion show event security contributes to the overall success and positive experience of the event.

Fashion Show Event Skill Building

A fashion show event is a curated production that showcases the latest designs and trends in fashion. It is an organized event where designers, models, stylists, and other industry professionals come together to present their collections to an audience of buyers, media, and fashion enthusiasts. The primary purpose of a fashion show event is to promote and market the featured designs and brands. It serves as a platform for designers to showcase their creativity and craftsmanship, allowing them to establish their brand identity and gain exposure in the industry. Fashion shows typically take place during fashion weeks, which are held in major fashion capitals around the world, such as Paris, Milan, New York, and London. During a fashion show event, designers present their collections through a carefully choreographed runway presentation. Models walk down the runway wearing the designs, displaying them to the audience, photographers, and media. The clothing, accessories, and styling elements are meticulously chosen to reflect the designer's vision and convey the desired aesthetic. The models' movements and expressions are coordinated to highlight the garments and create a visually captivating experience for the viewers. Aside from showcasing the designs, fashion show events also serve as a networking and business opportunity for designers. They often attract buyers, retailers, and industry professionals who attend to discover new talent and potential collaborations. Designers may receive feedback, establish connections, and even secure orders for their collections during these events. Furthermore, fashion show events contribute to the overall cultural exchange and development of the fashion industry. They inspire and influence trends, allowing designers and consumers to stay in touch with the ever-changing world of fashion. By bringing together diverse talents, perspectives, and styles, fashion shows contribute to the continuous growth and evolution of the fashion landscape.

Fashion Show Event Slow Fashion Movement

The Slow Fashion Movement is a concept within the fashion industry that promotes a more sustainable and ethical approach to clothing production and consumption. It aims to counter the negative environmental and social impacts of fast fashion by encouraging slower production processes, higher quality garments, and mindful consumer choices. The movement emphasizes the importance of reducing waste, pollution, and exploitation in the fashion supply chain. It advocates for practices such as recycling and upcycling materials, using organic and sustainable fabrics, and supporting fair trade and local production. Slow fashion designers prioritize long-lasting design and craftsmanship, creating garments that are meant to be cherished and worn for years rather than discarded after a few uses.

Fashion Show Event Social Change

A Fashion Show Event for Social Change in the context of fashion design refers to a specialized fashion event that aims to promote and support social causes and bring about positive change in society. Such events leverage the power of fashion, creativity, and style to raise awareness, address social issues, and contribute to various charitable endeavors. Through the medium of fashion, designers, models, and organizers collaborate to create a platform that advocates for social causes and encourages individuals to make a difference.

Fashion Show Event Social Impact

A Fashion Show Event is a curated showcase of fashion designs and garments, featuring a collection of clothing and accessories created by fashion designers. It is an event that brings together industry professionals, fashion enthusiasts, and the general public to celebrate and appreciate the artistry and creativity of fashion design. With a strong emphasis on visual presentation and artistic expression, a Fashion Show Event serves as a platform for fashion designers to showcase their collections to a wider audience. These events are often organized by fashion houses, brands, or fashion schools, and are typically held in prestigious venues such as theaters, galleries, or other designated spaces. The main purpose of a Fashion Show Event is to provide a stage for designers to present their work in a visually captivating way, using models to display their creations on a runway or stage. The garments are carefully styled and accessorized to convey the designer's vision and highlight the unique features and details of each piece. In addition to showcasing the latest trends and designs, a Fashion Show Event also has social impact. It serves as a platform for promoting diversity, inclusivity, and body positivity within the fashion industry. By featuring models of different sizes, ethnicities, and abilities, fashion shows can challenge traditional beauty standards and promote a more inclusive and accepting society. Fashion Show Events also have the power to raise awareness and support for various social causes. Many fashion shows collaborate with charitable organizations or non-profits to raise funds and promote awareness for specific issues such as sustainability, human rights, or disease research. These collaborations allow fashion designers to use their creative platforms to make a positive impact and contribute to important social causes.

Fashion Show Event Social Justice

A fashion show event with a social justice theme aims to use fashion as a platform for promoting awareness and addressing social issues. In the context of fashion design, it involves the creation and showcasing of garments that convey meaningful messages and advocate for social change. Through the use of fashion, designers participating in a social justice fashion show event aim to challenge societal norms, expose injustice, and spark conversations about important topics. This event serves as a platform for designers to express their creativity while using their designs as a form of activism.

Fashion Show Event Social Responsibility Initiatives

Social responsibility initiatives in the context of a fashion show event refer to the actions and efforts taken by fashion designers, brands, and organizers to address and contribute positively to social, environmental, and ethical concerns associated with the fashion industry. These initiatives aim to promote sustainability, inclusivity, and ethical practices throughout the entire fashion show event process, from production to presentation. They involve implementing strategies and practices that prioritize the well-being of people, animals, and the environment, while also striving to make a positive impact on society as a whole.

Fashion Show Event Social Responsibility

Social responsibility in the context of fashion design for a fashion show event refers to the duty and obligation of fashion designers to consider the environmental, ethical, and societal impact of their designs and practices. It encompasses the emphasis on sustainability, fair labor practices, inclusivity, and community engagement in the fashion industry. When organizing a fashion show event, fashion designers need to be socially responsible by making conscious choices to minimize their carbon footprint and reduce waste. This can be achieved by using environmentally friendly materials, such as organic fabrics or recycled materials, and adopting sustainable production processes and techniques.

Fashion Show Event Sponsorships

Fashion show event sponsorships refer to the financial support provided by an organization or brand to a fashion show event in exchange for various promotional opportunities and benefits. These sponsorships enable fashion designers to showcase their collections on a public platform while receiving financial backing and marketing assistance. Sponsorships typically involve a formal agreement between the fashion show organizers and the sponsoring party, outlining the terms and conditions of the partnership. The sponsor may provide financial resources to cover the costs associated with organizing the event, such as venue rental, stage setup, lighting, sound, and marketing expenses. In addition to providing financial support, sponsors also benefit from the exposure and brand recognition associated with the fashion show. They gain visibility among the target audience attending the event, as well as through various media channels covering the show, including print, online, and social media platforms. The sponsoring organization's logo and branding are prominently displayed throughout the event, increasing brand awareness and establishing a positive association with the fashion industry. Sponsorships often include additional promotional opportunities, such as product placements, exclusive backstage access, and the possibility of collaborating with fashion designers on future projects. Sponsors may showcase their products or services during the event, allowing attendees to experience and interact with their offerings firsthand. These partnerships contribute to a mutually beneficial relationship, where the fashion show gains essential financial support, and the sponsor gains exposure and connects with potential customers. Some fashion show event sponsorships go beyond financial support and offer mentorship programs for emerging fashion designers. These programs provide aspiring designers with valuable guidance, industry knowledge, and networking opportunities, helping them establish their careers in the fashion industry. In conclusion, fashion show event sponsorships play a vital role in the success of fashion shows by providing financial support, marketing assistance, and promotional opportunities for designers. They facilitate the presentation of new collections to a wider audience and contribute to the growth and exposure of both the fashion show and the sponsoring organization.

Fashion Show Event Sustainability Initiatives

Fashion Show Event Sustainability Initiatives refer to the various measures and actions taken by fashion designers, brands, and event organizers to minimize the negative environmental and social impact of fashion shows. These initiatives aim to drive sustainable practices throughout the entire fashion show event, from the design and production of garments to the execution of the show itself.One key aspect of fashion show event sustainability initiatives is the use of eco-friendly materials and production processes. Designers are encouraged to choose sustainable fabrics, such as organic cotton, hemp, or recycled materials, and avoid using materials derived from endangered or non-renewable resources. Additionally, the production process should prioritize energy and water efficiency, waste reduction, and emissions reduction, minimizing the carbon footprint of the garments.

Fashion Show Event Sustainability In Fashion

A Fashion Show Event is an organized presentation of fashion designs and clothing collections, typically held to showcase new trends and styles to a targeted audience, such as industry professionals, buyers, media, and consumers. Fashion shows provide a platform for fashion designers and brands to display their creative work, generate interest in their collections, and ultimately drive sales. Sustainability in fashion refers to the adoption of environmentally and socially responsible practices throughout the entire fashion production cycle, from design and sourcing to manufacturing and distribution. It involves minimizing the negative impact of the fashion industry on the environment, conserving natural resources, reducing waste and pollution, and ensuring fair and safe working conditions for all those involved in the production process.

Fashion Show Event Sustainability

A fashion show event sustainability in the context of fashion design refers to the incorporation of environmentally friendly practices and ethical considerations into the planning, production, and execution of a fashion show. It encompasses the use of sustainable materials, responsible sourcing, waste reduction, and the promotion of fair trade practices within the fashion industry. Sustainability in fashion shows starts with careful selection of materials used in the creation of garments. Designers must opt for sustainable fabrics such as organic cotton, hemp, bamboo, or recycled materials to minimize their environmental impact. Additionally, the use of natural and non-toxic dyes promotes sustainability and reduces pollution. By prioritizing these choices, designers contribute to the preservation of natural resources and reduce the negative effects of traditional textile production. Furthermore, sustainability entails responsible sourcing of materials. Designers should prioritize working with suppliers that adhere to ethical practices and support fair trade. This includes ensuring that workers involved in the production process receive fair wages and work in safe conditions. Supporting fair trade helps promote social justice within the fashion industry, creating a positive impact on the lives of workers and their communities. Waste reduction is also a crucial aspect of fashion show event sustainability. Designers can minimize waste by carefully planning their collections, avoiding overproduction, and utilizing materials efficiently. By embracing techniques such as upcycling and recycling, designers can breathe new life into existing fabrics and reduce the demand for new resources. Additionally, embracing a "less is more" approach encourages longevity and quality in garments, reducing the frequency of disposable consumption. In the execution of a sustainable fashion show event, various factors come into play. This includes the efficient use of energy and water during production and the event itself. Designers should also consider the carbon footprint generated by transportation and strive to minimize it by choosing local and eco-friendly means of travel whenever possible. Considerations should also be made to reduce paper waste by utilizing digital invitations, programs, and other communications. In conclusion, fashion show event sustainability encompasses the integration of environmentally friendly practices, responsible sourcing, waste reduction, and ethical considerations into the planning, production, and execution of fashion shows. By embracing these principles, fashion designers can contribute to the goal of a more sustainable and socially conscious fashion industry.

Fashion Show Event Sustainable Development Goals

Sustainable Development Goals (SDGs) are a set of global targets adopted by the United Nations to address various social, economic, and environmental challenges facing the world. In the context of fashion design, the SDGs serve as a framework for promoting sustainable practices and responsible consumption within the industry. The fashion industry is known for its significant environmental and social impacts, such as waste generation, pollution, and poor working conditions. By aligning with the SDGs, fashion designers and brands can contribute to a more sustainable and equitable future by implementing strategies that address these challenges.

Fashion Show Event Thought Leadership

A Fashion Show Event Thought Leadership in the context of fashion design refers to a highly influential and knowledgeable individual who spearheads and guides the creative direction, innovation, and strategic vision of a fashion show event. This thought leader possesses a deep understanding of the fashion industry, trends, and consumer preferences, and uses their expertise to shape the overall experience and narrative of the fashion show. The Fashion Show Event Thought Leader plays a pivotal role in curating collections, selecting designers, models, and stylists, and creating a cohesive and engaging showcase of fashion. They are responsible for conceptualizing the theme or concept of the fashion show, ensuring that it aligns with the brand's identity and objectives, while also capturing the interest and attention of the target audience. This thought leader brings a fresh perspective and innovative ideas to the table, constantly pushing boundaries and redefining traditional fashion show formats. They possess a keen eye for detail and a strong sense of aesthetics, enabling them to curate a visually stunning and impactful event that leaves a lasting impression on attendees. In addition to their creative prowess, the Fashion Show Event Thought Leader also possesses strong leadership and communication skills. They collaborate closely with designers, stylists, and other key stakeholders to effectively translate their vision into reality. They are adept at fostering strong relationships with industry professionals and key influencers, leveraging these connections to create strategic partnerships and generate buzz around the fashion show. Furthermore, the Fashion Show Event Thought Leader stays abreast of the latest fashion trends, consumer insights, and technological advancements, allowing them to incorporate cutting-edge elements into the event. This thought leader understands the importance of integrating digital platforms and social media engagement to amplify the reach and impact of the fashion show, ensuring that it resonates with a wider audience beyond the physical event space. Overall, the Fashion Show Event Thought Leadership in fashion design combines creativity, strategic thinking, and industry knowledge to shape and elevate the fashion show experience. They encapsulate the essence of the brand and bring to life a captivating event that not only showcases the latest fashion trends but also leaves a lasting impression on attendees, industry professionals, and the fashion community as a whole.

Fashion Show Event Traceability

A fashion show event traceability refers to the process of tracking and documenting the various elements and stages involved in the organization and execution of a fashion show, specifically in the context of fashion design. It encompasses the systematic recording of the different components such as garments, accessories, models, and backstage operations from the initial planning to the final runway presentation. The purpose of implementing fashion show event traceability is to ensure a smooth and well-coordinated event that meets the desired objectives and standards. By maintaining a comprehensive record of all the key aspects, designers and event organizers can effectively manage and coordinate each step, minimizing errors, delays, and inconsistencies.

Fashion Show Event Transparent Supply Chains

A fashion show event with transparent supply chains is a showcase of fashionable garments and accessories that are created and produced with full disclosure and visibility of their supply chains. In the context of fashion design, a transparent supply chain refers to the process and journey of a fashion product from its conception to its final delivery to the consumer. In a fashion show event with transparent supply chains, designers and brands emphasize and value the importance of transparency by providing detailed information about the sourcing of materials, the manufacturing processes involved, and the social and environmental impact of their products. This includes disclosing the origins of the raw materials, such as cotton or silk, and the ethical standards followed in their production.

Fashion Show Event Vegan Fashion

Fashion Show Event Volunteer Programs

A fashion show event volunteer program is a structured initiative that allows individuals to contribute their time, skills, and energy to support the planning and execution of a fashion show. These programs provide opportunities for individuals with an interest in fashion design to gain practical experience, network with industry professionals, and contribute to the success of the event. Volunteers in a fashion show event program may assist with various tasks such as event setup and breakdown, backstage management, model dressing, guest coordination, or any other activities essential to the smooth running of the fashion show. They are typically assigned specific roles and responsibilities based on their skills and interests.

Fashion Show Event Waste Reduction

Fashion Show Event Waste Reduction refers to the implementation of practices and strategies aimed at minimizing and managing waste during fashion shows. It involves adopting sustainability measures to reduce the environmental impact associated with the production and execution of fashion events. Waste reduction in the context of fashion design encompasses various aspects, including material choices, production processes, and event organization. Firstly, it involves the selection of eco-friendly and sustainable fabrics, such as organic cotton, recycled materials, and innovative alternatives like Tencel or Piñatex. By opting for these materials, designers can contribute to reducing the pollution and resource depletion caused by conventional textile production.

Fashion Show Event Worker Rights

The Fashion Show Event Worker Rights refer to the set of rules and regulations designed to protect the rights and ensure the well-being of workers involved in fashion show events. These rights encompass various aspects of their working conditions, fair treatment, and safety. Firstly, one crucial aspect of worker rights is the fair treatment and non-discrimination policy. All workers, regardless of their gender, race, religion, or other personal characteristics, should be treated fairly and equally. They should not face any form of harassment or discrimination based on these factors, ensuring a safe and inclusive working environment for everyone involved. Secondly, the rights of fashion show event workers also include fair compensation and reasonable working hours. Workers should receive fair wages that comply with the industry standards and regulations. They should be provided with clear and transparent contracts that outline their working hours, breaks, and overtime policies. The maximum working hours and minimum rest breaks should adhere to the labor laws of the respective country to prevent exploitation and promote work-life balance. Thirdly, health and safety regulations form an essential part of worker rights in the context of fashion shows. Employers must ensure that workers have access to a safe and healthy working environment. This includes adequate lighting, ventilation, and suitable amenities such as restrooms and break areas. Employers should also implement measures to prevent accidents, provide proper training, and supply necessary personal protective equipment (PPE) where required. In addition, workers should have the right to organize and join labor unions to collectively bargain for their rights and negotiate better working conditions. Employers should respect this right and not impede or discriminate against workers who exercise their freedom of association. Overall, the Fashion Show Event Worker Rights aim to protect workers' dignity, provide fair treatment, ensure proper compensation, promote occupational health and safety, and protect their right to organize. These rights contribute to creating a more ethical and sustainable fashion industry by ensuring the well-being of the workers who bring the artistic visions of designers to life on the runway.

Fashion Show Front Of House

A Fashion Show Front of House refers to the area of a fashion show that is accessible to the general public and is responsible for managing all aspects related to the audience experience. It is the face of the fashion show and sets the tone for the entire event. The Front of House team is responsible for various tasks, including ticketing, crowd control, and ensuring the smooth flow of the show. They work closely with designers, models, and production teams to create a well-organized and visually appealing experience for the attendees. The ticketing aspect of the Front of House involves managing the sales and distribution of tickets to the show. They may handle both pre-sale and on-site ticketing, ensuring that the process is efficient and all attendees have valid tickets. Crowd control is another crucial responsibility of the Front of House team. They are responsible for maintaining order and managing the flow of people entering and exiting the venue. This may involve coordinating with security personnel and ensuring that the audience follows the designated pathways. The Front of House also plays an important role in creating a visually appealing experience for the attendees. They collaborate with the production team to design the layout and setup of the venue, including the placement of seats, stage, and runway. Additionally, they may handle the decoration and styling of the entrance and other designated areas. Overall, the Fashion Show Front of House is the central point of contact for attendees and acts as a bridge between the audience and the behind-the-scenes elements of the fashion show. They ensure that the event runs smoothly, with a focus on providing an enjoyable and visually captivating experience for all attendees.

Fashion Show Guest List

A fashion show guest list is a carefully curated roster of individuals who are invited to attend a fashion show. The guest list is created by fashion designers and event organizers to ensure that the right audience, industry professionals, and influential personalities are present at the event. The fashion show guest list serves several important purposes. First and foremost, it helps create buzz and excitement about the fashion show. By inviting industry professionals, journalists, bloggers, and fashion influencers, designers can generate media coverage, reviews, and social media posts that showcase their designs and increase brand visibility. Secondly, the guest list allows designers to target specific individuals or demographics that align with their brand image and target market. For example, if a designer specializes in high-end luxury fashion, they would invite high-profile celebrities, wealthy clients, and fashion editors from prestigious magazines. On the other hand, a designer focusing on sustainable fashion might invite eco-conscious celebrities, activists, and journalists who promote ethical and environmentally-friendly practices. Furthermore, the guest list is also used as a networking tool. Fashion shows provide an opportunity for industry professionals, such as buyers, stylists, and photographers, to connect with designers, models, and other key players in the fashion industry. By carefully selecting and inviting influential guests, designers can foster valuable relationships and collaborations that can benefit their future projects and career growth. Creating a fashion show guest list requires careful consideration and research. Designers and event organizers need to identify individuals who have the potential to make an impact on the success of the show. They often consult with public relations agencies, fashion consultants, and industry insiders to ensure that the right mix of guests is invited. In conclusion, the fashion show guest list plays a crucial role in the success of a fashion show. It helps generate buzz, target specific audiences, and facilitate networking opportunities. By inviting the right individuals, designers can maximize the exposure of their brand and create long-lasting connections in the fashion industry.

Fashion Show Holograms

Fashion Show Holograms is a pioneering concept in the realm of fashion design that utilizes holographic technology to display virtual garments and runway presentations. It revolutionizes the traditional runway show by replacing physical garments and models with holographic projections, creating a visually stunning and immersive experience for the audience. In a Fashion Show Holograms, designers leverage advanced digital techniques to create lifelike 3D representations of their designs. These holographic garments are then projected onto a runway or any other designated space, allowing viewers to see the clothing in its full glory without the need for physical prototypes or models. This innovative technology opens up endless possibilities for fashion designers. They can experiment with unconventional materials, intricate patterns, or even futuristic designs that would be challenging to achieve in traditional fashion presentations. Fashion Show Holograms allows designers to push the boundaries of creativity and redefine what is possible in the fashion industry. The virtual nature of Fashion Show Holograms also enables designers to showcase their collections to a global audience, regardless of geographical restrictions or venue limitations. These holographic displays can be livestreamed or recorded, making it accessible to anyone with an internet connection. It enhances inclusivity by democratizing the fashion industry and widening the audience base. Moreover, Fashion Show Holograms provides designers with the opportunity to curate personalized and unique experiences for each viewer. With interactive features, users can manipulate the holographic garments, change colors, or even mix and match pieces to create their own customized looks. This interactive element promotes engagement and allows fashion enthusiasts to become active participants in the fashion show experience. Overall, Fashion Show Holograms merges technology and fashion to create a captivating and futuristic display of design. It represents an evolution in the way fashion is showcased, challenging traditional norms and offering exciting possibilities for both designers and viewers.

Fashion Show Live Streaming

Fashion Show Live Streaming refers to the process of broadcasting a fashion show in real-time over the internet, allowing viewers to watch the event from anywhere in the world. It involves capturing the runway event using cameras and transmitting the footage to online platforms, where it can be accessed by a wide audience. This technology has revolutionized the fashion industry by breaking down geographical barriers and making fashion shows accessible to a global audience. It allows designers to showcase their collections to a wider demographic, including fashion enthusiasts, industry professionals, and potential buyers who may not have the opportunity to physically attend the event.

Fashion Show Model Fittings

A fashion show model fitting is a crucial step in the process of preparing for a fashion show. It is an appointment that takes place prior to the show where the models try on the various garments that they will be wearing on the runway. The purpose of these fittings is to ensure that the clothes fit properly and look impeccable on the models, while also allowing the designers to make any necessary adjustments or alterations. During a fashion show model fitting, the models are typically asked to try on each outfit they will be wearing in the show. This includes clothes, shoes, accessories, and any other elements of the outfit. The fitting provides an opportunity for the designers to see how the garments look on the models and how they move and flow when worn. It also allows the designers to assess the overall aesthetic of the collection and make any necessary adjustments to achieve the desired look. In addition to the designers, there are often other key individuals present during the fittings. This may include stylists, fashion show directors, and members of the design team. Their input and feedback are valuable in ensuring that the final looks meet the vision of the designer and are cohesive with the overall theme of the show. During the fittings, the models may be asked to walk or pose in the outfits to simulate the runway experience. This helps the designers to visualize how the garments will look in motion and make any necessary modifications to enhance the overall presentation. The models may also be asked to provide feedback on the fit and comfort of the garments, as their input is valuable in ensuring that they feel confident and comfortable while wearing the outfits. Overall, fashion show model fittings play an integral role in the success of a fashion show. They allow the designers to perfect the fit and appearance of their garments and ensure that they are showcased to their full potential on the runway. These fittings are a collaborative process that involves the input and expertise of various individuals, and they contribute to creating a visually stunning and cohesive fashion show.

Fashion Show Pop-Up Shops

A fashion show pop-up shop is a temporary retail space that is set up specifically to showcase and sell a designer's collection immediately following a fashion show. These pop-up shops are typically located near the venue where the fashion show took place or in popular shopping areas to attract the attention of fashion enthusiasts and potential customers. Unlike traditional retail stores, fashion show pop-up shops are designed to create a unique and immersive shopping experience for customers. The temporary nature of these shops allows designers to experiment with innovative store layouts, decor, and atmospheres that align with the theme or aesthetic of their collection. This helps to create a cohesive brand experience for customers, strengthening the designer's brand identity. Fashion show pop-up shops often feature limited edition or exclusive items that are not available in regular retail stores. This scarcity and exclusivity can create a sense of urgency in customers, encouraging them to make a purchase immediately. Additionally, designers may offer special promotions or discounts during the pop-up shop to incentivize sales and create a buzz around their brand. These pop-up shops also serve as a platform for designers to directly interact with their customers. Designers or brand representatives are often present at the pop-up shops to provide styling advice, share the inspiration behind the collection, and connect with customers on a personal level. This direct interaction not only enhances the overall shopping experience but also allows designers to receive valuable feedback and insights from their target audience. Overall, fashion show pop-up shops are an effective strategy for designers to generate brand awareness, engage with customers, and drive sales. By creating a unique shopping experience and offering exclusive products, these temporary retail spaces help designers differentiate themselves in the competitive fashion industry and establish a strong connection with their target audience.

Fashion Show Press Release

p{font-weight:normal;} A fashion show press release is a formal document that provides information to the media and the public about an upcoming fashion show. It is usually written by the event organizers or public relations team and serves as a promotional tool to generate buzz and excitement for the show. The press release typically includes key details about the fashion show, such as the date, time, and location, as well as information about the featured designers and their collections. It may also highlight any special guests or celebrities who will be attending the event.

Fashion Show Production

A fashion show production is the intricate process of planning and executing a live event that showcases various designs and collections created by fashion designers. This event, often referred to as a runway show or fashion presentation, is a platform for designers to display their creations to the public, industry professionals, and potential buyers. The production of a fashion show involves several key components that work together to create a visually captivating and cohesive experience. These components include venue selection, set design, lighting and sound arrangements, model casting, choreography, hair and makeup styling, as well as overall event management and coordination.

Fashion Show Projection Mapping

Fashion Show Projection Mapping is a dynamic and innovative technology-driven concept that combines fashion design and projection mapping techniques to create a visually captivating and immersive runway experience. Projection mapping is a method of mapping 3D visuals onto 2D surfaces, in this case, the garments and accessories presented on the runway. It involves using specialized software to precisely align projected images with the contours and details of the clothing, creating an illusion of movement and transformation. By utilizing projection mapping in a fashion show, designers can push the boundaries of traditional runway presentations and elevate their collections to new heights of artistic expression. One of the main advantages of fashion show projection mapping is its ability to transform static garments into dynamic and interactive pieces of art. Through the use of visuals projected onto the clothing, designers can add animated patterns, textures, and colors that enhance the overall aesthetic and story of the collection. This technology allows for a seamless integration of digital elements into the physical world, blurring the line between fashion design and digital artistry. Furthermore, fashion show projection mapping offers designers endless creative possibilities. They can experiment with various visual effects, such as morphing shapes, illusionary textures, and virtual embellishments, that would be impossible to achieve solely with fabric manipulation. This technology opens up a realm of exploration where designers can push the boundaries of their designs and challenge the norms of traditional fashion shows. Moreover, fashion show projection mapping enables designers to create immersive and engaging narratives for their collections. They can transport the audience into different worlds, settings, and moods by projecting scenic backgrounds, atmospheric lighting, or even virtual models onto the runway. This allows viewers to experience fashion in a multi-dimensional and fantastical way, elevating the emotional connection between the audience and the designer's vision. In conclusion, Fashion Show Projection Mapping is a cutting-edge technology in the world of fashion design. It merges the realms of fashion and digital art, offering designers limitless possibilities to create visually captivating and immersive runway experiences. By combining projection mapping techniques with innovative garment designs, fashion shows become interactive, dynamic, and unforgettable events that redefine the boundaries of traditional runway presentations.

Fashion Show Rehearsals

Fashion Show Rehearsals are practice sessions in the field of fashion design where models, designers, stylists, and other members of the fashion industry prepare for an upcoming fashion show. These rehearsals are crucial for ensuring a seamless and visually appealing showcase of the designer's collection on the runway. During Fashion Show Rehearsals, models are guided through their movements, poses, and overall presentation on the catwalk. The choreographer or creative director instructs the models on how to walk, turn, and interact with props or other elements of the show. This ensures that the models are synchronized and showcase the clothes in the best possible way, capturing the essence and vision of the designer. In addition to the models, Fashion Show Rehearsals also involve the participation of hair stylists, makeup artists, and dressers. These professionals work together to create the desired look for each model, ensuring that their appearance complements the garments they are wearing. The dressers are responsible for assisting the models in quick changes backstage, ensuring that they appear in different looks at various stages of the show. The rehearsals also involve the fitting of garments on the models. This allows the designers to make any necessary adjustments to the clothes, ensuring a perfect fit and proper functionality on the runway. It is a collaborative process between the designer, models, and dressers to ensure that the outfits are worn effortlessly and look stunning during the show. Fashion Show Rehearsals are not solely focused on the models and their movements. They also include technical run-throughs where lighting, music, sound effects, and any special effects are tested and adjusted to create the desired mood and atmosphere for the show. The rehearsals allow the production team to fine-tune these elements, ensuring that they enhance the overall presentation of the designs. In summary, Fashion Show Rehearsals are the practice sessions that take place before a fashion show to ensure that all aspects of the show, including the models, clothing, styling, and technical elements, are flawlessly executed. They are crucial in creating a visually captivating and cohesive showcase of the designer's collection on the runway.

Fashion Show Run Of Show

A fashion show run of show is a comprehensive document that outlines the sequence and timing of events during a fashion show. It serves as a detailed guide for the designers, models, production team, and other key individuals involved in the show, ensuring that everything runs smoothly and according to plan. The run of show typically includes information such as the order of the fashion presentations, the models assigned to each look, the music and lighting cues, and any special effects or set changes. It also includes important backstage details such as the hair and makeup schedule, dress rehearsals, and any technical requirements. The purpose of the run of show is to maintain organization and coordination throughout the fashion show. By providing a clear timeline and precise instructions, it helps everyone involved understand their roles and responsibilities, ensuring that they are in the right place at the right time. This document acts as a blueprint for the entire production, allowing for a seamless execution of each segment. Fashion designers rely on the run of show to present their collections in the most effective and impactful way. It allows them to strategically plan the order of their designs, taking into consideration factors such as color schemes, styles, themes, and moods. By carefully arranging the looks, designers can create a coherent narrative or visual progression that highlights the unique aspects of their collections. Models also benefit from the run of show, as it provides them with the necessary information to prepare for their appearances on the runway. It specifies the outfits they will be wearing, the order in which they will walk, and any specific movements or poses they need to execute. This ensures that the flow of the show remains uninterrupted and that each model knows exactly what is expected of them. In summary, a fashion show run of show is a detailed plan that outlines the sequence and timing of events during a fashion show. It is a crucial tool that allows designers, models, and production teams to effectively organize and execute the show, ensuring a smooth and impactful experience for both the audience and the participants.

Fashion Show Set Design

Fashion Show Set Design is a crucial aspect of fashion design that focuses on creating the overall aesthetic and atmosphere for a fashion show. It involves the thoughtful and strategic arrangement of various elements, including props, lighting, staging, and scenery, to ensure a visually captivating and cohesive presentation. The set design serves as a backdrop that complements and enhances the fashion collection being showcased. It sets the mood and tone, while also providing a narrative and context for the clothing and accessories. Whether it's a simple minimalist stage or an elaborate, immersive environment, the set design helps create a memorable experience for the audience that aligns with the designer's creative vision.

Fashion Show Ticketing

Fashion Show Ticketing refers to the process of selling tickets for a fashion event or show, which allows individuals to attend and witness the display of new collections and designs by fashion designers. The ticketing system is an essential component in managing the audience and ensuring a smooth and organized event. The primary purpose of fashion show ticketing is to facilitate the reservation, sale, and distribution of tickets to members of the public who wish to attend the fashion show. The process typically involves various steps, including ticket creation, pricing, sales, and validation.

Fashion Show VIP Seating

Fashion Show VIP Seating refers to the exclusive and premium seating arrangement at a fashion show event specifically designed for distinguished guests, celebrities, influential personalities, industry professionals, and high-profile individuals. These attendees, often referred to as VIPs, are granted special privileges and luxuries that enhance their overall fashion show experience. The VIP seating area is strategically positioned and adorned with opulent furnishings to provide an elevated level of comfort, sophistication, and privacy.

Fashion Show Venue Selection

A fashion show venue is a carefully selected location where designers showcase their latest collections to industry professionals, media, and potential buyers. It serves as a platform for designers to display their creativity, craftsmanship, and overall brand image. The selection of a fashion show venue is crucial as it sets the tone and atmosphere for the collection presentation. The venue should align with the designer's brand identity and complement the overall aesthetic of the collection. It should also be able to accommodate the desired number of guests, provide appropriate lighting and sound systems, and offer sufficient space for runway setup and seating arrangements. Designers often choose unique and unconventional venues to create a memorable and immersive experience for the audience. These venues can range from art galleries, historical buildings, industrial warehouses, or even outdoor spaces. By selecting an unconventional venue, designers can add an element of surprise and novelty to their show, enhancing the overall impact of their collection. Factors such as location, accessibility, and logistics are also important considerations when selecting a fashion show venue. It should be easily accessible for guests arriving from different parts of the city or even from other countries. Additionally, the venue should have ample parking facilities or be well-connected to public transportation options. Moreover, the backstage area of the venue is equally important as it serves as the nerve center for the models, hairstylists, makeup artists, and dressers. It should have adequate space for changing rooms, hair and makeup stations, and storage for garments and accessories. The backstage area should be organized and efficient to ensure smooth transition between different segments of the fashion show. In conclusion, the selection of a fashion show venue plays a crucial role in the success of a collection presentation. It sets the stage for designers to showcase their work and create a lasting impression on the audience. A well-chosen venue should align with the designer's brand identity, provide adequate space and facilities, and contribute to an overall immersive experience for the attendees.

Fashion Show Video Mapping

Fashion Show Video Mapping is a creative technique used in fashion design to enhance the experience of a runway show through the use of digital projections onto the garments and the surrounding space. By incorporating video mapping technology into a fashion show, designers have the opportunity to transform the traditional runway presentation into a visually captivating and immersive experience. Video mapping involves projecting customized images, animations, and visual effects onto three-dimensional surfaces, such as garments, walls, or props, creating a dynamic and interactive spectacle.

Fashion Show Virtual Reality

Virtual Reality (VR) fashion shows are immersive and interactive digital experiences that showcase the latest fashion designs in a simulated environment. In these virtual showcases, designers can present their collections to a global audience without the limitations of physical space, time, or budget constraints. VR fashion shows allow viewers to navigate and explore the virtual environment, experiencing the collection from various angles and perspectives. Users can interact with the digital avatars or models, zoom in on the garments, and even change the colors or patterns of the outfits. Through the use of VR headsets, users can feel as if they are sitting in the front rows of a real fashion show, creating a sense of presence and engagement.

Fashion Show

A fashion show is a platform that showcases various clothing designs and accessories created by fashion designers. It is a visually stunning event where models walk on a runway, presenting the latest trends and styles to the audience. Fashion shows are an integral part of the fashion industry, serving as a medium to connect designers, retailers, and consumers. The primary purpose of a fashion show is to display and promote the designer's collection. Fashion designers create unique and innovative clothing pieces, often following a specific theme or inspiration. The fashion show allows them to present their creations in a controlled and choreographed environment, ensuring that every detail is highlighted. The models, dressed in the designer's collection, walk down the runway, allowing the audience to witness the garments' form, fit, and movement. In addition to showcasing the designer's collection, a fashion show also serves as a platform for networking and publicity. Fashion shows attract a diverse audience, including industry professionals, fashion enthusiasts, celebrities, and the media. Designers get the opportunity to interact with potential buyers, retailers, and other key players in the industry. They can build connections, negotiate contracts, and form partnerships that can help grow their brand and business. Fashion shows also create a buzz and generate publicity for the designers and their collections. The media covers these events extensively, providing exposure and visibility to the brands. News outlets, fashion magazines, and social media platforms share images and videos from the show, creating a ripple effect of promotion for the designers. Moreover, fashion shows play a crucial role in setting trends and shaping the fashion landscape. Designers use these events to introduce new styles, fabrics, colors, and silhouettes to the audience. The fashion industry closely follows these shows to predict the upcoming trends and incorporate them into their own designs. Fashion critics and influencers analyze and dissect the collections, providing feedback and commentary that influences consumer preferences. In conclusion, a fashion show is a prestigious event in the fashion industry that showcases a designer's collection, provides networking opportunities, generates publicity, and sets trends. It is a creative and dynamic platform that brings together designers, models, retailers, and fashion enthusiasts to celebrate and appreciate the art of fashion design.

Fashion Showroom

A Fashion Showroom is a physical space or a virtual platform that showcases and displays the latest collections and designs of fashion brands. It serves as a presentation platform where fashion designers and brands can exhibit their creations to potential buyers, industry professionals, and the general public. Within a fashion showroom, designers or brands create visually appealing displays that highlight their clothing, accessories, and other fashion items. These displays are carefully curated to reflect the brand's aesthetic and overall vision. The showroom may include various elements such as mannequins, racks, shelves, and props to enhance the presentation of the garments and accessories.

Fashion Silk

Fashion Silk refers to a luxurious and versatile fabric that is commonly used in fashion design. It is made from the natural fibers of the silkworm's cocoon, which are spun into a fine thread. Known for its lustrous appearance and smooth texture, silk has been highly valued for centuries and is associated with elegance and sophistication. Silk is considered one of the most sought-after fabrics in the fashion industry due to its numerous desirable qualities. Firstly, it is known for its natural sheen, which gives garments a luxurious and glamorous look. The fabric also drapes beautifully and has a soft, lightweight feel, allowing for comfortable and effortless movement. Additionally, silk has excellent temperature-regulating properties, keeping the wearer cool in warm weather and warm in cool weather. One of the key characteristics of fashion silk is its versatility. It can be used in a wide range of garments and accessories, including dresses, blouses, skirts, scarves, ties, and even lingerie. Silk can be woven or knitted into various patterns, allowing designers to create intricate and unique designs. Moreover, silk can be easily dyed, enabling the production of garments in a vast array of vibrant colors. Due to its high demand and rich history, silk has become a symbol of luxury and exclusivity in the fashion world. It is often used in high-end and couture fashion, where attention to detail and craftsmanship are paramount. Silk garments are typically associated with special occasions and formal events, as they exude an air of elegance and opulence. However, silk can also be incorporated into more casual, everyday outfits to add a touch of sophistication. In conclusion, fashion silk is a luxurious and versatile fabric made from the natural fibers of the silkworm's cocoon. It is renowned for its lustrous appearance, smooth texture, and excellent draping properties. With its wide range of uses and association with elegance, silk continues to be a highly prized fabric in the fashion industry.

Fashion Sketch

A fashion sketch is a two-dimensional representation of a garment or fashion design, usually created by hand or digitally. It serves as a visual blueprint for designers, allowing them to communicate their ideas and concepts to clients, manufacturers, and team members involved in the production process.The purpose of a fashion sketch is to convey the overall look, structure, and details of a garment before it is constructed. It showcases the designer's creativity, style, and vision, presenting a preview of the final product. The sketch includes important elements such as the silhouette, style lines, fabric choices, embellishments, and proportions.When creating a fashion sketch, designers use various techniques and materials to bring their ideas to life. They may use pencils, markers, watercolors, or digital software to draw the outline of the garment and add color and texture. The sketch may also feature additional elements like accessories, hairstyles, and makeup to complete the overall look.A fashion sketch typically focuses on the front view of the garment, showcasing its key features and design elements. However, designers may also include side or back views to provide a more comprehensive understanding of the design. The sketch may be accompanied by brief descriptions or notes that explain the designer's intentions, fabric choices, or construction techniques.Fashion sketches are essential tools in the fashion design process, serving as a visual language that enables designers to express their ideas accurately and convincingly. They facilitate effective communication between designers, clients, and manufacturers, ensuring that everyone involved in the production process has a clear understanding of the desired design. Fashion sketches help streamline the development process, minimize misunderstandings, and provide a reference point throughout the various stages of production.In conclusion, a fashion sketch is a visual representation of a garment or fashion design, created to communicate the designer's ideas, style, and vision. It showcases the overall look and details of the garment, serves as a blueprint for production, and facilitates effective communication in the fashion design industry.

Fashion Sketching

Fashion sketching is a fundamental skill in the field of fashion design that involves drawing and illustrating clothing designs to visually communicate the creative ideas of a designer. It is a crucial step in the design process as it allows designers to convey their concepts and bring their visions to life, serving as a blueprint for the creation of garments. Utilizing a range of artistic techniques and tools, fashion sketching involves the use of pencil, pen, markers, or digital software to create sketches that showcase various design elements such as silhouettes, fabrics, patterns, and details. These sketches serve as a visual representation of the designer's ideas, capturing the overall aesthetic and feel of the design.

Fashion Smart Casual

Smart casual is a dress code that effortlessly combines elements of both formal and casual attire. It represents a stylish and sophisticated way of dressing that is suitable for various social and professional settings. Fashion designers often create collections that incorporate the smart casual style, as it allows individuals to express their personal style while maintaining a polished and put-together look. Smart casual outfits typically consist of a combination of dressy and more relaxed garments. For men, this may include a well-fitted blazer or sports coat paired with tailored trousers or chinos. A button-down shirt or a polo shirt is often worn underneath, along with leather shoes or clean sneakers. It is essential to choose fabrics that are of high quality and in good condition to ensure a polished appearance. Women can opt for a variety of stylish options within the smart casual dress code. This may include a tailored blazer or cardigan paired with a blouse or a sweater. Skirts and dresses are also acceptable, as long as they are not too revealing or overly formal. Trousers or well-fitted jeans are often chosen along with stylish footwear such as pumps or fashionable flats. Accessories play a significant role in completing a smart casual outfit. For men, this may include a dress watch, a stylish belt, and a pocket square. Women can accessorize with statement jewelry, a belt to cinch the waist, and a stylish handbag. It is important to choose accessories that enhance the outfit without overpowering it. One of the key aspects of smart casual fashion is the ability to balance comfort and style. While the attire may be less formal than business or cocktail attire, it is still important to maintain a level of professionalism and refinement. Cleanliness, proper fit, and attention to detail are crucial elements in achieving a successful smart casual look. With its versatility and timeless appeal, smart casual fashion has become increasingly popular in modern society. It offers individuals the opportunity to express their personal style while adhering to the expectations of a particular dress code. By combining formal and casual elements in a harmonious way, smart casual fashion allows individuals to look effortlessly stylish and polished in any situation.

Fashion Socks

Fashion Socks: Fashion socks, also known as designer socks or statement socks, are a type of hosiery that is designed to showcase unique and fashionable patterns, colors, and styles. These socks have gained popularity as a trendy and expressive accessory in the world of fashion design. Fashion socks are created by fashion designers who incorporate their creative ideas and unique designs into the sock's aesthetic. These socks often feature bold patterns, intricate designs, and vibrant colors that make them stand out when worn. They are made using a variety of materials such as cotton, wool, nylon, and synthetic blends, which provide both comfort and durability. The primary purpose of fashion socks is to add a touch of personality and style to an outfit. They are often worn to make a fashion statement or to complement and enhance the overall look. Fashion designers utilize various techniques like jacquard knitting, embroidery, and digital printing to achieve intricate and eye-catching designs on the socks. These socks are versatile and can be styled in different ways to create various fashion looks. They can be paired with different types of footwear, such as sneakers, loafers, or even heels, depending on the desired style and occasion. Fashion socks are often worn with cropped pants, skirts, or dresses to draw attention to the legs and add visual interest to the overall ensemble. With the emergence of street-style fashion and the rise of fashion influencers on social media platforms, fashion socks have become a prominent trend. They are often featured in fashion editorials, runway shows, and street-style photography, contributing to their growing popularity. Overall, fashion socks serve as a unique and fashionable accessory that allows individuals to express their personal style. They have become an essential element in contemporary fashion design, offering endless possibilities for self-expression and creativity.

Fashion Sourcing Specialist

A Fashion Sourcing Specialist is a professional who plays a crucial role in the fashion design industry. This specialist is responsible for identifying, evaluating, and selecting the suppliers and manufacturers that will produce the materials and finished products needed for a fashion brand. The Fashion Sourcing Specialist collaborates with designers, merchandisers, and production teams to ensure that the brand's vision is translated into high-quality, cost-effective, and timely products. They have a deep understanding of the fashion industry's supply chain and stay updated on the latest trends, materials, and production techniques.

Fashion Sourcing Trips

Fashion sourcing trips refer to organized visits or tours undertaken by fashion designers or industry professionals to physically assess, evaluate, and select materials, fabrics, suppliers, and manufacturers for their fashion design creations. These trips often involve travel to different regions or countries known for their expertise in specific aspects of the fashion industry, such as textile production, leather goods, or jewelry.During fashion sourcing trips, designers aim to identify the best quality materials, innovative designs, and skilled artisans or factories that can bring their creative vision to life. These trips provide an opportunity for designers to establish direct contacts with suppliers and manufacturers, negotiate pricing and terms, and ensure the execution of their designs meets their desired standards of quality and craftsmanship.

Fashion Spandex

Fashion Spandex refers to a type of fabric commonly used in the field of fashion design. It is known for its stretchability, elasticity, and form-fitting nature. Fashion designers often incorporate spandex into their creations to achieve a tight, body-hugging fit, allowing garments to accentuate the curves of the wearer's body. Spandex, also known as elastane, is a synthetic fiber that was first developed in the late 1950s. Its unique properties make it an ideal choice for garments that require a high degree of stretch and recovery. The fabric is made by combining spandex fibers with other fibers, such as nylon or polyester, to create a blend that balances stretch with comfort.

Fashion Startup Incubator

A fashion startup incubator is a specialized program or organization that provides resources, guidance, and support to emerging fashion designers and entrepreneurs in order to help them successfully establish and grow their fashion-based businesses. Through an incubator, aspiring fashion designers can access a range of services and amenities designed to assist them in various aspects of their business development. These resources may include mentorship and advisory services, access to industry networks and contacts, workspace and studio facilities, educational workshops and training programs, funding opportunities, and exposure to potential investors or buyers.

Fashion Startup

A fashion startup refers to a newly established business in the fashion industry that aims to introduce innovative designs and ideas to the market. It is a venture driven by creativity, passion, and a vision for transforming the world of fashion. Typically, a fashion startup begins with a small team of designers, marketers, and entrepreneurs who come together to create a unique brand identity and product line. They strive to fill a gap in the market by offering garments, accessories, or services that are distinct from what established fashion brands provide. This differentiation can be through the use of unconventional materials, avant-garde design techniques, or by targeting an untapped niche market. One of the key aspects of a fashion startup is its emphasis on innovation and disruption. Startups in this industry aim to challenge traditional norms and push boundaries by introducing fresh perspectives and ideas. They often incorporate technology and sustainability into their processes, leveraging advancements in fabric development or implementing eco-friendly manufacturing practices. Furthermore, fashion startups are driven by the desire to capture the attention and loyalty of consumers who appreciate uniqueness and individuality in their clothing choices. They aim to inspire self-expression and personal style, enabling individuals to stand out from the crowd and make a statement through their apparel. In line with this ethos, many fashion startups also prioritize inclusivity and diversity, designing for a wide range of body types, genders, and cultural backgrounds. The success of a fashion startup depends on its ability to navigate the highly competitive fashion landscape and establish a strong brand presence. This includes effective marketing strategies, efficient supply chain management, and the cultivation of a loyal customer base. In conclusion, a fashion startup is a dynamic and innovative business venture in the fashion industry that aims to disrupt the market with inventive designs, unique branding, and a commitment to individual expression and diversity.

Fashion Streetwear

Fashion streetwear encompasses a style of clothing that emerged from urban culture and blends elements of sports, street fashion, and casual wear. It is characterized by its distinctive and unique designs, which often incorporate bold graphics, vibrant colors, and oversized or relaxed silhouettes. Fashion streetwear draws inspiration from the streets and subcultures such as skateboarding, hip-hop, and graffiti. It represents a rebellious and nonconformist attitude, challenging traditional fashion norms and embracing individuality and self-expression.

Fashion Studio Lighting

Fashion Studio Lighting refers to the specific lighting techniques used in a studio setting to enhance and create visually appealing images of fashion designs. It involves careful placement and manipulation of lighting equipment to highlight the details, colors, and textures of the garments or accessories being photographed. The goal of fashion studio lighting is twofold: to accurately represent the designer's vision and to create captivating images that will capture the attention of the target audience. Proper lighting can make the fabrics appear more luxurious, the colors more vibrant, and the overall design more eye-catching.

Fashion Styling

Fashion Styling is a crucial aspect of the fashion design industry, responsible for curating garments, accessories, and makeup to create visually appealing and cohesive looks. It is an art form that involves combining different elements of fashion, such as clothing, colors, patterns, textures, and silhouettes, to convey a specific style or message. As a fashion stylist, one must possess a deep understanding of current fashion trends, cultural influences, and the target audience to create a unique and visually striking aesthetic. They are tasked with selecting and coordinating outfits for various purposes, including editorial photoshoots, fashion shows, advertising campaigns, and celebrity appearances. The process of fashion styling begins with thorough research and analysis of the desired concept or theme. This includes studying fashion magazines, watching runway shows, and observing street style to gather inspiration and keep up with emerging trends. The stylist then carefully handpicks garments, accessories, and props that align with the chosen concept, taking into consideration factors such as color palettes, fabric textures, and stylistic details. Once the garments are selected, the fashion stylist focuses on creating harmonious outfits by combining different pieces in a way that flatters the human body and reflects the desired aesthetic. They pay attention to proportions, fit, and silhouette to ensure that the clothing enhances the wearer's physique and communicates the intended message. To complete the overall look, a fashion stylist also takes into account hairstyling and makeup. They collaborate with hair stylists and makeup artists to create hairstyles and makeup looks that complement the chosen outfits. This holistic approach to styling enhances the overall visual impact and elevates the concept to a higher level. Furthermore, a fashion stylist must possess excellent communication and interpersonal skills to effectively collaborate with photographers, models, designers, and other creative professionals involved in a fashion production. They should be detail-oriented and have a keen eye for aesthetics, as even the smallest details can significantly impact the final outcome. In essence, fashion styling is a transformative process that uses clothing, accessories, and makeup to create visually captivating looks. It is an integral part of fashion design, allowing designers to showcase their creations in a way that evokes emotions, tells a story, and captures the attention of the audience.

Fashion Stylist

A fashion stylist is a professional who works in the field of fashion design and is responsible for creating and executing the overall visual appearance of individuals or groups in various fashion contexts. Their role involves selecting and coordinating clothing, accessories, and other visual elements to create a desired aesthetic and convey a specific message or style. As a fashion stylist, their primary goal is to enhance the appearance and image of their clients by carefully curating outfits and creating cohesive looks that are in line with current fashion trends or specific themes. They must have a keen eye for detail and an ability to understand and interpret the individual style preferences and aesthetic goals of their clients. One of the key responsibilities of a fashion stylist is wardrobe selection. They meticulously choose clothing items, shoes, and accessories that complement the client's body shape, skin tone, and overall style. This requires a deep understanding of color palettes, silhouettes, and fabric textures, as well as knowledge of the latest fashion trends and designers. In addition to wardrobe selection, a fashion stylist also plays a crucial role in coordinating the overall visual concept for fashion shoots, runway shows, or editorial spreads. They collaborate with photographers, makeup artists, hair stylists, and other creative professionals to ensure that the desired aesthetic is achieved. This involves creating mood boards, selecting locations, and styling models or clients for the shoot or event. Furthermore, a fashion stylist is often called upon to provide fashion advice and consultation to clients, including celebrities, public figures, or individuals seeking personal style guidance. They may assess their clients' current wardrobe, offer suggestions for improvement, and provide recommendations for clothing and accessory purchases. In summary, a fashion stylist is a highly skilled professional who possesses a deep understanding of fashion design and trends. They are responsible for creating and executing visually appealing and cohesive looks, whether it be for individual clients, fashion events, or editorial shoots. Their role involves wardrobe selection, concept development, and providing fashion advice, all with the aim of enhancing the image and personal style of their clients.

Fashion Summit

A Fashion Summit is an event or gathering that brings together professionals, experts, and enthusiasts in the fashion industry to discuss and explore various topics related to fashion design, sustainability, and industry practices. During a Fashion Summit, attendees have the opportunity to participate in panel discussions, workshops, and lectures that cover a wide range of subjects, such as sustainable fashion, ethical manufacturing, innovation in design, and the future of the industry. The summit aims to create a platform for collaboration, education, and exchange of ideas, with the ultimate goal of driving positive change within the fashion industry.

Fashion Sunglasses

fashion sunglasses are a type of eyewear that are specifically designed to enhance and complement a person's overall fashion style. They are not only functional in terms of protecting the eyes from harmful UV rays, but also serve as a fashion accessory that can elevate an individual's look and make a style statement. When it comes to fashion design, sunglasses play a significant role in completing an outfit and adding a touch of personality. They come in a variety of shapes, sizes, colors, and materials, allowing designers to incorporate them into their collections and create unique and fashionable looks.

Fashion Supply Chain Management

Fashion Supply Chain Management refers to the strategic planning, coordination, and control of the activities involved in the production, distribution, and retailing of fashion products. It encompasses all the processes that take place from the conception of a fashion design to its delivery to the end consumer. In the context of fashion design, Fashion Supply Chain Management involves the management and coordination of various functions and stakeholders to ensure a smooth flow of materials, information, and products throughout the entire supply chain. This includes activities such as sourcing of raw materials, product development and design, production planning and manufacturing, logistics, distribution, and retailing. The key objective of Fashion Supply Chain Management is to meet the ever-changing demands of the fashion market while minimizing costs, maximizing efficiency, and ensuring timely delivery of fashion products. It requires effective collaboration and communication among designers, manufacturers, suppliers, distributors, and retailers. In the design phase, Fashion Supply Chain Management involves the selection of materials, suppliers, and manufacturing processes that align with the design concept and its target market. It also aims to optimize the use of resources and minimize waste in the production process. Once the design is finalized, Fashion Supply Chain Management ensures that the production is efficiently planned, coordinated, and monitored to meet the desired quality, quantity, and delivery timelines. It involves the sourcing of materials, management of production facilities and workforce, and implementation of quality control measures. The distribution and retailing phase of Fashion Supply Chain Management focuses on the efficient movement of fashion products from the manufacturing facility to the retail outlets or directly to the end consumer. This includes transportation, warehousing, inventory management, and customer service. Overall, Fashion Supply Chain Management plays a vital role in the success of fashion design by ensuring the availability of fashionable products in the right place, at the right time, and in the right quantity. It requires careful planning, coordination, and monitoring of all activities involved in the fashion supply chain to meet the ever-changing demands of the fashion industry.

Fashion Supply Chain

A fashion supply chain refers to the entire process and network of activities involved in the production and distribution of fashion products, from the initial design concept to the final delivery to the end customer. It encompasses various stages, including sourcing of raw materials, production, distribution, and retail. At the sourcing stage, fashion designers and companies identify and select the raw materials needed to create their products. This may involve working with suppliers and manufacturers to ensure the quality and availability of materials. The sourcing stage also includes considerations such as sustainability, ethical sourcing practices, and cost efficiency. The production stage involves transforming the raw materials into finished fashion products. This may include designing and pattern making, fabric cutting, sewing, and quality control. Production can take place either in-house or through outsourcing to manufacturers or factories, depending on the company's resources and strategies. The distribution stage focuses on the transportation and logistics involved in delivering the fashion products to the market. This includes activities such as warehousing, inventory management, and transportation. Companies need to consider factors like lead times, order quantities, and delivery schedules to ensure their products reach customers in a timely and efficient manner. Lastly, the retail stage involves the selling of fashion products to consumers through various channels, including physical stores and e-commerce platforms. Retail operations may involve store layout and merchandising, sales strategies, and customer service. Retailers need to keep up with changing fashion trends, manage inventory, and create engaging shopping experiences to attract and retain customers.

Fashion Sustainability Metrics

Fashion sustainability metrics refer to the methods and tools used to measure and evaluate the environmental, social, and economic impact of fashion design and production processes. These metrics enable fashion designers and industry stakeholders to assess and improve the sustainability performance of their products throughout their lifecycle. In the context of fashion design, sustainability metrics provide a framework for quantifying and analyzing the sustainability aspects of garments, accessories, and textiles. They help designers understand and assess the environmental impacts of raw material sourcing, manufacturing processes, transportation, use, and end-of-life disposal. Social aspects such as labor conditions, worker rights, and community impacts are also considered under these metrics. The key purpose of fashion sustainability metrics is to promote more sustainable practices by providing a standardized and measurable way to compare the sustainability performance of different fashion products and production methods. By using these metrics, fashion designers can identify areas for improvement and make informed decisions about materials, suppliers, manufacturing techniques, and design choices. Some commonly used sustainability metrics in fashion design include: - Water footprint: Measures the amount of water consumed and polluted during the production of textiles and garments. - Carbon footprint: Quantifies the greenhouse gas emissions associated with the entire lifecycle of a fashion product, including raw material extraction, manufacturing, transportation, use, and disposal. - Waste generation: Assesses the amount of waste generated at different stages of the fashion supply chain, from raw material extraction to end-of-life disposal. - Chemical usage: Evaluates the types and quantities of chemicals used in textile processing, dyeing, and finishing, considering their potential environmental and human health impacts. - Social impact: Considers the working conditions, fair wages, and social welfare of workers involved in the production of fashion products. By using these sustainability metrics, fashion designers can measure their progress towards sustainability goals, identify areas of improvement, and communicate transparently about their sustainability performance to industry stakeholders and consumers.

Fashion Sustainability Panel

A fashion sustainability panel refers to a group of experts, professionals, and stakeholders who come together to discuss and address the environmental, social, and economic impacts of the fashion industry. The panel aims to explore and promote sustainable practices, policies, and solutions in the field of fashion design.The fashion industry is notorious for its negative impact on the environment and society. It is the second largest polluter in the world, contributing to carbon emissions, water pollution, and waste generation. In addition, it often perpetuates labor exploitation and poor working conditions in its supply chains.The fashion sustainability panel plays a crucial role in advocating for change and fostering dialogue among key players in the industry. The panel members may include fashion designers, industry executives, policymakers, environmental activists, academics, and representatives from non-governmental organizations (NGOs).Through their collective expertise, the panel aims to assess the existing problems and challenges in the fashion industry and propose innovative solutions to address them. They focus on promoting sustainable practices throughout the entire lifespan of a garment - from design and production to distribution and consumption.The panel's discussions may cover a wide range of topics, including eco-friendly materials and manufacturing processes, waste reduction and recycling initiatives, supply chain transparency, fair labor practices, and promoting circular fashion models.Furthermore, the panel engages in knowledge-sharing activities to increase awareness and understanding of sustainability issues within the fashion industry and among consumers. This can include organizing conferences, workshops, and exhibitions, as well as collaborating with educational institutions to integrate sustainability into fashion design curricula.By bringing together diverse perspectives and expertise, the fashion sustainability panel acts as a catalyst for change, encouraging collaboration and cooperation among industry stakeholders. Their goal is to create a more sustainable and responsible fashion industry that considers environmental, social, and economic factors in its decision-making processes.The work of the fashion sustainability panel is essential for driving the necessary transformation towards a more sustainable and ethical fashion industry. Through their collective efforts, they can influence trends, policies, and consumer behavior, ultimately leading to positive change and a more sustainable future for fashion design.

Fashion Sustainable Fashion

Fashion Sustainable Fashion is a design approach that seeks to minimize the negative impact of the fashion industry on the environment, while also considering social and ethical factors. It involves the development, production, and consumption of fashion items in ways that are environmentally friendly, socially responsible, and economically viable. At its core, Fashion Sustainable Fashion aims to achieve a balance between fashion and sustainability. It takes into account the entire life cycle of a fashion product, from the sourcing of materials to the final disposal. This approach emphasizes the use of eco-friendly materials, such as organic fibers, recycled fabrics, and low-impact dyes, which are less harmful to the environment and human health. In addition to eco-conscious materials, Fashion Sustainable Fashion promotes responsible manufacturing practices. This can include reducing waste, conserving energy and water, and implementing fair labor standards. It also encourages transparency and traceability throughout the supply chain, ensuring that workers are treated ethically and paid fair wages. Furthermore, Fashion Sustainable Fashion encourages mindful consumption by promoting longer product lifecycles and reducing the amount of clothing that ends up in landfills. This can be achieved through the design of timeless and durable pieces, as well as by encouraging repair, recycling, and upcycling of garments. It also encourages consumers to make informed choices and prioritize quality over quantity. Overall, Fashion Sustainable Fashion acknowledges the environmental and social impacts of the fashion industry and seeks to address them through responsible design practices. It recognizes that fashion can be a powerful force for positive change and advocates for a more holistic and conscious approach to creating and consuming fashion items.

Fashion Swimwear

Fashion Swimwear refers to a type of clothing designed specifically for use in water-based activities such as swimming, sunbathing, and water sports. It is a subset of the wider fashion industry that focuses on creating stylish and functional swimwear garments for both men and women. The design of fashion swimwear takes into consideration various factors such as comfort, fit, style, and durability. It aims to provide individuals with clothing that not only allows them to move freely in the water but also enhances their appearance and boosts their confidence. Fashion swimwear designers often incorporate innovative materials, patterns, and techniques to create unique and eye-catching designs. When designing fashion swimwear, designers carefully choose fabrics that are suitable for contact with water. These fabrics are typically chosen for their ability to dry quickly and resist fading and stretching. Additionally, designers consider the level of sun protection provided by the swimwear, as exposure to harmful ultraviolet (UV) rays can be detrimental to the skin. Another important aspect of fashion swimwear design is the consideration of body types and individual preferences. Designers create swimwear styles that cater to various body shapes and sizes, ensuring that everyone can find a flattering garment that suits their personal style. They may incorporate features such as adjustable straps, padding, and underwire to provide additional support and enhance the wearer's natural curves. Furthermore, fashion swimwear designs are influenced by current trends and the latest fashion movements. Designers take inspiration from runway shows, street style, and popular culture to create swimwear designs that are both trendy and timeless. This allows individuals to express their personal style while enjoying water-based activities. In conclusion, fashion swimwear is a specialized category within the fashion industry that focuses on creating stylish and functional garments for water-based activities. Designers consider factors such as comfort, fit, style, durability, sun protection, and body types when creating swimwear designs. By incorporating innovative materials and following current trends, fashion swimwear designers cater to the diverse needs and preferences of individuals seeking fashionable swimwear options.

Fashion Symposium

A Fashion Symposium is an organized discussion or conference that focuses on various aspects of fashion design. It provides a platform for industry professionals, designers, scholars, and students to exchange ideas, showcase their work, and engage in critical dialogue about fashion. During a Fashion Symposium, experts present their research, insights, and experiences related to fashion design, including but not limited to fashion history, trends, sustainable practices, cultural influences, and innovation. These presentations may be in the form of lectures, panel discussions, presentations, or visual demonstrations. The purpose of a Fashion Symposium is to foster collaboration, encourage interdisciplinary dialogue, and challenge traditional notions of fashion design. It serves as a space for creative individuals to explore new perspectives, push boundaries, and address pressing issues within the fashion industry. In addition to presentations, Fashion Symposiums often feature exhibitions, fashion shows, and workshops that allow participants to engage with fashion design in a practical and immersive manner. These events provide opportunities for networking, mentoring, and career development. Furthermore, a Fashion Symposium plays a crucial role in documenting and preserving fashion heritage. It allows for the exchange of knowledge and expertise, enabling the sharing of best practices and the development of innovative approaches in fashion design. Overall, a Fashion Symposium serves as a platform for creative exchange, critical discourse, and community building within the field of fashion design. It contributes to the growth and evolution of the fashion industry by fostering collaboration, inspiring innovation, and promoting sustainability and inclusivity.

Fashion Tailored Suit

A fashion tailored suit is a type of formal attire that is custom-made to fit an individual's body measurements and specifications. It is designed and crafted by skilled fashion designers and tailors to ensure a precise and flattering fit. The process of creating a fashion tailored suit involves several steps, starting with taking precise measurements of the individual's body. These measurements are then used as a guide to cut and shape the fabric, ensuring that it will fit the individual perfectly. The fabric used for a tailored suit is typically of high quality, such as fine wool or silk, chosen for its durability, drape, and luxurious look and feel. Once the fabric is cut, it is stitched together using traditional sewing techniques or modern methods, depending on the designer's preference. The stitching is done with great attention to detail, ensuring that the seams are strong and invisible, and that the garment will hold its shape and structure over time. One of the key features of a fashion tailored suit is its ability to enhance the wearer's silhouette and accentuate their best features. Tailoring techniques such as darts, pleats, and shaping seams are used to create a flattering silhouette that highlights the individual's body shape. A fashion tailored suit is typically composed of several pieces, including a jacket, trousers or skirt, and sometimes a vest or waistcoat. The jacket is usually single-breasted or double-breasted, with a variety of lapel styles to choose from, such as notch, peak, or shawl lapels. The trousers or skirt are tailored to fit the individual's waist and hips, with options such as pleats or flat fronts. In addition to the fit and construction, the design of a fashion tailored suit can be customized to reflect the individual's personal style. Various options for colors, patterns, and fabrics are available, allowing the individual to create a unique and stylish look that suits their taste and occasion. Overall, a fashion tailored suit is a sophisticated and timeless garment that exudes elegance and professionalism. With its impeccable fit and attention to detail, it is a go-to choice for formal events such as weddings, business meetings, or any occasion where a polished and refined appearance is desired.

Fashion Tailoring

Fashion tailoring is a specialized technique in fashion design that involves the creation and alteration of garments to ensure a perfect fit for an individual's body shape and size. The process of fashion tailoring starts with taking precise measurements of the client's body, including the bust, waist, hips, and length of various body parts. These measurements serve as a blueprint for creating or altering the garment to achieve the desired fit and look. Fashion tailors are skilled artisans who have a deep understanding of how different fabrics drape and conform to the body. They use their expertise to manipulate fabric and stitch it together in a way that accentuates the wearer's best features while minimizing any flaws or imperfections. In addition to creating or altering clothing, fashion tailoring also involves the selection of appropriate fabrics, buttons, zippers, and other embellishments to enhance the overall design and functionality of the garment. One of the key principles of fashion tailoring is attention to detail. Tailors meticulously sew each seam, ensuring that it is aligned and maintains the structural integrity of the garment. They also meticulously finish edges, add linings where necessary, and apply any necessary trim or embellishments to achieve a polished and professional look. Throughout the process, fashion tailors may need to make adjustments and alterations to ensure a proper fit. This may involve taking in or letting out seams, shortening or lengthening sleeves or hems, and reshaping the garment to conform to the client's body shape. These alterations are done with precision and care to ensure that the final result is a garment that fits the client's unique body proportions perfectly. In summary, fashion tailoring is a specialized technique in fashion design that involves the creation and alteration of garments to achieve a perfect fit. By utilizing precise measurements, skilled craftsmanship, and attention to detail, fashion tailors create garments that not only flatter the wearer's body but also reflect their personal style and taste.

Fashion Tapes

Fashion tapes are an essential tool utilized in fashion design to secure garments in place, enhance the overall appearance, and provide a seamless finish. These tapes are commonly made of adhesive materials that have been specially designed to be gentle on the skin yet strong enough to withstand the movements and strains associated with wearing clothing. Unlike traditional pins or stitching, fashion tapes offer a temporary solution for quick adjustments and modifications without causing any damage or leaving visible marks on the fabric. Fashion tapes are frequently employed in various fashion scenarios such as runway shows, photoshoots, red carpet events, or simply for everyday wear. They serve multiple purposes, including preventing wardrobe malfunctions by keeping garments in place, creating smooth silhouettes by seamlessly adhering fabrics together, and providing added support to ensure a comfortable and secure fit. Designers and stylists often rely on fashion tapes to maintain the desired shape and structure of garments. They can be strategically applied to neckline edges, shoulder seams, side slits, or any area that requires discreet attachment. By using fashion tapes, fashion professionals can effortlessly achieve clean lines, eliminate visible straps or bra outlines, and prevent fabrics from slipping or bunching up during movement. Furthermore, fashion tapes also offer practical solutions for individuals who wish to tailor their clothing to their specific measurements or preferences. They enable users to temporarily adjust hem lengths, secure oversized or loose fabrics, or create unique draping effects, all without the need for permanent alterations. Overall, fashion tapes are a versatile and indispensable accessory for fashion designers, stylists, and individuals alike. They provide a quick, convenient, and non-invasive method for securing garments, ensuring a flawless and polished appearance. By utilizing fashion tapes, individuals can confidently wear their chosen outfits without worrying about slip-ups or the need for last-minute adjustments.

Fashion Tech Conference

A fashion tech conference is an event that brings together fashion designers, technology experts, industry professionals, and fashion enthusiasts to explore the intersection of fashion and technology. This conference serves as a platform for showcasing innovative ideas, discussing the latest trends and advancements in fashion technology, and fostering collaborations between fashion and tech communities. At a fashion tech conference, attendees have the opportunity to attend panel discussions, workshops, and presentations led by industry experts. These sessions cover various topics such as wearable technology, digital fashion, sustainability in fashion, e-commerce, virtual reality, augmented reality, and artificial intelligence in fashion.

Fashion Tech Integration

Fashion Tech Integration refers to the incorporation of technology into the field of fashion design to enhance and innovate the products, processes, and experiences associated with fashion. It involves the utilization of various technological tools, materials, and concepts to integrate technology seamlessly into the design and production of garments, accessories, textiles, and other fashion-related products. This integration allows for the creation of novel designs, improved functionality, and enhanced user experiences in the fashion industry. Fashion Tech Integration encompasses a wide range of technologies, including but not limited to wearable electronics, 3D printing, virtual reality, augmented reality, fabric technology, and smart textiles. Wearable electronics involve the integration of electronic components, such as sensors, lights, and displays, into clothing and accessories to add functionality or create interactive experiences. 3D printing technology enables the creation of complex and customizable fashion items with reduced waste and increased efficiency. Virtual reality allows designers and consumers to explore and visualize virtual environments, facilitating the design process and enhancing the shopping experience. Augmented reality overlays digital content onto real-world environments, enabling virtual try-on and enhancing customer engagement. Fabric technology and smart textiles incorporate advanced materials and manufacturing techniques that provide performance-enhancing properties, such as moisture-wicking, temperature regulation, or embedded sensors for health monitoring.

Fashion Technology

Fashion technology refers to the integration of technology and fashion design processes for creating innovative and functional clothing and accessories. It encompasses the use of various technologies such as computer-aided design (CAD) software, 3D printing, smart fabrics, wearable technology, and digital manufacturing techniques to revolutionize the fashion industry. The main objective of fashion technology is to combine the principles of fashion design with technological advancements to enhance creativity, efficiency, and sustainability in the production and consumption of fashion products. With the integration of CAD software, fashion designers can now easily create digital sketches and patterns, minimizing the need for manual drafting and reducing production time. This technology also allows for accurate measurements, scaling, and modifications, resulting in better fitting garments. 3D printing plays a significant role in fashion technology by enabling designers to transform their virtual designs into tangible prototypes. This technology allows for the creation of complex and customized pieces, reducing waste and cost in the production process. Smart fabrics and wearable technology have revolutionized the fashion industry by incorporating functionality and interactivity into clothing. These technologies enable the integration of sensors, electronics, and connectivity, resulting in garments that can monitor the wearer's health, adapt to environmental changes, and enhance performance. Digital manufacturing techniques, such as laser cutting and robotic sewing, are being increasingly adopted in fashion technology to automate and streamline production processes. These techniques not only enhance efficiency but also reduce material waste and human labor. In conclusion, fashion technology is the fusion of fashion design and technological advancements. It allows for the creation of innovative, functional, and sustainable fashion products by leveraging tools such as CAD software, 3D printing, smart fabrics, wearable technology, and digital manufacturing techniques.

Fashion Textile Design

Fashion Textile Design refers to the process of creating textile designs specifically for the fashion industry. It involves the application of various artistic and technical skills to produce unique and innovative patterns and prints that are used in the production of garments and accessories. The field of fashion textile design requires a combination of creativity, technical proficiency, and understanding of the fashion market and trends. Fashion designers, textile artists, and printmakers collaborate to develop textiles that are not only visually appealing but also functional and appropriate for the intended clothing or accessory. The process of fashion textile design begins with extensive research into trends, colors, and themes that are relevant to the target market. Designers gather inspiration from various sources such as fashion shows, art exhibitions, nature, and cultural references. They analyze and interpret these inspirations, and then develop concepts and mood boards to guide the creation of their textile designs. Once the concept is established, fashion textile designers experiment with different techniques and materials to create unique patterns and textures. They may employ traditional methods such as hand-dyeing, screen printing, or embroidery, as well as utilize modern digital printing technologies. It is essential for designers to have a thorough understanding of different textile materials, their properties, and the effects that can be achieved through different techniques. After the initial designs are created, fashion textile designers collaborate with manufacturers, garment designers, and stylists to ensure that the textile designs seamlessly integrate with the overall fashion collection. They consider factors such as scale, placement, and color harmony to ensure that the textiles enhance the aesthetics and functionality of the garments or accessories. The role of fashion textile design extends beyond the creation of patterns and prints. It also involves exploring sustainable and eco-friendly materials and processes, as well as continually staying updated on technological advancements in the field. By combining artistic vision, technical expertise, and market awareness, fashion textile designers play a crucial role in the creation of visually striking and commercially successful fashion products.

Fashion Tights

Fashion tights are a type of hosiery specifically designed for fashion purposes in the field of fashion design. They are similar to regular tights in terms of their structure and material composition, but they are distinguished by their unique patterns, colors, and textures. Fashion tights are worn as a statement piece to enhance the overall aesthetic appeal of an outfit and add a touch of style and creativity. These tights are crafted using various materials such as nylon, polyester, spandex, and cotton. The choice of material depends on the desired texture, elasticity, and durability. Fashion tights can be opaque, translucent, or sheer, allowing for different levels of coverage and skin exposure. One of the key features of fashion tights is their wide range of patterns and designs. They can be found in solid colors, prints, stripes, polka dots, animal prints, geometric shapes, and many other artistic motifs. These patterns are applied through various techniques such as screen printing, digital printing, or jacquard weaving. Fashion tights are a versatile accessory that can be worn with various types of clothing. They can be paired with skirts, dresses, shorts, or even layered under ripped jeans for a bold and fashionable look. The choice of color and pattern should complement the overall outfit and create a harmonious visual balance. When it comes to styling, fashion tights offer endless possibilities. They can be the focal point of an ensemble, drawing attention to the legs, or they can be used to create a cohesive and coordinated look by matching them with other elements of the outfit, such as shoes, handbags, or belts. Fashion tights can also be used to highlight specific body parts or add an element of contrast to an otherwise monochromatic outfit. In conclusion, fashion tights are a type of hosiery that serves as a fashion statement in the field of fashion design. They are characterized by their unique patterns, colors, and textures, which are used to enhance the aesthetic appeal of an outfit. Fashion tights offer versatility in terms of material, density, and styling, making them a popular accessory for those who seek to express their personal style and creativity.

Fashion Trade Association

The Fashion Trade Association is an industry organization comprised of fashion designers, manufacturers, retailers, and other professionals involved in the fashion design and trade sector. Its main objective is to foster collaboration and promote the growth and success of its members in the highly competitive and constantly evolving fashion industry. The association provides a platform for its members to network, share knowledge and ideas, and access resources and support to enhance their professional development and business operations. Through various initiatives and programs, the Fashion Trade Association aims to facilitate the exchange of information and expertise among its members, as well as provide opportunities for professional development and education. It organizes workshops, seminars, and conferences to address industry trends, technologies, and best practices. These events also serve as forums for members to showcase their designs, products, and innovations, thus enabling potential partnerships and business opportunities to flourish. Moreover, the Fashion Trade Association serves as an advocate for its members' interests and concerns, acting as a collective voice on important issues affecting the fashion design and trade sector. It actively engages with governmental bodies, industry regulators, and other relevant stakeholders to influence policy, legislation, and regulations in favor of its members and the industry as a whole. In addition to its networking and advocacy efforts, the Fashion Trade Association collaborates with other industry organizations and institutions to foster collaboration and knowledge-sharing. It establishes partnerships with educational institutions to support the development of future fashion designers and professionals, providing scholarships, internships, and mentorship programs to aspiring talents. Overall, the Fashion Trade Association plays a vital role in shaping the fashion industry by bringing together professionals, facilitating knowledge-sharing and collaboration, advocating for industry interests, and nurturing the next generation of fashion designers and professionals. Its activities contribute to the growth, innovation, and sustainability of the fashion design and trade sector.

Fashion Trade Show

A fashion trade show is a specialized event in the fashion industry where designers, brands, retailers, and other industry professionals come together to showcase and promote their latest collections, products, and services. It serves as a platform for networking, business transactions, and trend analysis. At a fashion trade show, various participants set up booths or exhibition spaces to display their offerings. These can include clothing, accessories, footwear, jewelry, textiles, and other fashion-related items. The booths are often designed in a visually appealing and unique manner to attract visitors and create a memorable brand experience. The primary purpose of a fashion trade show is to enable designers and brands to connect with potential buyers. Retailers, boutique owners, and department store representatives attend trade shows to discover new brands, establish relationships with designers, and place orders for their stores. These face-to-face interactions are crucial for building business partnerships and expanding market reach. In addition to buyer interactions, fashion trade shows also provide a platform for industry professionals to gain insights into the latest fashion trends and market developments. Designers can gather feedback on their collections and receive industry recognition through various awards and competitions held during the event. They can also connect with media representatives and influencers, potentially leading to increased media coverage and brand exposure. Fashion trade shows are often organized by professional event management companies or fashion industry associations. These organizations ensure that the trade show runs smoothly by coordinating logistics, managing exhibitor registrations, and promoting the event to ensure maximum participation. In conclusion, a fashion trade show is a crucial event in the fashion industry where designers, brands, and retailers gather to showcase their collections, connect with buyers, and gain insights into the latest trends. It serves as a platform for business transactions, networking, and industry recognition.

Fashion Trade Shows

Fashion trade shows are events specifically organized for fashion designers, retailers, buyers, and other industry professionals to showcase and promote their latest collections, products, and services.These trade shows provide a platform for fashion designers to exhibit their creations, ranging from clothing, accessories, footwear, and jewelry, to potential buyers and retailers who are actively seeking new trends and designs to enhance their product offerings.During fashion trade shows, designers set up booths or spaces where they display their products and interact with potential buyers. They use various marketing techniques and strategies to attract attention, such as creative displays, visual merchandising, and informative catalogs or lookbooks.Additionally, fashion trade shows often feature runway shows or presentations, where designers can showcase their collections on models, giving buyers and attendees a firsthand look at the garments' fit, fabric, and overall aesthetic. This live experience allows buyers to assess the quality and design of the garments before making purchasing decisions.Trade shows also serve as a networking opportunity for fashion industry professionals. Designers can connect with other designers, manufacturers, suppliers, and industry experts, fostering collaborations and partnerships that can help them grow their business.Furthermore, fashion trade shows offer valuable market insights and industry trends. Attendees have the opportunity to participate in panel discussions, seminars, or workshops conducted by industry leaders, which provide valuable knowledge about the current market, consumer preferences, and emerging trends.In conclusion, fashion trade shows are important events in the fashion industry, providing designers with a platform to showcase their latest collections, connect with buyers, and gain valuable market insights. These events play a significant role in shaping the fashion industry and driving business growth for designers and retailers alike.

Fashion Trend Analysis

A fashion trend analysis is a systematic process of studying and interpreting the evolving patterns and shifts in the fashion industry. It involves analyzing various elements such as clothing styles, color palettes, fabric choices, and design techniques that dominate the fashion landscape. Fashion designers and industry professionals conduct trend analysis to understand the present market scenario and anticipate future consumer demands. By keeping abreast of the latest fashion trends, they gain insights into what styles and aesthetics are preferred by consumers, helping them design and create products that have a higher likelihood of success in the market.

Fashion Trends Symposium

A fashion trends symposium is a gathering or conference in the field of fashion design where experts, professionals, and enthusiasts come together to discuss and analyze current and emerging fashion trends. It serves as a platform for individuals to exchange ideas, gain insights, and deepen their understanding of the ever-evolving world of fashion. During a fashion trends symposium, participants engage in various activities such as presentations, panel discussions, workshops, and exhibitions. These activities are designed to provide attendees with valuable information about the latest fashion trends, including the colors, silhouettes, fabrics, styles, and cultural influences that are shaping the industry.

Fashion Trends

Fashion Trendsetter

A fashion trendsetter is an individual or entity that establishes and popularizes new fashion styles or influences existing ones. They are often at the forefront of the fashion industry, showcasing their unique sense of style and creativity through their designs and personal fashion choices. Trendsetters can be fashion designers, celebrities, influencers, style icons, or even fashion brands. They have a discerning eye for fashion and possess the ability to identify emerging styles, create innovative designs, and introduce them to the wider public. Their influence extends beyond their own fashion choices, as they shape the direction of the industry and inspire others to follow their lead.

Fashion Trendspotting

Fashion trendspotting is the practice of observing and analyzing current and emerging trends in fashion design in order to identify new and popular styles, ideas, and concepts. It is a crucial aspect of fashion forecasting, which involves predicting and anticipating upcoming trends to guide the design and production of clothing and accessories. Trendspotting is both a creative and analytical process that requires a deep understanding of fashion history, cultural influences, and societal shifts. Through trendspotting, fashion designers and industry professionals can gain insights into consumer preferences, create innovative designs, and stay ahead of the competition. Trendspotters primarily rely on their sensory perception, intuition, and aesthetic sensibilities to identify emerging trends. They closely observe street style, fashion shows, magazines, social media, and other sources of inspiration to detect recurring motifs, color palettes, silhouettes, and materials.

Fashion Tulle

Fashion tulle is a lightweight, fine netting fabric that is commonly used in the fashion design industry. It is known for its delicate appearance and ability to add volume and texture to garments. Tulle is made from various fibers including silk, nylon, polyester, or rayon, and it can be found in a variety of colors and patterns. Tulle is often used in the construction of skirts, dresses, and veils, where it is layered or gathered to create a voluminous effect. Its airy and translucent quality adds a romantic and ethereal touch to garments, making it a popular choice for formal and bridal wear. Tulle is versatile and can be used in a variety of ways in fashion design. It can be layered over other fabrics to add dimension, used as an overlay to create a sheer effect, or used as a decorative element in the form of ruffles or bows. It can also be used to create accessories such as gloves, scarves, or headpieces. In addition to its aesthetic appeal, tulle also has practical uses in fashion design. Its lightweight nature and soft drape make it comfortable to wear, allowing for ease of movement. Tulle is also relatively easy to work with, as it can be sewn, gathered, and manipulated without a lot of effort. When working with tulle, fashion designers often consider its texture, color, and weight to achieve the desired effect. The texture of tulle can vary depending on the type of fiber used and the construction of the fabric. It can range from soft and flowing to stiff and structured. The color of tulle can be chosen to complement or contrast with the other fabrics in a garment, adding visual interest. The weight of tulle can also be adjusted depending on the desired volume and drape. Overall, fashion tulle is a versatile and aesthetically pleasing fabric that adds texture, dimension, and a touch of romance to garments. Its lightweight nature and ease of manipulation make it a popular choice for designers in the fashion industry.

Fashion Tuxedo

A fashion tuxedo is a formal attire designed for men, typically worn for special occasions such as weddings, galas, or black tie events. It is a symbol of elegance, style, and sophistication, representing the pinnacle of men's formalwear. The tuxedo is characterized by its distinct features, including a tailored jacket, trousers, and matching accessories. The jacket of a fashion tuxedo is tailored to fit the wearer's body shape, usually made from high-quality materials like wool, silk, or velvet. It typically features a satin lapel, which adds a touch of luxury and elegance. The jacket can be single-breasted or double-breasted, depending on the wearer's personal preference. It may also have one or two buttons, with the buttons often covered in satin or matched to the fabric of the jacket. The trousers of a fashion tuxedo are designed to complement the jacket, usually made from the same material. They are tailored to fit properly, ensuring a sleek and polished look. The trousers often have a satin stripe along the sides, adding a stylish element to the overall ensemble. In addition to the jacket and trousers, a fashion tuxedo is complete with several matching accessories. These include a formal dress shirt, typically made from cotton or silk, with a wingtip or spread collar. A bow tie or a formal necktie is worn around the collar, either in a matching fabric or a contrasting color for added flair. Other accessories that complete the look of a fashion tuxedo include a cummerbund or a waistcoat, worn around the waistline to add a touch of formality. A pocket square made from silk or linen is often placed in the jacket's breast pocket, adding a subtle pop of color. Additionally, formal shoes, usually patent leather Oxford or Derby shoes, complete the ensemble with their polished finish. A fashion tuxedo is a timeless and classic choice for men's formalwear, exuding confidence and elegance. It is a staple in any man's wardrobe, allowing him to stand out and make a statement at formal events. Whether worn with a traditional black and white color combination or in more modern variations with different colors and patterns, the fashion tuxedo embodies refinement and refinement in the world of fashion design.

Fashion Upcycled Fashion

Fashion Upcycled Fashion refers to a design approach in the fashion industry that focuses on creating and reinventing garments or accessories using discarded or unused materials. It is a sustainable and innovative practice that aims to reduce waste and environmental impact while showcasing unique and creative designs. Upcycling involves taking existing materials or items and transforming them into new, high-quality products with improved value. In the context of fashion design, upcycled fashion involves the repurposing of textiles, fabrics, and various clothing items that would otherwise be discarded or considered waste.

Fashion Vegan Fashion

Vegan fashion refers to the practice of designing and creating clothing and accessories that are made without the use of any animal products or by-products. It is a form of ethical and sustainable fashion that promotes the well-being and protection of animals, as well as the environment. In vegan fashion design, designers utilize materials that are free from animal-derived components, such as leather, fur, silk, wool, and feathers. Instead, they opt for alternatives like plant-based fabrics (such as cotton, linen, hemp, bamboo, and pineapple leather), synthetic textiles, recycled materials, and innovative cruelty-free alternatives.

Fashion Velvet

Fashion Velvet is a luxurious fabric commonly used in fashion design. It is characterized by its soft and smooth texture, as well as its rich and vibrant colors. Velvet is created by weaving a blend of synthetic or natural fibers in a specific way that creates a dense pile on the surface of the fabric, giving it a unique sheen and plushness. This fabric has been used in fashion for centuries and is often associated with elegance, sophistication, and glamour. It is commonly used to create dresses, skirts, jackets, and other garments that require a touch of luxury and opulence. Velvet is also used for accessories such as handbags, shoes, and hats, adding a touch of richness to any outfit. One of the key features of Fashion Velvet is its ability to reflect light in a unique way, creating a subtle shimmer that adds depth and dimension to the fabric. This makes it a popular choice for evening wear and formal attire, as it has a flattering effect in low-light settings. The richness of the colors also contributes to its versatility, allowing it to be easily incorporated into both casual and high-end fashion designs. In addition to its aesthetic appeal, Fashion Velvet also offers practical benefits. The dense pile of the fabric provides warmth, making it a popular choice for winter and cooler climates. It is also durable and resistant to wrinkles, making it a practical choice for garments that require frequent wear and use. When it comes to caring for Fashion Velvet, it is important to handle it delicately. The fabric should be spot cleaned or dry cleaned to maintain its luxurious appearance and texture. Ironing should be done on the reverse side of the fabric or with a cloth in between to prevent crushing the pile. In conclusion, Fashion Velvet is a luxurious and versatile fabric that adds a touch of elegance and richness to any fashion design. Its soft and smooth texture, vibrant colors, and unique light-reflecting properties make it a popular choice for formal and evening wear. Whether used for garments or accessories, Fashion Velvet is a timeless and sophisticated choice in the world of fashion.

Fashion Vintage Fashion

Fashion Vintage Fashion refers to the style of clothing and accessories that were popular between the 1920s and the 1980s. It is a form of fashion design that draws inspiration from the past, incorporating garments and accessories that are either authentic vintage pieces or contemporary reproductions. The use of the term "vintage" in fashion is often misunderstood. True vintage clothing refers to garments and accessories that were produced in a different era and have stood the test of time. These pieces are typically of high quality, made with attention to detail and craftsmanship. They are often unique and possess a certain charm and character that is hard to find in modern clothing. Vintage fashion enthusiasts often value the historical and sentimental significance of these pieces. Fashion designers who specialize in vintage fashion draw inspiration from various decades, incorporating elements from iconic eras such as the glamorous 1920s flapper style, the elegant 1950s pencil skirts, the mod and psychedelic 1960s, and the bold and exaggerated styles of the 1980s. They may also take inspiration from specific subcultures or movements, such as the bohemian hippie style of the 1970s or the punk rock aesthetic of the 1980s. When creating vintage-inspired designs, fashion designers carefully study the silhouettes, fabrics, prints, and details of the past. They aim to recreate the essence of a particular era while adapting it to suit modern tastes and trends. This may involve incorporating vintage-inspired elements into contemporary designs or reimagining and updating vintage pieces with a modern twist. Vintage fashion has gained popularity in recent years due to its ability to stand out in a world of mass-produced fast fashion. It offers individuals a chance to express their unique style and personality through clothing that tells a story and carries a sense of nostalgia. Vintage fashion celebrates the beauty and timelessness of fashion history, allowing individuals to connect with the past while staying relevant and fashionable in the present.

Fashion Visual Display

Fashion Visual Display refers to the art and technique of arranging and presenting merchandise in a visually appealing manner to enhance the overall shopping experience and promote sales in the fashion retail industry. It involves the creative use of space, lighting, color, props, and various display techniques to effectively showcase fashion products, convey brand identity, and create a captivating atmosphere that engages customers and drives their desire to purchase. Fashion visual display plays a crucial role in attracting attention, arousing interest, and influencing buying decisions. The goal of fashion visual display is to create visually appealing and immersive spaces that effectively communicate the brand's message, evoke emotions, and entice customers to explore and engage with the showcased products. It requires a deep understanding of the target audience, brand identity, and current fashion trends, as well as a keen eye for aesthetics and composition. Through careful arrangement and organization of merchandise, fashion visual display aims to highlight the unique features, quality, and style of the products, while also creating a sense of aspiration and desirability. It involves the strategic placement of mannequins, props, and signage to create engaging product stories and visual narratives that reflect the brand's image and story. In addition, fashion visual display also includes the thoughtful consideration of lighting and color schemes, as they have a significant impact on the overall perception and mood of the space. The use of appropriate lighting can enhance the details and texture of garments, while colors can evoke certain emotions and create a cohesive and harmonious visual experience. Overall, fashion visual display is a vital aspect of fashion design and retail, as it serves as a powerful marketing tool that helps brands differentiate themselves, establish an emotional connection with customers, and ultimately drive sales. It requires a combination of creativity, strategic thinking, and an understanding of consumer behavior to create visually stunning displays that effectively communicate the brand's message and inspire customers to make a purchase.

Fashion Vlog

A fashion vlog, short for fashion video blog, is a digital platform where individuals share their personal style, trends, and fashion advice through video format. It is a form of online content creation that focuses specifically on fashion-related topics. A fashion vlog typically features a fashion influencer or enthusiast who records and edits videos to showcase their sense of style, fashion hauls, outfit ideas, and fashion-related experiences such as attending events or trying out new trends. These videos are often accompanied by commentary, tips, and recommendations to guide viewers in their own fashion journey.

Fashion Wallet

A fashion wallet is a small, typically flat and compact accessory designed to store and organize essential items such as cash, cards, and identification in a fashionable and stylish manner. As a key component of the fashion industry, fashion wallets go beyond mere functionality and serve as a statement piece that reflects personal style and complements the overall outfit or ensemble. They come in a wide variety of materials, colors, patterns, and designs to cater to diverse fashion tastes and preferences.

Fashion Watch

A fashion watch is a type of wristwatch that is designed with a focus on style and trendiness, rather than just functionality. Fashion watches are created by fashion designers or fashion houses, who bring their unique sense of style and design to the watch industry. These watches often incorporate the latest fashion trends, materials, and colors, allowing wearers to make a fashion statement while also keeping track of time.

Fashion Webinar

A fashion webinar is a virtual event that focuses on providing educational and informative content related to fashion design. It offers a platform for fashion enthusiasts, aspiring designers, and industry professionals to gain knowledge, insights, and inspiration from experts in the field. During a fashion webinar, participants can expect to learn about various aspects of fashion design, including fashion history, garment construction techniques, textile selection, trend forecasting, and styling. The content is typically presented through live or pre-recorded video sessions, accompanied by supporting slides or visuals. One of the key benefits of a fashion webinar is its accessibility. Participants can join the event from anywhere in the world, as long as they have an internet connection. This eliminates the need for travel and allows individuals to attend the webinar from the comfort of their own homes or offices. Furthermore, fashion webinars often provide opportunities for interaction and engagement. Participants can ask questions, share their opinions, and network with other attendees through live chat features or dedicated Q&A sessions. This fosters a sense of community and allows for a more dynamic learning experience. Another important aspect of fashion webinars is their ability to cater to a wide range of interests and skill levels. Whether someone is a beginner looking to learn the basics of fashion design or a seasoned professional seeking advanced techniques and industry insights, there are webinars available to suit their needs. In conclusion, a fashion webinar offers a convenient and interactive way for individuals to expand their knowledge and skills in fashion design. By leveraging the power of technology, these virtual events provide valuable educational content to fashion enthusiasts and aspiring designers worldwide.

Fashion Week

Fashion Week is a highly anticipated event in the world of fashion design. It is a series of runway shows, presentations, and exhibitions that showcase the latest collections of designers and fashion houses. This event takes place bi-annually in various fashion capitals around the world, including New York, Paris, London, and Milan. During Fashion Week, designers have the opportunity to display their creations to a wide audience, including influential industry professionals, buyers, journalists, and celebrities. The shows are typically held in prestigious venues and are meticulously choreographed to create a visually stunning and memorable experience for attendees.

Fashion Weeks

Fashion Weeks are highly anticipated and prestigious events that showcase the latest trends and designs in the world of fashion. They are organized biannually in fashion capitals around the globe, such as New York, Paris, Milan, and London, to name a few. Fashion Weeks serve as a platform for designers, brands, and industry professionals to present their collections and creations to a global audience, including buyers, journalists, celebrities, and fashion enthusiasts. During Fashion Weeks, designers showcase their collections through runway shows, presentations, or installations. These events are meticulously planned and orchestrated to create a captivating experience that highlights the creativity, craftsmanship, and innovation in fashion design. Fashion Weeks not only provide a glimpse into the seasonal trends but also serve as a reflection of the cultural, social, and artistic influences shaping the fashion industry.

Fashion White Tie

White Tie is a formal dress code in fashion design, typically reserved for upscale and prestigious events. It is considered the most formal attire for evening wear, and it represents the epitome of elegance and sophistication. This dress code is commonly associated with diplomatic and state events, royal occasions, high-class parties, and ceremonies. White Tie attire for men consists of a tailcoat, vest, and bow tie, while women are required to wear a full-length ball gown or evening dress. Every aspect of the White Tie ensemble is meticulously chosen to create a harmonious and refined look.

Fashion Wholesaler

A fashion wholesaler is a company or individual that buys clothing and accessories directly from manufacturers and sells them in bulk to retailers. They serve as intermediaries between clothing manufacturers and retailers, facilitating the distribution process and ensuring a steady supply of fashionable products for retail stores. Fashion wholesalers play a crucial role in the fashion industry by connecting manufacturers with retailers. They have a deep understanding of the fashion market and trends, allowing them to curate collections that appeal to different target markets. By purchasing clothing and accessories in large quantities, they can negotiate better prices with manufacturers and pass on those cost savings to retailers.

Fashion Wool

Fashion wool refers to the use of wool fiber in the creation of clothing and accessories that are designed to be stylish and trendy. Wool is a natural fiber that comes from sheep and is known for its warmth, softness, and durability. It is a popular choice in fashion design due to its unique properties and versatility. When used in fashion design, wool can be woven, knitted, or felted to create a wide range of garments and accessories. Wool fabrics can be textured, such as tweed or herringbone, or smooth and fine, such as merino wool. The natural crimp and elasticity of wool make it suitable for creating garments with a good drape and fit. Fashion wool is often used in the creation of winter wear, such as coats, jackets, and sweaters, as it provides excellent insulation and warmth. Wool fibers are capable of trapping air pockets, retaining heat, and wicking away moisture, making it ideal for cold weather garments. Additionally, wool is naturally fire-resistant, adding an extra layer of safety and practicality. In addition to its practical advantages, wool is also a versatile material in terms of design. It can be dyed easily and holds colors well, allowing for a wide spectrum of hues and patterns. Wool can be blended with other fibers, such as silk or cashmere, to enhance its softness, sheen, and drape. It can also be treated and processed in various ways to achieve different textures, finishes, and weights. Furthermore, fashion wool is a sustainable choice. Wool is a renewable resource, and sheep are shorn annually without harm. It is biodegradable and breaks down naturally without releasing harmful substances into the environment. In recent years, there has been a growing demand for eco-friendly and ethical fashion, and wool fits into this ethos. In conclusion, fashion wool is a natural fiber that is highly regarded in the world of fashion design. Its warmth, durability, versatility, and sustainability make it a favored choice for creating stylish and trendy clothing and accessories. The unique properties of wool allow for endless possibilities in terms of design, texture, and color. From winter coats to cozy sweaters, fashion wool is a timeless and practical option for fashion-conscious individuals.

Fashion Workshop

A fashion workshop is a structured learning environment where individuals can gain knowledge and develop skills in the field of fashion design. It provides a platform for aspiring designers to engage in hands-on activities, collaborate with industry professionals, and enhance their understanding of various aspects of the fashion industry. During a fashion workshop, participants are exposed to a wide range of topics that are relevant to the field of fashion design. These topics can include garment construction, pattern making, fabric selection, fashion illustration, fashion business management, and trend forecasting. Through practical exercises and demonstrations, participants are able to learn the techniques and methods involved in creating clothing and accessories. A fashion workshop typically offers a combination of theoretical and practical sessions, allowing participants to simultaneously gain knowledge and apply it in a creative manner. This hands-on approach allows individuals to explore their creativity and develop their unique design aesthetic. By engaging in practical exercises, participants can also gain a deeper understanding of the technical aspects of fashion design, such as the use of different sewing techniques and the manipulation of fabric. Additionally, fashion workshops often provide opportunities for networking and collaboration. Participants have the chance to interact with industry professionals, including established designers, fashion buyers, and fashion journalists. This exposure can be invaluable for aspiring designers, as it allows them to gain insights into the industry and build valuable connections. Overall, a fashion workshop is a dynamic learning environment that provides individuals with the necessary skills and knowledge to pursue a career in fashion design. By offering a combination of theoretical and practical sessions, it enables participants to develop their creativity, technical skills, and business acumen in the field of fashion. Through collaborative opportunities and exposure to industry professionals, fashion workshops provide aspiring designers with a stepping stone to success in the highly competitive fashion industry.

Fashionista

Fashionista is a term commonly used in the world of fashion design to describe an individual who has a deep passion and keen interest in fashion. A fashionista is someone who not only follows the latest trends and styles but also possesses an innate ability to effortlessly put together chic and stylish outfits. They have a thorough understanding of different fabrics, patterns, colors, and silhouettes, and can creatively combine these elements to create unique and fashion-forward looks. A fashionista's sense of style is often admired and emulated by others, as they have a natural flair for selecting garments and accessories that suit their body type, personality, and the occasion. They are not afraid to take risks and experiment with different styles, embracing both classic and cutting-edge fashion to create a one-of-a-kind look.

Faux Fur Vest

A faux fur vest is a type of garment in the field of fashion design that is designed to resemble the appearance and texture of real fur, but it is made without using any animal products. It is typically made from synthetic materials such as acrylic, polyester, or modacrylic fibers, which are constructed to imitate the look and feel of natural fur. Faux fur vests are popular in the fashion industry due to their versatility and ethical appeal. They can be worn as a stylish outerwear piece or used as a statement accessory to enhance an outfit. The design of a faux fur vest usually features a sleeveless silhouette, allowing it to be layered over various clothing items like long-sleeved tops or dresses. When it comes to the design details, faux fur vests can vary in length, from hip-length options to longer, knee-length versions. They can also come with various closure options, such as front zippers, hook-and-eye fastenings, or even open-front designs. Some faux fur vests may also include additional elements like pockets or decorative accents such as belts or buckles. The versatility of faux fur vests allows them to be styled in numerous ways. They can be paired with jeans and a basic top for a casual yet chic look, or dressed up with a skirt or trousers for a more elevated ensemble. Faux fur vests can be layered over a variety of garments, from turtlenecks and sweaters to blouses and dresses, making them suitable for both colder and milder weather. In conclusion, a faux fur vest is a fashionable garment that mimics the appearance and texture of real fur while using only synthetic materials. Its sleeveless design and various length options make it a versatile piece that can be styled in numerous ways. With its ethical appeal and ability to add a touch of glamour to any outfit, the faux fur vest has become a popular choice in the fashion industry.

Flapper Dress

A flapper dress is a type of women's dress that was popular in the 1920s, during the era known as the Roaring Twenties. This style of dress was characterized by its loose and straight silhouette, which was a departure from the more fitted and structured styles of the previous decade. Flapper dresses were typically made from lightweight materials such as silk or chiffon, which allowed for ease of movement and a fluid drape. The defining features of a flapper dress were its dropped waistline and short hemline. The waistline of the dress was often positioned at the hips or just below, creating a more boyish and androgynous silhouette. The hemline, called the "shocking length" at the time, fell above the knee, which was considered scandalously short in comparison to the ankle-length skirts of the past. This shorter hemline allowed for more freedom of movement and reflected the changing social attitudes of the time. Flapper dresses were also known for their embellishments and decorative details. The dresses were often adorned with sequins, beads, or fringe, adding movement and sparkle to the garment. These embellishments were often concentrated around the hemline, neckline, or sleeves, creating a visual focal point and drawing attention to the wearer. In terms of color and pattern, flapper dresses embraced bold and vibrant choices. Art Deco motifs, geometric shapes, and exotic prints were popular during this time period. Bold colors such as red, blue, and gold were frequently seen, as well as contrasting color combinations and color blocking techniques. Flapper dresses were a reflection of the changing societal norms and attitudes of the Roaring Twenties. The style became associated with the flapper lifestyle, which was characterized by women challenging traditional gender roles, embracing independence, and participating in the newfound freedoms and opportunities of the post-World War I era. The flapper dress encapsulated the spirit of this era, with its unconventional silhouette, short hemline, and bold embellishments, making it an iconic symbol of the 1920s.

Flare Jeans

Flare jeans, also known as bell-bottoms or bootcut jeans, are a style of jeans that are characterized by their wide and bell-shaped leg openings. They were originally popularized in the 1960s and 1970s as a fashion statement and signify a sense of retro nostalgia in contemporary fashion design. The defining feature of flare jeans is the exaggerated width of the leg openings, which gradually widens from the knee down. This flared shape creates a visually striking silhouette that accentuates the wearer's legs and adds a sense of drama to their overall appearance. The leg openings are typically wide enough to cover or skim over the wearer's footwear, such as heels or boots, hence the name "bootcut."

Fleece Jacket

A fleece jacket is a type of outerwear garment that is constructed using a soft and fuzzy synthetic fabric called fleece. It is designed to provide warmth and insulation to the wearer, making it a popular choice for outdoor activities or as a layering piece in colder weather. Characterized by its lightweight and breathable nature, fleece jackets are highly versatile and can be worn in a variety of settings. They can be found in various styles, including full-zip, half-zip, or pullover designs, allowing for easy on and off and the ability to adjust the level of ventilation. Fleece jackets are known for their exceptional thermal properties. The fabric's unique construction traps air within its fibers, effectively creating a layer of insulation that helps to retain body heat. This makes fleece jackets an excellent choice for maintaining warmth without sacrificing mobility or comfort. When it comes to design, fleece jackets often feature a range of functional elements. These may include zippered pockets for storage, adjustable cuffs or hemlines for a customizable fit, and a high collar or hood for added protection against wind and cold. Additionally, they may have reinforced panels or overlays on high-wear areas to enhance durability. One of the key advantages of fleece jackets is their moisture-wicking properties. Unlike natural fibers such as cotton, fleece has the ability to pull moisture away from the body, keeping the wearer dry and comfortable during physical activities or in damp weather conditions. In terms of aesthetics, fleece jackets can be found in an array of colors and patterns, catering to various style preferences. From solid neutrals to vibrant hues or even prints inspired by nature, there are options to suit every individual's taste. Overall, a fleece jacket is a practical and functional garment that offers warmth, insulation, and comfort. Whether worn as a standalone piece or as a layering component, it is a staple in many wardrobes, particularly in regions with cold or unpredictable weather.

Floral Romper

A floral romper is a type of clothing item that combines the characteristics of a romper and floral patterns to create a unique and versatile fashion piece. A romper, also known as a playsuit, is a one-piece garment that combines a top and shorts. It is typically made of lightweight and casual materials, making it perfect for warm weather and casual occasions. Rompers are popular among both men and women, although floral rompers are usually designed for women. The defining feature of a floral romper is the incorporation of floral patterns or prints. These patterns can range from small, delicate flowers to bold and vibrant blooms. Floral prints are often inspired by nature, and they can add a feminine and playful touch to any outfit. Floral rompers come in various colors and designs, allowing individuals to express their personal style. Floral rompers are popular during the spring and summer seasons when floral patterns are typically associated with blooming flowers and warmer weather. They are versatile pieces that can be dressed up or down depending on the occasion. For a casual look, floral rompers can be paired with sandals or sneakers. To create a more formal outfit, they can be styled with heels or wedges and accessorized with statement jewelry. When designing a floral romper, fashion designers consider factors such as fabric choice, pattern scale, and silhouette. The choice of fabric can impact the overall look and feel of the romper, with lightweight and breathable materials being preferred for warm weather. Pattern scale refers to the size of the floral prints, with larger prints often making a bolder statement. Silhouette choices include fitted, loose, or tailored designs, allowing for various levels of comfort and flexibility. Overall, a floral romper is a fashion-forward and versatile clothing item that combines the practicality of a romper with the timeless beauty of floral patterns. Its popularity during the spring and summer seasons makes it a must-have piece for individuals looking to add a touch of femininity and playfulness to their wardrobe.

Fray Check

Fray Check is a liquid product used in fashion design to prevent fabric from unraveling or fraying. It is typically applied to the raw edges of fabric, such as hems, seams, or cut edges, to reinforce the fibers and prevent them from fraying over time. The purpose of Fray Check is to ensure the longevity and durability of garments by preventing loose threads and frayed edges. It acts as a sealant by creating a clear, flexible barrier that binds the fabric fibers together, effectively preventing them from unraveling or fraying. When working with delicate or fraying fabrics, such as chiffon, silk, or satin, or when creating garments with raw edges or fringed details, Fray Check is an essential tool in a fashion designer's arsenal. By applying it to the exposed edges of the fabric, designers can prevent unraveling and maintain the overall quality and appearance of the garment. One of the main advantages of Fray Check is its ease of use. It comes in a small bottle with an applicator tip, allowing for precise and controlled application. To use Fray Check, designers simply squeeze the bottle gently and apply a thin line of the liquid along the edge of the fabric. It dries quickly, forming a clear and invisible protective barrier. It is important to note that Fray Check should be used sparingly and only on the edges that require reinforcement. Overuse of the product can create stiffness or discoloration in the fabric. Additionally, it is advisable to test Fray Check on a small, inconspicuous area of the fabric before applying it to the entire garment. Overall, Fray Check is a valuable tool for fashion designers, providing a reliable solution to prevent fabric fraying and ensure the longevity of their creations. By using this product, designers can achieve professional-quality finishes and maintain the integrity of their garments.

Frayed Hem Jeans

Frayed Hem Jeans are a type of denim pants characterized by their intentionally unravelled or fringed bottom edge. This distinctive feature sets them apart from regular jeans and adds a touch of edginess and individuality to any outfit. Frayed hems are achieved by cutting off the original hemline of the jeans and allowing the fabric to naturally fray over time. This creates a raw, unfinished look that is often associated with a casual and relaxed aesthetic. The fraying effect can vary in length and intensity, ranging from a few loose threads to a more substantial fringed edge. Frayed hem jeans provide a versatile and trendy option for the fashion-forward individual. They can be found in various styles and cuts, including skinny, straight, flared, or wide-legged. Additionally, they are available in different washes, from light blue to dark indigo, allowing for a wide range of outfit possibilities. These jeans can effortlessly elevate a casual look and add a touch of effortless coolness. They are often paired with simple t-shirts, blouses, or sweaters, making them an easy choice for everyday wear. Frayed hem jeans can also be dressed up by combining them with statement tops, blazers, or heels for a more sophisticated and polished ensemble. In terms of footwear, these jeans can be worn with a variety of shoe styles. Sneakers and sandals can create a relaxed and laid-back vibe, while ankle boots or high heels can add a touch of elegance and sophistication. The versatility of frayed hem jeans makes them suitable for any season and occasion. When it comes to accessorizing, frayed hem jeans give fashion enthusiasts the opportunity to express their personal style. They can be paired with belts, scarves, or hats to add an extra layer of detail and visual interest. Additionally, they can be combined with different types of jewelry, such as layered necklaces or statement earrings, to complete the look. Overall, frayed hem jeans are a fashion staple that adds a modern and distinctive twist to any wardrobe. Their unique detailing and effortless style make them a popular choice among fashion-forward individuals who seek to make a statement with their outfits.

Fraying Tools

Fraying tools, in the context of fashion design, refer to a set of instruments or equipment used to intentionally create frayed or worn-out edges on fabric or garments. This technique is often employed to achieve a distressed or vintage look in clothing or accessories, adding a touch of authenticity and character. The basic premise of fraying tools revolves around the concept of unraveling or loosening the fibers of a fabric, resulting in a fringed or frayed appearance. These tools typically include but are not limited to: - Seam rippers: Seam rippers are small, sharp tools with a pointed end and a curved blade. They are primarily used for removing stitches, but can also be used to create deliberate fraying by gently pulling on the fabric threads. - Tweezers: Tweezers with a fine tip are often employed to carefully tease and separate individual threads and fibers, helping to create a more controlled and precise frayed effect. - Sandpaper: Sandpaper, typically a medium to coarse grit, can be used to manually distress the edges of fabric by rubbing it against the surface. This action weakens the threads and fibers, resulting in a frayed appearance. - Wire brushes: Wire brushes with firm bristles are commonly used to roughen up the surface of fabrics, causing the fibers to become unraveled and creating a distressed or frayed look. Fraying tools empower fashion designers with the ability to experiment and push the boundaries of traditional garment construction. By utilizing these tools, designers can introduce an element of deconstruction and individuality to their creations. The intentional fraying of fabric edges not only adds visual interest but can also evoke a sense of nostalgia or a worn-in aesthetic, which has become a popular trend in contemporary fashion.

Fringe Cutters

A fringe cutter is a tool used in fashion design to create fringes on fabric or trim. It consists of a sharp blade attached to a handle, which allows the user to easily cut precise and even strands of fabric. Fringes are decorative elements made by cutting several parallel strands of fabric, often in a straight line or pattern. The fringe cutter is an essential tool for designers who want to add texture and movement to their garments or accessories. Fringes can be used on various types of fabrics, such as silk, satin, chiffon, or suede, to create a range of different looks and effects.

Fringe Sweater

A fringe sweater is a type of sweater that features fringed trim or detailing. The fringe is typically made from strands of fabric or yarn that are attached to the edges or hemline of the garment. The fringe can be short or long, and may hang loosely or be tightly woven. Fringe sweaters are popular in fashion design for their unique and bohemian-inspired look. The fringe trim adds texture and movement to the sweater, creating a visually interesting and playful effect. It can also give the sweater a more relaxed and casual vibe, making it a versatile and stylish addition to any wardrobe.

Fur Stole

A fur stole is a luxurious accessory in fashion design that is typically made from fur and worn draped around the shoulders and neck. It is a long and narrow piece, often with pointed ends, that adds elegance and warmth to an outfit. Fur stoles have a long history and have been a popular fashion choice for centuries. They were originally worn by women as a way to display wealth and social status. In the early 20th century, fur stoles became particularly fashionable, and they were commonly worn by Hollywood starlets and socialites.

Fusible Interfacing

Fusible interfacing is a fabric material used in the field of fashion design to provide structure, stability, and reinforcement to various types of garments and accessories. It is commonly used in areas such as collars, cuffs, waistbands, and buttonholes to add strength and support. Fusible interfacing is typically made of polyester or cotton fibers that have been coated with a thin layer of adhesive on one side. When applied with heat and pressure, the adhesive side of the interfacing bonds to the main fabric, creating a firm and stable surface. This bonding process eliminates the need for stitching the layers together, resulting in a clean and seamless finish. Fusible interfacing is available in various weights and thicknesses, allowing designers to choose the most appropriate option for their specific garment or accessory.

Garment Bags

Garment bags, in the context of fashion design, refer to protective bags specifically designed to store and transport clothing items. These bags are commonly used by fashion designers, stylists, and individuals who want to keep their garments organized and well-preserved. The primary purpose of garment bags is to protect clothing from dust, dirt, and other potential damages. By providing a barrier between the garments and the external environment, these bags help to prevent stains, wrinkles, and discoloration. They are especially useful for preserving delicate and expensive fabrics, such as silk, lace, and cashmere, which can easily get damaged or snagged during transportation or storage.

Garment Construction

Garment construction refers to the process of creating wearable garments through the assembly of fabric pieces using various sewing techniques. It is an essential aspect of fashion design that requires technical expertise and precision to bring a designer's vision to life. The garment construction process involves multiple stages, starting from pattern-making to the final finishing touches. Designers begin by creating a pattern, which serves as a blueprint for the garment. They take measurements, draft the patterns, and then cut the fabric accordingly. Accuracy in pattern-making is crucial as it determines the fit and shape of the garment. Next, the fabric pieces are stitched together using different sewing techniques. This may include techniques like straight stitching, zigzag stitching, and overlocking, depending on the design and fabric type. Seams are carefully created to ensure durability and a clean finish. Additionally, designers may incorporate decorative elements like pleats, ruffles, or topstitching to enhance the aesthetic appeal of the garment. During the construction process, designers also consider proper garment fitting. This involves making adjustments to the garment's shape and size to ensure it flatters the wearer's body. Common fitting alterations include taking in or letting out seams, shortening or lengthening hems, and adjusting sleeve lengths. Finishing touches play a crucial role in garment construction. These include tasks like hemming, adding closures (such as buttons, zippers, or hooks), attaching linings or interfacings, and applying trims or embellishments. Finishing ensures that the garment appears polished and ready for use. Garment construction requires a deep understanding of fabric properties, sewing techniques, and construction methods. It is a combination of technical skills and artistic vision, as designers must not only create garments that are visually appealing but also functional and comfortable to wear. The construction process should result in a well-constructed garment with proper finishing, impeccable stitching, and precise fit. In conclusion, garment construction is an integral part of fashion design that involves transforming fabrics into finished garments through pattern-making, cutting, stitching, fitting, and finishing. It requires meticulous attention to detail, technical proficiency, and a creative flair to bring a designer's vision to life.

Garment Fit And Alterations

Garment fit refers to the way a piece of clothing conforms to the body when worn, taking into account the body's size, shape, and proportions. It is an integral aspect of fashion design, as the fit of a garment can greatly affect its overall aesthetics and comfort. Achieving the perfect fit involves careful consideration of various factors such as pattern design, fabric choice, and the use of alterations.Alterations, on the other hand, are modifications made to a garment to ensure a better fit. They can involve minor adjustments or more significant changes to the garment's structure and silhouette. Alterations are typically performed by skilled tailors or seamstresses who possess the technical knowledge and expertise to manipulate the fabric and construction of a garment.

Garment Labels

Garment Labels in the context of fashion design are small pieces of fabric or other materials that are attached to clothing items to provide essential information about the garment. They serve as a form of communication between the brand and the consumer, conveying important details about the product's composition, care instructions, size, and origin. Garment labels are typically sewn into the inside of the clothing, near the collar or waistline. They can also be found on clothing tags or hangtags, depending on the brand's preference and design. These labels are crucial for both the brand and the consumer, as they offer valuable information that affects the overall experience and use of the garment.

Garment Steamers

A garment steamer is a device commonly used in the field of fashion design to remove wrinkles and creases from clothing and fabrics without the necessity of an ironing board or iron. This innovative tool primarily uses steam to relax the fibers within the garments, allowing for easy manipulation and restoration of their original shape. Unlike traditional irons, garment steamers offer a gentler and more efficient method of removing wrinkles, particularly on delicate fabrics such as silk, chiffon, and satin. The steamer's nozzle emits a continuous flow of steam, which penetrates the fabric and relaxes the fibers. As a result, the garment regains its smoothness and natural form, eliminating the need for harsh ironing or pressing.

Godet Skirt

A godet skirt is a type of skirt that features triangular or oval-shaped insertions of fabric, known as godets, which are sewn into the garment. These godets are strategically placed along the hemline of the skirt, allowing it to flare out and create additional volume and movement. The godet skirt is characterized by its unique and stylish design, which sets it apart from other types of skirts. It is often chosen by fashion designers for its ability to add drama and flair to an outfit, making it a popular choice for special occasions or red carpet events.

Grommet Kits

Grommet kits are essential tools used in fashion design for adding decorative and functional metal eyelets, called grommets, to fabric or leather garments and accessories. These kits typically consist of various components, including a grommet setter, an anvil, and a selection of grommets in different sizes and finishes. The grommet setter is a handheld tool with a metal rod or mandrel that is used to secure the grommets to the fabric or leather. It typically has a handle for comfortable grip and may feature interchangeable mandrels to accommodate different grommet sizes. The anvil, on the other hand, is a flat metal surface against which the fabric or leather is placed during the grommet-setting process. It provides support and stability to ensure clean and precise grommet installation. Grommet kits are available in various sizes and formats to suit different fashion design needs. They are commonly used in the construction of garments such as corsets, belts, shoes, and handbags. Grommets not only add a decorative element but also serve functional purposes, such as creating openings for lacing, cording, or other closure methods. They can also reinforce stress points in a garment and prevent fabric or leather from fraying or tearing. The selection of grommets included in a kit may differ in terms of size, material, and finish. Common materials used for grommets include metal alloys such as brass, nickel, or stainless steel. These materials provide durability and resistance to corrosion. Grommet finishes can range from polished or matte to antique or colored options, allowing for customization and coordination with the overall design aesthetics. In fashion design, grommet kits provide designers and makers with the necessary tools to add professional and polished finishing touches to their creations. They allow for precise and consistent placement of grommets, ensuring a high-quality final product. Whether used for functional purposes, such as adding corset lacing or creating adjustable straps, or for purely decorative purposes, grommet kits offer versatility and control in fashion design.

Hairstylist

A hairstylist in the context of fashion design is a professional who specializes in creating hairstyles that complement and enhance the overall aesthetic of a fashion collection or an individual's style. They possess the skills and expertise to interpret the designer's vision and create hairstyles that align with the desired look and feel of the fashion garments or the individual's personality. Hairstylists in fashion design are responsible for conceptualizing and executing hairstyles that are in sync with the overall theme and concept of a fashion collection.

They collaborate closely with fashion designers, makeup artists, and other members of the creative team to ensure a cohesive and unified vision. Their role goes beyond simply creating hairstyles; they contribute to the storytelling and narrative of the collection through their hairstyling choices.

Halter Neck Dress

A halter neck dress is a type of dress that features a strap or fabric strip that wraps around the neck, providing support and closure for the garment. The strap is typically secured with a tie or fastening at the back, creating an open back design. The halter neck dress is a popular choice in fashion design for its unique and eye-catching neckline. The halter neck dress is known for its versatility and ability to flatter a variety of body types. The neckline draws attention to the shoulders and collarbone, creating an elegant and elongating effect. This style of dress can be found in a range of lengths, from mini to maxi, and is suitable for both casual and formal occasions.

Harem Pants

Hat Blocking Pins

Hat blocking pins are essential tools used in fashion design for shaping and forming hats. These pins are specifically designed to securely hold and manipulate hat materials, such as straw, felt, or fabric, during the blocking process. The blocking process in hat making involves reshaping a hat's crown and brim to achieve a desired style or silhouette. Hat blocking pins play a crucial role in this process by carefully pinning the hat material onto a hat block or mold. Hat blocks or molds are wooden or metal forms that help shape the hat as it dries and sets into its final shape.

Hat Blocks

Hat blocks are tools used in fashion design to create and shape hats. They are typically made of wood or metal and come in various shapes and sizes to produce different styles of hats. Hat blocks serve as a mold for the hat, allowing the designer to manipulate the material and shape it precisely to achieve the desired look. When designing a hat, the first step is to select a suitable hat block that corresponds to the desired style. The block is then used as a guide to shape the material, whether it's felt, straw, or fabric. The material is draped over the hat block and secured in place, allowing the designer to work on shaping the hat.

Hat Stands

Hat stands, also known as hat racks or hat holders, are fixtures used in fashion design to display and store hats. They are essential in organizing and presenting hats in a visually appealing and accessible manner. Typically made of wood or metal, hat stands come in various shapes, sizes, and designs to accommodate different styles and types of hats. They often consist of a central pole or post, sometimes adjustable in height, with a rounded or flat top where the hat is placed. Some hat stands also include additional hooks or arms to hang hat accessories such as scarves or gloves.

Haute Couture

Haute Couture refers to the highest level of fashion design and production. The term, which is French for "high sewing" or "high dressmaking," specifically applies to garments that are custom-made to fit individual clients, using intricate techniques and luxurious fabrics. In order for a fashion house to be considered Haute Couture, it must be a member of the Syndicate of Haute Couture, an industry trade association based in Paris. This prestigious designation is reserved for a select few designers who meet strict criteria, ensuring that the garments they produce are of exceptional quality and craftsmanship.

Hemming Tapes

refer to a type of adhesive material that is used in fashion design to create neat and professional-looking hems on garments. These tapes are typically made from a durable fabric or thermoplastic material, and are designed to be applied to the fabric using heat or pressure. offer a quick and convenient alternative to traditional sewing methods of hemming, as they eliminate the need for time-consuming hand stitching or machine sewing. They are particularly useful for hemming lightweight or delicate fabrics that may be difficult to sew with a needle and thread. The application of is relatively simple. First, the fabric is folded and pressed to create the desired hem. Then, the tape is placed between the folded edge and the main body of the fabric, and heat or pressure is applied to activate the adhesive. This causes the tape to bond the folded fabric securely, creating a clean and streamlined hemline. One of the main advantages of using is that they provide a strong and durable bond, ensuring that the hem remains intact even after repeated wear and washing. They also help to prevent fraying and unraveling of the fabric edges, enhancing the overall longevity and appearance of the garment. Furthermore, offer versatility in terms of the types of fabrics they can be used on. They can be applied to various fabrics such as cotton, polyester, silk, and even stretchy materials like jersey or spandex. This makes them suitable for a wide range of fashion design projects, from basic alterations to intricate couture creations. In addition to their practical applications, also contribute to the aesthetic aspects of fashion design. They provide a seamless and invisible finish to hems, as the tape is hidden between the fabric layers. This helps to maintain the clean lines and desired silhouette of the garment, without any visible stitching or bulkiness. Overall, are an essential tool in the fashion designer's toolkit, offering a quick, convenient, and professional solution for creating beautifully finished hems. Whether used for basic alterations or high-end couture, these adhesive tapes provide a reliable and versatile alternative to traditional sewing methods, ensuring that garments are both durable and aesthetically pleasing.

Hemming Tools

Hemming tools are essential implements used in fashion design to create a neat and professional finish on the edges of garments. These tools are specifically designed to facilitate the process of hemming, which involves folding up and sewing the lower edge of a fabric to give it a clean and polished appearance. One commonly used hemming tool is the hem gauge, which is a small ruler-like device with multiple measurements marked on it. This tool allows fashion designers to accurately measure and mark the desired hem length on the fabric. By adjusting the hem gauge to the desired length and sliding it along the fabric edge, designers can create consistent and even hems across the garment. Another popular hemming tool is the hemming foot, which is a specialized sewing machine attachment. The hemming foot helps to guide the fabric and ensure a straight and uniform stitching line as the fabric is folded and sewn. This foot is particularly useful for creating narrow hems or curved hems, where precision is crucial to achieve a professional result. Additionally, fashion designers may also use hem tapes or adhesives as tools for hemming. Hem tapes are narrow strips of fabric with a heat-activated adhesive on one side. These tapes are placed between the fabric layers, and when heated, the adhesive bonds the layers together, effectively securing the hem. This technique is especially useful for delicate fabrics or when a temporary hem adjustment is required. In conclusion, hemming tools are integral to the process of fashion design as they enable designers to create tidy, well-finished hems on garments. Whether it's using a hem gauge for precise measurements, a hemming foot for accurate stitching, or hem tapes for temporary adjustments, these tools ensure that the edges of the fabric are neatly folded and secured, resulting in a refined and professional look.

Henley Sweater

A Henley sweater, also known as a Henley, is a type of sweater that is characterized by its unique collar style. It is named after the town of Henley-on-Thames in England, where it is said to have originated. The Henley sweater is a popular choice in fashion design due to its versatility and timeless appeal. The collar on a Henley sweater is different from a regular sweater in that it has a row of buttons or a single button at the front, usually extending halfway down the chest. This buttoned placket on the collar adds a touch of elegance and sophistication to the sweater, making it suitable for both casual and semi-formal occasions.

High-Waisted Jeans

High-waisted jeans are a style of pants that are designed with a waistline that sits above the natural waist of the wearer. This style has gained popularity in the fashion industry and has become a staple in many people's wardrobes. The key feature of high-waisted jeans is the placement of the waistline, which typically falls above the belly button or higher. This design choice creates the illusion of longer legs and a more defined waist, making it a flattering option for various body types. High-waisted jeans often have a fitted or tapered silhouette, accentuating the curves of the wearer's body.

Hooded Cardigan

A hooded cardigan is a type of garment that combines the design elements of both a cardigan and a hooded sweatshirt. It typically features a button-down or zip-up front closure and a hood attached to the neckline. The hooded cardigan is considered a versatile and practical piece of clothing that can be worn in a variety of settings, ranging from casual to more formal occasions. The cardigan is a classic style of sweater that originated in the 19th century and is characterized by its open front and button-down or zip-up closure. It is commonly made from knit fabric, although variations in materials and designs exist. The addition of a hood to the traditional cardigan design creates the hooded cardigan, adding an extra layer of functionality and style.

Hoodie

A hoodie is a type of sweatshirt or jumper that has a hood attached to it. It is a popular article of clothing in fashion design, known for its casual and comfortable style. The hoodie is typically made of a soft and thick fabric, such as cotton or fleece, which provides warmth and insulation. The design of a hoodie usually includes a hood with adjustable drawstrings, long sleeves, and a large front pocket, known as a kangaroo pocket. The hood can be worn up or down, providing versatility and customization to the wearer. The kangaroo pocket serves both functional and aesthetic purposes, allowing for storage of small items and adding visual interest to the garment. Originally, hoodies were primarily worn as athletic or leisurewear, associated with sports teams and hoodlum subcultures. However, the hoodie has since become a prominent fashion statement, embraced by both streetwear enthusiasts and high-end fashion designers. The versatility and comfort of the hoodie make it a go-to choice for many individuals, regardless of age or gender. In fashion design, the hoodie has been adapted and reinvented in various ways. Designers experiment with different fabrics, colors, and prints to create unique and innovative hoodies. They often incorporate branding elements, such as logos or slogans, to enhance the overall aesthetic and convey a sense of identity. Hoodies can be styled in numerous ways, making them suitable for a range of occasions. They can be dressed up or down, paired with jeans or skirts, and layered with other garments. The relaxed fit of the hoodie provides a comfortable and effortless look, while also allowing for freedom of movement. Overall, the hoodie is a versatile and iconic piece of fashion design. Its combination of practicality, comfort, and style has made it a staple in many wardrobes. Whether worn casually or as a fashion statement, the hoodie continues to be a timeless and popular choice in the world of fashion.

Hook And Eye Closures

Hook and eye closures are small, discreet fastening devices commonly used in fashion design to secure fabric openings such as those found on garments, accessories, or even home furnishings. These closures consist of two parts, a hook and an eye, which interlock to hold the fabric edges together. The hook portion of the closure is typically made of a small metal or plastic piece shaped like a hook. It features a curved or bent end that is designed to catch onto the opposite component, known as the eye. The eye is usually a small metal or plastic loop with an opening that allows the hook to be inserted and secured. When properly aligned, the hook and eye interlock, creating a secure fastening that keeps the fabric edges in place.

Hook And Loop Tape

Hook and Loop tape, also known as Velcro tape, is a versatile fastening system commonly used in fashion design. It consists of two components: the hook side and the loop side. The hook side is made up of small, stiff hooks that interlock with the soft, fuzzy loops on the loop side. When both sides are pressed together, the hooks catch onto the loops, creating a secure bond. This bond can be easily separated by pulling the two sides apart.

Hot Pants

A hot pant refers to a type of short, tight-fitting shorts that are typically worn by women. This fashion garment typically has a high waistline and is characterized by its short length, usually extending no longer than mid-thigh. Hot pants are designed to be form-fitting, emphasizing the curves and shape of the wearer's lower body. Hot pants gained popularity in the 1960s and 1970s as a symbol of female liberation and empowerment. They were often associated with the free-spiritedness and boldness of the era. The fashion trend originated from shorts worn by dancers in the 1940s and 1950s, which gradually became shorter and more revealing over time.

Iron And Ironing Board

Iron: An essential tool used in fashion design for the purpose of pressing and removing wrinkles from garments. It is typically made of metal and consists of a flat, heated surface with adjustable temperature settings. The iron is used in conjunction with an ironing board to achieve smooth and crisp fabric finishes. Ironing Board: A support surface designed specifically for ironing garments in the fashion design process. It is typically constructed with a sturdy metal or wooden frame and a padded, heat-resistant surface. The ironing board provides a stable platform for positioning garments, allowing for easy access to all areas of the fabric. It is height-adjustable to accommodate individual comfort and ergonomics during ironing.

Jammer Swimsuit

A jammer swimsuit is a type of swimsuit that is designed specifically for competitive swimmers. It is typically worn by male swimmers and is known for its tight fit and longer length. The primary function of a jammer swimsuit is to enhance performance in the water by reducing drag and providing muscle compression. The design of a jammer swimsuit is sleek and aerodynamic, with a form-fitting shape that hugs the body. It is made from a blend of fabrics that are specifically chosen for their hydrodynamic properties. The most commonly used fabric is a combination of nylon and spandex, which provides a snug and stretchy fit. A key feature of a jammer swimsuit is its longer length compared to other types of swimsuits. It extends from the waist to just above the knee, providing additional coverage and reducing drag in the water. The longer length also helps to enhance muscle compression, which is important for swimmers as it can improve endurance and performance. The tight fit of a jammer swimsuit is another important aspect of its design. It molds to the body and reduces drag by eliminating excess fabric that can slow swimmers down in the water. The compression provided by the tight fit is also beneficial, as it helps to support and stabilize the muscles during intense physical activity. In addition to its functional aspects, a jammer swimsuit is also stylish and visually appealing. It often features bold colors and patterns to add a touch of personality to the swimmer's look. Some jammer swimsuits may also include additional design elements such as a drawstring waist for a secure and customizable fit. In conclusion, a jammer swimsuit is a form-fitting, longer length swimsuit designed specifically for competitive male swimmers. It is made from a blend of fabrics that provide hydrodynamic properties and muscle compression. The tight fit and longer length of a jammer swimsuit help to reduce drag and enhance performance in the water. Despite its functional design, it is also visually appealing with various color and pattern options. Overall, a jammer swimsuit is a go-to choice for serious swimmers looking to maximize their performance in the pool.

Jodhpur Pants

Jodhpur pants, also known as Jodhpurs, are a style of trousers that originate from Jodhpur, a city in the Rajasthan state of India. These pants are a popular fashion choice, particularly among equestrians and fashion enthusiasts. Jodhpur pants are characterized by their unique design, which sets them apart from other types of trousers. The distinguishing feature of Jodhpur pants is the reinforced panel that extends from the waistband down to the knees. This panel, often called the "Jodhpur patch," provides additional support and durability to the pants, making them suitable for various activities, including horse riding. The patch is typically made from a heavier material, such as suede or leather, which adds protection and a distinctive visual element to the pants. In addition to the Jodhpur patch, these pants feature a close-fitting silhouette. They are designed to sit high on the waist, providing a flattering and streamlined look. Jodhpur pants are typically tailored to fit snugly around the hips and thighs, gradually tapering down to a narrower leg opening. This design creates a sleek and elegant appearance, suitable for both casual and formal occasions. Traditionally, Jodhpur pants were made from lightweight and breathable materials, such as cotton or linen. However, modern variations may incorporate a wider range of fabrics, including denim, twill, and synthetic blends. The choice of fabric depends on the intended use and desired aesthetic. For example, equestrians may opt for Jodhpur pants made from stretchy and moisture-wicking materials that enhance comfort and performance. Another characteristic of Jodhpur pants is the presence of straps or buckle closures at the ankle. These straps, often referred to as "stirrups," help to keep the pants in place and prevent them from riding up during movement. Additionally, these ankle straps add a distinctive equestrian-inspired detail to the overall design of the pants. Jodhpur pants have gained popularity not only among horse riders but also in the fashion industry. They offer a unique and stylish alternative to traditional trousers, combining functionality with a touch of vintage charm. Whether paired with a tailored blazer for a formal look or matched with a simple blouse for a more casual ensemble, Jodhpur pants add a subtle yet sophisticated flair to any outfit.

Kaftan

A kaftan is a loose-fitting, full-length garment that is often associated with Middle Eastern and North African fashion. It originated in ancient Mesopotamia and has since been adopted by various cultures throughout history, becoming a popular style in contemporary fashion. The kaftan is typically made from lightweight, flowing fabrics such as silk, chiffon, or cotton, offering comfort and ease of movement. It is characterized by its loose, kimono-style sleeves, wide V-neckline, and a straight, unstructured silhouette that drapes loosely over the body.

Keyhole Top

A keyhole top is a fashion design element that features a small, narrow cutout or opening near the neckline of a garment. The cutout resembles the shape of a keyhole, hence the name. This design detail adds a touch of elegance, femininity, and allure to a top, making it a popular choice for both casual and formal wear. The keyhole can be placed in various positions, such as in the center of the neckline, off to the side, or even at the back of the garment. It can be simple and small, or it can be larger and more intricate, depending on the desired aesthetic. The opening is often shaped and finished with a bound edge or a small facing to ensure a neat and polished look.

Kick-Flare Jeans

Kick-flare jeans are a type of denim trousers that combine the elements of both bootcut and cropped jeans. The term "kick-flare" refers to the shape of the jeans, which feature a fitted waist and hips that gradually widen from the knee down to the ankle, creating a slight flare or kick at the bottom of the leg. These jeans are known for their versatility and ability to flatter various body types. The fitted waist and hips accentuate the curves of the body, while the flared leg creates a balanced and elongating effect. The kick-flare silhouette is also often used to create a retro or vintage-inspired look. Paired with the right top and accessories, these jeans can be dressed up or down for different occasions.

Kimono Cardigan

A kimono cardigan is a loose-fitting, open-front garment that draws inspiration from the traditional Japanese kimono. It features wide sleeves and a flowing silhouette, giving it a relaxed and comfortable feel. The kimono cardigan is often made from lightweight and breathable fabrics such as cotton, silk, or rayon, making it suitable for warmer weather. The design of the kimono cardigan is characterized by its simplicity and versatility. It is typically unstructured and does not have any fastenings or closures, allowing it to be easily thrown on over other clothing. The lack of fastenings also adds to its effortless and laid-back aesthetic. The length of the kimono cardigan can vary, ranging from just below the hip to ankle-length, providing options for different styling preferences. The kimono cardigan has become a popular choice in contemporary fashion due to its ability to add a touch of elegance and sophistication to any outfit. Its loose and flowing silhouette creates graceful movement, while the wide sleeves add a sense of drama and flair. The kimono cardigan can be worn as a statement piece or used as a layering item to enhance an ensemble. One of the key features of the kimono cardigan is its versatility in styling. It can be paired with a variety of bottoms, such as jeans, skirts, or shorts, to create different looks. For a casual and bohemian vibe, it can be worn over a basic tank top and denim shorts. On the other hand, it can be paired with tailored pants and a blouse for a more polished and sophisticated outfit. In terms of accessorizing, the kimono cardigan can be styled with belts to cinch in the waist and create a more defined silhouette. It can also be layered with scarves, statement necklaces, or hats to add extra visual interest. The versatility of the kimono cardigan allows it to be worn in various settings, from casual outings to formal events, making it a versatile and practical wardrobe staple.

Kimono Dress

A kimono dress is a traditional garment that originated in Japan. It is known for its loose and flowing silhouette, which is inspired by the traditional Japanese kimono. The dress typically features wide sleeves, a wrap-style closure, and a belted waist. Kimono dresses are often made from luxurious fabrics such as silk or satin, and they can be adorned with intricate patterns or embroidery. The length of the dress can vary, ranging from mini to maxi, but it typically falls below the knee.

Kimono Top

A kimono top is a loose-fitting, T-shaped garment that is inspired by traditional Japanese kimono robes. It is typically made from lightweight fabrics such as silk, chiffon, or cotton, and features wide, flowing sleeves and an open front. The design of the kimono top draws heavily from the traditional clothing of Japan, particularly the kimono. However, it has been adapted for modern fashion and often incorporates contemporary elements and trends. The kimono top is known for its effortless elegance and versatility, making it a popular choice for both formal and casual occasions.

Knitting Machines

A knitting machine, in the context of fashion design, refers to a device that automates the process of creating knitted fabrics, garments, or accessories. It is a mechanical or electronic tool that can produce various types of stitches and patterns, allowing fashion designers to rapidly create knitted pieces without the need for manual labor. These machines consist of a bed or needle bed, which holds the knitting needles, and a carriage that moves across the bed to form the stitches. The needles on the bed are positioned to create a specific stitch pattern, and as the carriage moves back and forth, it transfers the yarn between the needles to form the fabric.

Knitting Needles

Knitting needles are essential tools used in the art of fashion design. They are long, slender, and pointed rods typically made of metal, wood, or plastic, designed specifically for creating knitted fabrics. These needles are integral in the process of transforming yarn into various textiles and garments. When a fashion designer begins a knitting project, they rely on knitting needles to guide and manipulate the yarn as they craft intricate patterns and stitches. The needles provide the structure and support necessary to create tightly woven or loosely draped fabrics, depending on the desired outcome of the design.

Lace Blouse

A lace blouse is a garment characterized by its delicate and intricate lace fabric construction. It is typically designed as an upper-body garment, worn by women, that features lace as the main fabric or as an embellishment on certain parts of the blouse. Lace blouses can vary in style, design, and overall aesthetic. They can be sleeveless, short-sleeved, or long-sleeved, and can come in a variety of necklines such as scoop necks, V-necks, or high necks. The lace used in the construction of a blouse can be either machine-made or handcrafted, and the patterns and motifs can range from simple to intricate. These blouses are often considered feminine and elegant, with their delicate and romantic appearance. The lace fabric used in the construction of a blouse usually adds a sense of sophistication, refinement, and texture to the overall design. The sheer nature of the fabric also allows for glimpses of skin, creating a subtly alluring and sensual effect. Lace blouses can be versatile and can be styled for various occasions. They can be worn casually with a pair of jeans for a relaxed yet sophisticated look, or can be dressed up with a skirt or dress pants for a more formal and refined ensemble. They can also be paired with jackets or blazers for a polished and professional appearance. In terms of color, lace blouses are available in a wide range of options. They can be found in classic, neutral hues such as white, black, or beige, which are timeless and versatile. They can also be found in bold and vibrant colors, such as red, blue, or green, for those who prefer a more statement-making look. Overall, a lace blouse is a versatile and stylish garment that adds a touch of femininity, elegance, and delicacy to any outfit. Its intricate lace fabric construction creates an eye-catching and visually appealing design, making it a timeless and sophisticated choice in the world of fashion.

Lace Playsuit

A lace playsuit is a one-piece garment designed for women, typically made from lace fabric. It is a popular fashion choice for various occasions, including parties, weddings, and even casual outings. The playsuit features a combination of a top and shorts, merging them into a single, cohesive design. This fusion creates a stylish and fashionable look that is both elegant and playful. The lace playsuit offers a unique and feminine appeal, primarily due to the use of lace fabric. Lace is a delicate, openwork fabric characterized by intricate patterns and designs. It adds a touch of sophistication and elegance to the playsuit, making it appropriate for formal events or for those who want to make a fashion statement. The lace fabric also provides a sense of texture and depth, enhancing the overall aesthetic of the garment. Featuring a fitted bodice and shorts, the lace playsuit is designed to accentuate the woman's figure. It typically has a defined waistline, creating an hourglass silhouette. The fitted bodice emphasizes the upper body, while the shorts showcase the legs. This combination allows women to feel both stylish and comfortable, as the playsuit provides freedom of movement and ease of wear. With its versatile design, the lace playsuit can be styled in various ways to suit different occasions. For a formal event, it can be paired with heels and elegant accessories for a sophisticated look. Alternatively, it can be dressed down with flats and minimal accessories for a casual yet chic ensemble. The playsuit also allows for layering, making it suitable for different seasons. It can be worn with a blazer or jacket during colder months or simply on its own during warmer weather. In conclusion, a lace playsuit is a fashionable one-piece garment for women, combining a top and shorts into a single design. Made from lace fabric, it offers a unique and feminine appeal, suitable for formal occasions or making a fashion statement. With its fitted bodice and shorts, it accentuates the woman's figure while providing comfort and freedom of movement. Its versatility allows for various styling options, making it a versatile and trendy fashion choice.

Leather Burnishing Tools

A leather burnishing tool is a specialized tool used in fashion design for finishing and polishing leather edges. It is used to create a smooth and polished surface on leather edges, enhancing the overall appearance and durability of leather goods. The burnishing process involves applying pressure and friction to the leather edge using the burnishing tool, resulting in the smoothing and sealing of the raw edge. This technique helps to prevent fraying and unraveling of the leather, ensuring a clean and professional finish.

Leather Dye Kit

A leather dye kit is a set of materials and tools used in the fashion design industry to change the color of leather goods and enhance their appearance. It typically includes a variety of dye colors, a leather preparer, a sealer, and applicator tools. The purpose of a leather dye kit is to give fashion designers the ability to transform the color of leather products, such as shoes, bags, and accessories, to match their desired aesthetic or to rejuvenate old or worn-out pieces. By using a leather dye kit, designers have the flexibility to create unique and personalized designs, making their creations stand out in the fashion market.

Leather Edge Bevelers

A leather edge beveler is a tool commonly used in fashion design to create smooth and rounded edges on leather materials. It is a cutting instrument that is specifically designed to remove sharp edges or excess material from leather edges, resulting in a more polished and professional finish. The leather edge beveler operates by applying pressure to the edge of the leather, which causes the sharp blade of the tool to remove a thin strip of material. This process not only eliminates any rough or uneven edges but also helps to thin down the edge, making it easier to fold or attach to other pieces of leather.

Leather Hole Punch

A leather hole punch is a tool used in the field of fashion design to create precise holes in leather materials. It is commonly used by designers and artisans to add functionality and decorative elements to leather garments, accessories, and footwear. The primary purpose of a leather hole punch is to create holes of various sizes in leather, allowing for the attachment of closures such as buttons, snaps, buckles, and hooks. This tool is essential in the creation of belts, wallets, purses, shoes, and other leather goods that require secure fastenings.

Leather Sewing Machine

A leather sewing machine is a specialized stitching tool used in the field of fashion design that is designed specifically for sewing leather materials. It is equipped with unique features and capabilities that make it suitable for working with this particular type of fabric. Unlike regular sewing machines, a leather sewing machine has a more durable and powerful motor, as leather is a much thicker and tougher material to sew. It also features a heavier-duty construction with a robust frame and components to provide the necessary stability and strength to handle the demands of sewing leather.

Leather Skiving Tools

Leather skiving tools are specialized instruments used in fashion design to thin or shave down leather material. Skiving refers to the process of reducing the thickness of the leather, usually at the edges, to create a more aesthetically pleasing and functional finish. These tools allow fashion designers to create clean and precise edges on leather garments, bags, shoes, and other accessories. They work by removing layers of leather to achieve a desired thickness, ensuring that the final product is both visually appealing and comfortable to wear.

Leather Stamps

Leather stamps are essential tools used in the field of fashion design to create unique patterns and designs on leather surfaces. These stamps are made of various materials, such as metal or wood, and consist of engraved or embossed shapes, symbols, or patterns. The primary purpose of leather stamps in fashion design is to enhance the aesthetic appeal of leather goods, such as bags, belts, shoes, and accessories. By using leather stamps, designers can imprint intricate designs onto the surface of the leather, creating a visually appealing and personalized look. These stamps allow designers to add exquisite details, textures, and patterns that elevate the overall quality and design of the leather product.

Leather Tools

Leather tools, in the context of fashion design, refer to a set of specialized handheld instruments used specifically for working with leather in the process of creating leather garments, accessories, and other products. These tools are designed to enable fashion designers and artisans to manipulate and shape leather materials with precision and accuracy. Leather tools typically include various implements that aid in cutting, stitching, punching, and shaping leather. Some commonly used leather tools include: 1. Leather Cutting Tools: These tools are used to cut leather into desired shapes and sizes. They may include different types of knives, blades, and shears, each designed for specific cutting techniques and purposes. 2. Leather Punching Tools: Leather punching tools are used to create holes in leather for various purposes, such as attaching hardware, creating decorative patterns, and joining leather pieces together. They may include tools like hole punches, awls, and chisels of different sizes and shapes. 3. Leather Stitching Tools: These tools are essential for stitching leather pieces together to create seams, decorative details, and secure closures. Stitching tools for leather may include needles, thread, thimbles, leather punches, and stitching awls. 4. Leather Shaping Tools: Shaping tools are used to mold and shape leather into desired forms and patterns. They may include tools like leather mallets, leather molds, and specialized shaping boards or surfaces. 5. Leather Edge Finishing Tools: These tools are used to finish and refine the edges of leather to give them a polished and professional appearance. Edge finishing tools may include bevellers, slickers, burnishing tools, and specialized finishes or dyes. Overall, leather tools are essential for fashion designers and artisans working with leather materials. They allow for precise and intricate work, enabling the creation of beautifully crafted leather garments, accessories, and products with attention to detail and professional finish.

Leathercraft Needles

Leathercraft needles are essential tools used in the field of fashion design. These specialized needles are specifically designed to work with leather and other heavy fabrics, allowing fashion designers to create intricate and detailed designs. Unlike regular sewing needles, leathercraft needles have a thicker and stronger construction. This is necessary because leather is a much tougher and heavier material than most other fabrics. The thicker needle helps to penetrate through the leather without breaking or bending. Additionally, leathercraft needles have sharp points that enable them to pierce through the material with ease.

Leotard

A leotard is a one-piece garment that is typically worn by dancers, gymnasts, and other performers in the field of dance and athletics. It is designed to fit snugly against the body and is often made of stretchy fabric such as spandex or lycra. The leotard is named after Jules Léotard, a French acrobat who popularized the garment in the 19th century. The leotard is characterized by its sleeveless and legless design, which allows for maximum freedom of movement. It typically has a high neckline and is cut high on the hip for a streamlined and elongating effect. The absence of sleeves and legs helps to showcase the dancer's or athlete's muscles and physique while providing support and coverage.

Lingerie Romper

A lingerie romper is a one-piece garment that combines elements of lingerie and a romper. It is designed to be worn as sleepwear or as a sensual and playful fashion garment. The lingerie romper incorporates delicate and luxurious fabrics, such as lace, silk, or satin, and often features intricate details, such as cutouts, straps, or bows. The design of a lingerie romper typically includes a fitted bodice, which is often made with a stretchy fabric to ensure a flattering and comfortable fit. The bodice may feature underwire or padding to provide support and enhance the bust. The bottom part of the romper is usually loose-fitting, allowing for ease of movement and a relaxed, flirty look. Lingerie rompers are available in various styles and silhouettes, catering to different body types and personal preferences. Some lingerie rompers may feature a low-cut neckline or a plunging back for a bold and seductive look, while others may have a high neckline or long sleeves for a more modest and elegant appearance. The colors and patterns of lingerie rompers can range from classic shades like black, white, and red to vibrant hues and playful prints. These designs, along with the use of luxurious fabrics and intricate details, help create a sense of allure and sophistication. When designing a lingerie romper, fashion designers carefully consider the balance between functionality and aesthetics. They strive to create a garment that not only looks visually appealing but also provides comfort and support to the wearer. Lingerie rompers are versatile pieces that can be styled in different ways, depending on the occasion. They can be paired with a robe or a kimono for a luxurious loungewear look, or worn alone as a statement-making lingerie piece. In conclusion, a lingerie romper is a fusion of lingerie and romper design, creating a seductive, comfortable, and stylish garment that can be worn both as sleepwear and as a fashion piece. With their delicate fabrics, intricate details, and varied styles, lingerie rompers offer women a playful and enticing option for expressing their personal style and sensuality.

Lookbook

A Lookbook is a comprehensive and visually appealing collection of photographs or images that showcases various fashion designs and outfits created by a fashion designer or brand. In the context of fashion design, a Lookbook serves as a catalogue or portfolio that presents the overall aesthetic, style, and theme of a designer's collection. It allows the audience, such as buyers, stylists, or consumers, to preview and appreciate the designer's creative vision and fashion philosophy.

Lounge Romper

A lounge romper is a fashionable one-piece garment that is designed to provide comfort and style for women. It combines the casual elements of a romper with the relaxed and cozy features of loungewear, creating a versatile and trendy clothing option. The lounge romper typically features a loose-fitting silhouette with a relaxed bodice that is cinched at the waist, providing a flattering and comfortable fit. It is commonly made from soft and lightweight materials such as cotton, jersey, or linen, ensuring maximum comfort and breathability. The construction of the lounge romper often includes an elasticized waistband or drawstring, allowing for easy adjustment and ensuring a customized fit for different body types. One of the key design elements of a lounge romper is its versatility. It can be worn as a casual outfit for lounging at home, running errands, or hanging out with friends. The relaxed and effortless style of the romper makes it perfect for summer activities, beach trips, or even as a trendy alternative to pajamas. It can also be dressed up with accessories and paired with heels or sandals for a stylish and fashionable look. The lounge romper often features various neckline options, such as V-neck, scoop neck, or off-the-shoulder, providing different style possibilities. Another notable feature of the lounge romper is its functionality. Many lounge rompers are designed with practical details such as pockets, allowing for convenient storage of small items like keys or phones. Some lounge rompers may also incorporate adjustable straps or convertible designs, providing flexibility and versatility in styling. The length of the lounge romper can vary, with options ranging from short and flirty to long and flowy, catering to different preferences and occasions. In conclusion, a lounge romper is a fashionable one-piece garment that combines the comfort and style of loungewear with the trendy elements of a romper. Designed with a loose-fitting silhouette and made from soft materials, it offers both comfort and breathability. Its versatility allows it to be worn for various casual occasions, and its practical features enhance its functionality. The lounge romper is a fashionable and practical clothing option that embodies both style and comfort for women.

Low-Rise Jeans

Low-rise jeans are a style of denim pants that sit lower on the waist than traditional mid-rise or high-rise jeans. They are characterized by their low-cut design, which typically falls between the hips and the belly button. Low-rise jeans gained popularity in the late 1990s and early 2000s and have remained a staple in fashion ever since. These jeans are designed to accentuate the hips and create a more relaxed and casual aesthetic. They are often favored by younger demographics and individuals who embrace a more contemporary and trendy look. Low-rise jeans can be found in various styles, including bootcut, straight leg, skinny, and flare, allowing individuals to choose a silhouette that best suits their personal style and body shape.

Maillot

A maillot, in the context of fashion design, refers to a one-piece swimsuit that is worn by women. It is a classic style that has been popular since the early 20th century and continues to be a timeless option for swimwear. The maillot is known for its sleek and elegant design, offering full coverage while still maintaining a stylish and feminine look. The maillot typically features a fitted bodice that extends from the shoulders to the hips, with strategic seams and shaping to flatter the wearer's figure. It often has a high-cut leg and a low-cut back, adding to its sophisticated appeal. The neckline may vary, ranging from a sweetheart or halter style to a high neck or plunging V-neck. Some maillots also come with built-in cups or underwire for added support and shaping. Maillots can be made from a variety of materials, including nylon, spandex, and Lycra, which provide stretch and comfort for swimming and sunbathing. They may also feature embellishments such as ruching, shirring, or tummy control panels, aimed at enhancing the wearer's silhouette. Maillots come in a wide range of colors and patterns, from solid neutrals to vibrant prints, allowing women to express their personal style at the beach or pool. One of the advantages of wearing a maillot is its versatility. It can easily transition from the beach to other daytime activities, such as walking around the resort or grabbing a bite to eat. With the addition of a skirt or pair of shorts, a maillot can even be transformed into a stylish top for a casual summer outfit. Its simplicity and timelessness make the maillot a staple piece in any woman's swimwear collection. In conclusion, the maillot is a classic one-piece swimsuit for women, known for its sleek design and timeless appeal. It offers full coverage while still maintaining a stylish and feminine look. Made from stretchy and comfortable materials, maillots come in various styles, colors, and patterns to suit different tastes. They can be easily styled for both beach and casual wear, making them a versatile option for any woman's wardrobe.

Makeup Artist

A makeup artist in the context of fashion design is a professional who specializes in enhancing the appearance of individuals, models, or performers through the application of cosmetics, prosthetics, and other beauty products. The primary role of a makeup artist is to create visual transformations by utilizing a range of techniques, tools, and materials. The work of a makeup artist begins with a thorough understanding of the client's desired look or the artistic vision of the fashion designer. They collaborate closely with fashion designers, hairstylists, and photographers to ensure a cohesive and harmonious overall presentation. They carefully analyze the subject's features, skin tone, and facial structure to determine the most suitable makeup application techniques and products. Makeup artists skillfully manipulate colors, textures, and shading to create various effects, such as contouring, highlighting, and concealing. They may use liquid or powder foundations to even out the skin tone, employ eyeshadows, eyeliners, and mascaras to accentuate the eyes, and apply lipsticks and glosses to enhance the lips. In addition to these basic techniques, makeup artists are adept at implementing specialized techniques, like airbrushing or creating special effects makeup for editorial photo shoots or runway shows. As the fashion industry constantly evolves, makeup artists must stay abreast of the latest trends, products, and techniques. They continuously strive to innovate and push boundaries to create unique and impactful makeup looks. Additionally, they must possess excellent interpersonal skills as they often work in fast-paced and high-pressure environments, while maintaining attention to detail and ensuring the client's satisfaction. In conclusion, a makeup artist in the context of fashion design is a skilled professional who transforms the appearance of individuals by using cosmetics and beauty products. Their role is to collaborate with fashion designers and other professionals to create visually appealing and cohesive looks in line with the desired aesthetic. By combining their technical expertise, creativity, and knowledge of current trends, makeup artists contribute to the overall success of fashion shows, editorial photo shoots, and other fashion-related events.

Mannequins

A mannequin is a three-dimensional representation of the human body, commonly used in the fashion industry to display clothing and accessories. These life-sized figures are typically made of fiberglass or plastic and are designed to resemble the proportions and stance of an average human being. Mannequins serve as silent models, showcasing garments and providing a visual representation of how they would look on a real person. Mannequins are an essential tool for fashion designers, retailers, and visual merchandisers. They allow designers to showcase their creations in a realistic and dynamic way, helping customers visualize how the garments would fit and drape on a person. By providing a clear view from all angles, mannequins enable designers to highlight the unique features and details of their designs. In addition to their functional purpose, mannequins also contribute to the artistic presentation of fashion. They can be customized and styled to reflect different aesthetics and brand identities, creating an atmosphere that aligns with the intended image of the clothing line or store. From realistic mannequins that replicate the diversity of human body types to abstract forms that emphasize shape and movement, mannequins offer a versatile platform for creative expression in visual merchandising. Besides fashion design, mannequins are also prevalent in other industries such as film and television production, art, and medical education. In these fields, mannequins are used for various purposes, such as costume fittings, animation reference, artistic sculptures, and medical simulations. Overall, mannequins play a crucial role in fashion design by allowing designers to showcase their garments in a practical and visually appealing manner. By providing an accurate representation of the human body, mannequins help bridge the gap between the designer's vision and the customer's perception, facilitating the communication of style, fit, and overall aesthetic.

Maxi Dress

A maxi dress is a long, floor-length dress that typically has a loose and flowing silhouette. It is a versatile fashion garment that is popular among women for various occasions. Maxi dresses are designed to be comfortable and easy to wear, while still being stylish and fashionable. These dresses are often made from lightweight and flowy fabrics such as chiffon, silk, or jersey. They are known for their relaxed fit and often feature empire waistlines or elasticized waistbands to accentuate and define the waist. Maxi dresses can also come in a variety of styles, including strapless, halter neck, off-the-shoulder, or with different neckline designs. Maxi dresses are particularly favored during the warmer seasons, as they provide coverage and protection from the sun while still being breathable and lightweight. They are popular choices for outdoor events such as beach weddings, garden parties, or summer vacations. However, maxi dresses can also be styled for more formal occasions, depending on the fabric, design, and accessories paired with them. When it comes to accessorizing a maxi dress, the possibilities are endless. Adding a belt can help to accentuate the waist or create a more tailored look. Layering the dress with a jacket or cardigan can add warmth and create a more polished outfit. For a bohemian-inspired look, pairing a maxi dress with a floppy hat, layered jewelry, and sandals can create a free-spirited and carefree vibe. In conclusion, a maxi dress is a versatile and stylish garment that is loved by women for its comfort and elegance. Its long length and loose silhouette make it perfect for various occasions and can be styled in numerous ways. Whether it be for a casual day out or a formal event, a maxi dress is a go-to choice for fashion-forward women.

Maxi Skirt

A maxi skirt is a long skirt that typically reaches the ankles or floor. It is a popular and versatile piece of clothing in the fashion industry, often seen as a staple in many women's wardrobes. The design of a maxi skirt allows for comfortable and free movement while adding an elegant and feminine touch to an outfit. It is often made from lightweight and flowy fabrics such as chiffon, cotton, or silk, which contribute to its graceful appearance. Maxi skirts can be found in a variety of styles, including A-line, pleated, wrap, and tiered. These different styles offer various options for creating different looks, accommodating different body types, and catering to individual style preferences. One of the advantages of wearing a maxi skirt is its versatility. It can be dressed up or down, depending on the occasion. For a casual look, it can be paired with a simple t-shirt or tank top and sandals. To create a more formal ensemble, a maxi skirt can be combined with a fitted blouse or a tailored blazer, along with heels or boots. Maxi skirts can be worn throughout the year, making them suitable for both warm and cold weather. In the summer, they provide comfort and breathability, while in the colder months, they can be layered with tights, boots, and jackets for added warmth. Another appealing aspect of maxi skirts is their ability to flatter different body shapes. The longer length of the skirt can give the illusion of lengthening and slimming the figure, making it a popular choice for women of all sizes. In conclusion, a maxi skirt is a long, flowing skirt that is suitable for various occasions and can be styled in multiple ways. Its versatility, comfort, and flattering design make it a favored choice among fashion enthusiasts and a staple in women's fashion.

Measuring Tapes

Measuring tapes are essential tools used in fashion design to accurately determine the dimensions and proportions of garments. They are flexible, ribbon-like strips made of durable materials such as fiberglass or cloth, marked with printed measurements for precise sizing. These tapes typically have metric and imperial measurements printed on both sides, allowing fashion designers to work with international sizing standards. They commonly range from 60 to 150 inches (or 150 to 380 centimeters) in length, providing ample room to measure garments of various sizes.

Mermaid Dress

A mermaid dress, also known as a fishtail or trumpet dress, is a form-fitting style of dress that accentuates and enhances the curves of the wearer, particularly around the waist, hips, and thighs. Inspired by the mythical creature, the mermaid dress is designed to mimic the shape of a mermaid's tail, with a fitted bodice that extends into a flared skirt from the mid-thigh or knee down to the floor. This unique silhouette creates a striking and glamorous effect, making it a popular choice for formal events and red carpet appearances. The construction of a mermaid dress typically involves strategic seaming and tailoring techniques to ensure a close fit along the body and a seamless transition into the flared skirt. The bodice is often structured with boning or corsetry to provide support and enhance the wearer's shape. The skirt may feature layers of fabric, such as tulle or organza, to add movement and volume, or it can be made from a single fabric with a mermaid-style flare created through careful draping and pleating.

Mermaid Skirt

A mermaid skirt is a form-fitting skirt that is designed to closely follow the contours of the body, from the waist down to the mid-thigh or knees, before flaring out dramatically towards the hem. The silhouette of the skirt resembles the shape of a mermaid's tail, hence the name. This style of skirt is typically made from a fabric with a certain amount of stretch, such as satin or stretchy knits, to allow for ease of movement and to accentuate the curves of the wearer. It is commonly seen in formal and evening wear, as it creates a sleek and elegant look that is often associated with glamour and luxury.

Midi Dress

A midi dress is a type of dress that falls between the knee and ankle in length, typically hitting the mid-calf. It is a popular style in women's fashion and is known for its versatility and timeless elegance. The midi dress is characterized by its modest length, which sets it apart from shorter dresses like mini dresses and longer dresses like maxi dresses. This length is often considered more appropriate for formal occasions, making the midi dress a staple in many women's wardrobes for events such as parties, weddings, and cocktail parties. Midi dresses come in a wide range of styles, including fitted, flared, A-line, and wrap dresses. They can be made from various fabrics such as cotton, silk, chiffon, and satin, each giving the dress a different look and feel. The design of a midi dress can also vary, with options like strapless, sleeveless, cap sleeves, off-the-shoulder, and long sleeves. One of the key features of a midi dress is its ability to flatter a variety of body shapes and sizes. The length of the dress elongates the silhouette, making the wearer appear taller and slimmer. Additionally, the midi length offers a balance between showing off the legs and maintaining an element of sophistication. It is a versatile option that can be dressed up or down depending on the occasion. Midi dresses can be styled in numerous ways to create different looks. They can be paired with heels or sandals for a more formal appearance, or with flats or sneakers for a casual, daytime look. Accessories such as belts, statement jewelry, and handbags can also be added to enhance the overall outfit. In conclusion, a midi dress is a stylish and versatile piece of clothing that falls between the knee and ankle in length. It is a popular choice for formal events and can be found in a variety of styles, fabrics, and designs. The midi dress flatters different body shapes and can be dressed up or down depending on the occasion, making it a staple in every woman's wardrobe.

Midi Skirt

A midi skirt is a type of skirt that falls between the knee and the ankle, typically ending at or below the mid-calf. It is a popular fashion choice that has been embraced by designers and fashion enthusiasts alike. The midi skirt is known for its versatility and timeless appeal. It can be found in a variety of styles, including A-line, pencil, pleated, and flared. The skirt is typically made from lightweight fabrics such as cotton, chiffon, or silk, allowing for ease of movement and comfort.

Millinery Wire

Millinery wire, in the context of fashion design, refers to a flexible and lightweight material typically made from steel or copper, that is used in the construction of hats and other headpieces. It serves as a structural support, enabling the designer to create desired shapes and forms. Designed to be malleable and pliable, millinery wire is often covered with fabrics such as silk or velvet, or other materials like ribbon, to enhance its appearance and blend seamlessly into the overall design of the hat. It is commonly available in various gauges, which determine its thickness and strength, allowing designers to choose the appropriate wire for their specific needs.

Millinery

Millinery is a specialized discipline within the field of fashion design that focuses on creating and designing hats, headpieces, and other headwear accessories. It combines elements of art, culture, and fashion to craft unique and stylish pieces that enhance an individual's outfit and overall appearance. The practice of millinery dates back centuries and has evolved over time to reflect changing trends and societal norms. Milliners, the professionals who specialize in this craft, utilize various materials, techniques, and adornments to bring their designs to life. These materials can range from traditional textiles such as wool, straw, and silk to more unconventional choices like feathers, beads, and even metals. Millinery is not simply about creating functional headgear; it is an art form that allows designers to express their creativity and individual style. Each piece is carefully considered and crafted with attention to detail and impeccable craftsmanship. Milliners must have a keen eye for proportion, balance, and color, as well as an understanding of the wearer's personal style and desired aesthetic. In addition to designing hats and headpieces for everyday wear, milliners often create specialized pieces for occasions and events like weddings, royal ceremonies, and fashion shows. These designs are often more elaborate and can incorporate unique embellishments and intricate techniques such as pleating, draping, and sculpting. The impact of millinery extends beyond the fashion industry. Hats and headwear have long held cultural and social significance, representing wealth, status, and personal style. Millinery allows individuals to make a statement or convey a specific message through their choice of headwear. In recent years, millinery has experienced a resurgence in popularity, with more and more people appreciating the artistry and craftsmanship behind these unique accessories. Whether it's a classic wide-brimmed hat, a whimsical fascinator, or a retro-inspired headscarf, millinery offers endless possibilities for self-expression and style.

Mini Skirt

A mini skirt is a type of skirt that is designed to be short in length and typically falls above the knee. It is a popular fashion choice among women and is considered to be a trendy and fashionable garment. The mini skirt first gained popularity in the 1960s, during the era of the "Swinging Sixties" when youth culture and liberation became a significant influence on fashion. British fashion designer Mary Quant is often credited with creating the mini skirt, as she introduced this daring and revolutionary style to the masses. Mini skirts can be made from a variety of fabrics, including denim, cotton, wool, and synthetic materials. They can also feature a wide range of designs and details, such as pleats, ruffles, buttons, zippers, and embellishments. The versatility of mini skirts allows for endless possibilities in terms of styling and outfit combinations. Mini skirts can be worn for various occasions, ranging from casual day wear to more formal evening events. They can be paired with different types of tops, such as blouses, T-shirts, sweaters, or jackets, depending on the desired look. Mini skirts can also be combined with various footwear options, including heels, boots, flats, or sneakers, to complete the overall ensemble. The mini skirt has remained a timeless and iconic piece in the fashion industry, continuously evolving and adapting to current trends. It symbolizes youthfulness, femininity, and confidence, making it a staple in many women's wardrobes. In recent years, mini skirts have been reimagined with contemporary twists, such as asymmetrical hemlines, wrap styles, and bold prints. These modern updates have further reinforced the mini skirt's status as a must-have fashion item. Overall, the mini skirt is a design marvel that has stood the test of time. Its short length and youthful appeal continue to captivate fashion enthusiasts and empower wearers to embrace their individual style.

Mock Neck Top

A mock neck top is a type of clothing item that features a high neckline that extends up to the base of the neck, creating a snug fit around the neck without the need for a collar. The mock neck top is characterized by its sleek and sophisticated design, often used in both casual and formal wear. The mock neck top provides a modern and stylish alternative to traditional collared shirts or turtlenecks. It offers a more structured and polished look, while still maintaining a comfortable and relaxed feel. The neckline sits close to the base of the neck, providing extra warmth and protection during colder seasons, making it a versatile piece for year-round wear.

Model Agency

A model agency is a company that represents fashion models and connects them with clients in the fashion industry. It acts as a liaison between models and brands, designers, photographers, and other professionals in the fashion world. The main role of a model agency is to scout, train, and manage models, helping them to develop their careers and find opportunities in the fashion industry. They are responsible for promoting their models to potential clients and negotiating contracts on their behalf. One of the key functions of a model agency is scouting and discovering new talent. They have scouts who search for individuals with potential to become successful models. These scouts attend fashion shows, events, and even street casting to find new faces. Once a potential model is found, the agency provides training and guidance to help them develop their skills and make them marketable. Once a model is signed to an agency, the agency's job is to connect them with clients who need models for various fashion-related projects. This includes runway shows, fashion campaigns, editorial shoots, and commercials. The agency uses its network and industry contacts to secure bookings for their models. Model agencies also play a crucial role in managing the careers of their models. They help their models build a portfolio, develop their personal brand, and create a professional image. They also arrange meetings and auditions with clients, accompany models to castings and shoots, and provide support and guidance throughout their careers. In addition to connecting models with clients, model agencies also handle the financial aspects of their models' careers. This includes negotiating contracts, setting rates, and ensuring timely payment for the models' services. They also take a commission or a percentage from the models' earnings as their fee for providing representation and management services. In summary, a model agency is a company that represents fashion models and acts as a middleman between models and clients in the fashion industry. Its main functions include scouting and discovering new talent, connecting models with clients, managing their careers, and handling the financial aspects of their work.

Mom Jeans

The term "mom jeans" refers to a type of high-waisted, loose-fitting denim jeans that were popularized in the 1980s and 1990s, particularly among suburban middle-aged women. These jeans are characterized by their relaxed fit and straight leg, which often extends down to the ankle. Mom jeans are typically made from medium to heavyweight denim fabric, providing durability and structure to the garment. Mom jeans have a distinct design that sets them apart from other styles of jeans. The most defining feature is their high waist, which sits above the natural waistline and emphasizes the midsection. This high-rise design creates a more flattering silhouette for many body types, as it helps to visually elongate the legs and define the waist. Additionally, mom jeans often have a zip fly and button closure at the front, along with belt loops that allow for further customization and accessorizing. In terms of fit, mom jeans are known for their relaxed and comfortable nature. They typically have a roomy hip and thigh area, providing ample space for movement and ensuring a more relaxed feel compared to other styles of jeans. The leg of mom jeans is typically straight and slightly tapered, offering a timeless and classic look that can be easily dressed up or down. While mom jeans were initially associated with a more conservative and "mom-like" image, they have experienced a resurgence in popularity in recent years, particularly among younger individuals. The retro appeal of mom jeans, coupled with their comfortable fit and versatile styling options, has made them a staple in modern fashion. They can be effortlessly paired with a variety of tops, such as tucked-in t-shirts, cropped sweaters, or oversized blouses, allowing for endless outfit possibilities. In conclusion, mom jeans are a style of denim jeans that feature a high-waisted, relaxed fit with a straight leg. They offer a flattering silhouette, comfortable fit, and timeless design, making them a popular choice in contemporary fashion.

Monogramming Machines

A monogramming machine is a specialized device used in the field of fashion design to embroider personalized monograms onto various garments and accessories. It is an essential tool for creating unique and custom-made fashion items. This machine is equipped with advanced technology that allows designers to easily transfer intricate and detailed designs onto fabrics. By utilizing a combination of stitching techniques, such as satin and fill stitches, monogramming machines can produce stunning results that enhance the overall aesthetic appeal of a garment.

Monokini

A monokini is a one-piece swimsuit that combines the style of a bikini with the coverage of a traditional one-piece. It is a popular choice for women who want to show some skin while still maintaining modesty and comfort. The design of a monokini typically features cutouts or sheer panels, which expose parts of the body that would normally be covered by a traditional one-piece swimsuit. These cutouts can be located on the sides, front, or back of the garment, and they can vary in size and shape.

Mood Board

A Mood Board is a visual tool used in fashion design to convey the overall mood, aesthetic, and inspiration for a collection or design concept. It is a collage of images, textures, colors, and other visual elements that capture the desired atmosphere, emotions, and style that the designer intends to communicate through their designs. A Mood Board serves as a visual representation of the designer's creative vision and helps to establish a cohesive and consistent aesthetic for the collection. It acts as a guide throughout the design process, ensuring that all future design choices align with the initial concept. By visually organizing and presenting various elements, a Mood Board helps designers communicate their ideas effectively to others involved in the design process, such as clients, producers, and manufacturers. Composed of carefully curated images, a Mood Board allows the designer to express their inspiration, whether it be drawn from nature, art, culture, or any other source. The images may include photographs, magazine clippings, fabric swatches, color palettes, textures, illustrations, or even handwritten notes. These elements are thoughtfully arranged to create a visual narrative that conveys the desired feel, mood, and theme of the collection. The purpose of a Mood Board is to evoke a specific emotional response, translate abstract concepts into tangible visuals, and provide inspiration for the creative process. It helps the designer to establish a visual language and develop a clear direction for their designs, ensuring that they resonate with the intended audience. Ultimately, a well-executed Mood Board serves as a foundation for the entire design process, informing decisions about fabric selection, color schemes, garment silhouettes, and even marketing strategies. It serves as an invaluable tool for creating a cohesive and compelling collection that embodies the designer's vision and resonates with the target audience.

Needle Threaders

Needle threaders are small tools used in fashion design to assist in threading needles with ease and efficiency. They are typically made of metal or plastic and consist of a handle with a fine wire loop attached at one end. When designing garments, fashion designers often need to thread needles frequently to sew fabric pieces together, create intricate designs, or attach buttons and other accessories. Threading a needle can be a frustrating and time-consuming task, especially when working with delicate fabrics or using thin, fine needles. Needle threaders offer a simple solution to this problem.

Off-Shoulder Blouse

An off-shoulder blouse is a type of garment that is designed to expose the shoulders and collarbones, while covering the bust and torso. It is a popular choice in women's fashion, known for its elegant and feminine aesthetic. The off-shoulder blouse is characterized by its unique neckline, which sits below the shoulders and sometimes extends down the upper arms. This design feature creates a flattering and flirty look, as it accentuates the shoulder line and draws attention to the décolletage. The neckline of an off-shoulder blouse can vary in width and depth, allowing for different levels of exposure and versatility in styling. This type of blouse can be made from a variety of fabrics, including cotton, silk, chiffon, or lace, depending on the desired look and occasion. The choice of fabric can greatly affect the overall style and comfort of the blouse. For example, a cotton off-shoulder blouse may be more suitable for casual or daytime wear, while a silk or lace version can be dressed up for more formal or evening events. The off-shoulder blouse can be designed with various sleeve lengths or even sleeveless for different seasons and personal preferences. It can feature different types of sleeves, such as cap sleeves, flutter sleeves, or long sleeves, adding further interest to the garment. Additionally, off-shoulder blouses often incorporate other design elements, such as ruffles, pleats, or embroidery, to enhance their visual appeal. When styling an off-shoulder blouse, it is important to consider the overall proportions of the outfit. It pairs well with a variety of bottoms, such as high-waisted skirts, shorts, or pants, as it creates a balanced and flattering silhouette. Accessories like statement necklaces or earrings can complement the exposed neckline, while a belt can be added to define the waistline and create a more polished look. Overall, the off-shoulder blouse is a versatile and timeless piece that can be worn for a range of occasions, from casual outings to formal events. Its unique design and feminine charm make it a staple in many women's wardrobes, allowing them to exude elegance and confidence.

Off-Shoulder Bodysuit

An off-shoulder bodysuit is a fashion design garment that combines the elements of an off-shoulder top and a bodysuit. It is a one-piece garment that provides a seamless and streamlined look, with the neckline sitting just below the shoulders. The off-shoulder bodysuit is characterized by its unique neckline, which showcases the shoulders and collarbones while leaving the upper arms bare. This style creates an alluring and feminine silhouette, drawing attention to the neckline and upper body. The bodysuit aspect of the garment ensures a snug and form-fitting fit, making it perfect for pairing with high-waisted bottoms such as skirts or trousers.

Off-Shoulder Top

An off-shoulder top, also known as an off-the-shoulder top, is a fashion design garment that features a neckline that is positioned to expose the shoulders by sitting below the collarbone and baring the upper part of the shoulder. The top is designed in such a way that it showcases and emphasizes the shoulders while leaving the collarbone and neck area exposed, creating an elegant and fashionable look.Off-shoulder tops come in a wide variety of styles and designs, catering to different fashion tastes and preferences. They can either be loose-fitting or form-fitting, depending on the desired style and occasion. The neckline of the top can also vary, with some designs featuring an elasticized band that keeps the top in place on the shoulders, while others have a more relaxed fit that allows the top to naturally sit off the shoulders.

One-Shoulder Bodysuit

A one-shoulder bodysuit is a garment designed for women that combines the elements of a one-shoulder top and a bodysuit. It is a trendy and fashionable piece of clothing that has gained popularity in the world of fashion design. This type of bodysuit is characterized by its asymmetrical design, featuring a single shoulder strap or sleeve. The strap is usually wider than a typical spaghetti strap, creating a stylish and unique look. The bodysuit is designed to fit snugly against the body, providing a streamlined silhouette. The one-shoulder bodysuit is often made from stretchy materials such as spandex or elastane, which allows for a comfortable and flexible fit. It may also feature additional details such as ruffles, cut-outs, or embellishments that enhance the overall aesthetic of the garment. One-shoulder bodysuits can be versatile and can be styled in various ways to suit different occasions. They can be dressed up or down depending on the desired look. For a casual daytime outfit, it can be paired with high-waisted jeans or shorts and sandals. For a more formal or evening look, it can be paired with tailored trousers or a skirt and heels. This type of bodysuit is a popular choice for those who want to make a fashion statement and add a touch of glamour to their outfit. It is a flattering and feminine piece that accentuates the shoulders and collarbone, creating an elegant and alluring look. In conclusion, a one-shoulder bodysuit is a stylish and fashionable garment that combines the elements of a one-shoulder top and a bodysuit. It is characterized by its asymmetrical design and snug fit, making it a versatile choice for various occasions. With its unique and glamorous look, it is a trendy choice for those who want to make a fashion statement.

Oversized Shirt

An oversized shirt is a loose-fitting garment that is designed to be worn as a top. It is characterized by its generous dimensions, which typically extend beyond the usual proportions of a regular shirt. The oversized fit of the shirt allows for a relaxed and comfortable wearing experience, as it provides ample room for movement. The construction of an oversized shirt involves a slightly different pattern than that of a standard shirt. The length and width of the shirt are increased, resulting in a more voluminous silhouette. This oversized silhouette can be achieved through various design techniques, such as the inclusion of extra fabric or the use of exaggerated proportions. Oversized shirts are often made from lightweight and breathable materials, such as cotton or linen, to ensure optimum comfort. The loose fit of the shirt allows for better air circulation, making it ideal for warmer weather or casual occasions. Additionally, oversized shirts can be found in a variety of styles, including button-downs, tunic-style shirts, and even oversized t-shirts. When it comes to styling an oversized shirt, there are numerous options to consider. It can be worn as a standalone piece, paired with bottoms such as jeans or trousers, or layered with other garments for a more fashion-forward look. The versatility of the oversized shirt makes it a popular choice among both men and women. Overall, the oversized shirt is a trendy and comfortable addition to any wardrobe. Its relaxed fit and modern aesthetic make it a go-to piece for those seeking a casual yet stylish outfit. With its generous proportions and various styling options, the oversized shirt is a staple in contemporary fashion.

Palazzo Pants

Palazzo Pants, also known as wide-leg or culotte trousers, are a style of women's pants that have a loose and flowing silhouette. The term "palazzo" originates from Italian, meaning "palace," illustrating the luxurious and sophisticated nature of these pants. Palazzo pants are characterized by their wide leg opening, which starts from the waist and extends all the way to the hemline. They are typically made from lightweight, breathable fabrics such as silk, chiffon, or linen, allowing for maximum comfort and ease of movement. The fabric choice also adds to the elegant and airy drape of the pants, giving them a feminine and ethereal appearance. These pants are often high-waisted, sitting above the natural waistline, which elongates the legs and creates a flattering silhouette. The waistband is usually fitted with a zipper, hook-and-eye closure, or an elastic band for added comfort. Some versions of palazzo pants may feature a belt or waist tie for added detail and versatility. Palazzo pants have been a popular choice in fashion since the 1960s, when they first gained popularity as a symbol of women's liberation and empowerment. They offer a stylish alternative to restrictive and constricting clothing, allowing women to move freely and comfortably while still maintaining a polished and chic look. These pants can be dressed up or down, making them a versatile wardrobe staple. They can be paired with a fitted blouse or tailored blazer for a formal or professional look, or dressed down with a simple tank top or t-shirt for a more casual and relaxed ensemble. Palazzo pants are also often worn for special occasions or events, offering an elegant and unique alternative to traditional dresses or skirts. In recent years, palazzo pants have experienced a resurgence in popularity, with many fashion designers incorporating them into their collections. They have become a favorite among celebrities and fashion influencers, further solidifying their status as a trendy and fashionable choice. In conclusion, palazzo pants are wide-leg trousers that offer both style and comfort. Their flowy and relaxed silhouette, combined with a high-waisted design, creates a flattering and feminine look. Whether worn for a formal event or as part of a casual outfit, palazzo pants are a versatile and fashionable choice in women's fashion.

Paperbag Mini Skirt

A paperbag mini skirt is a type of skirt that is designed to have a gathered and bunched waistline, resembling the top of a paper bag when worn. It is typically short in length, falling above the knee, and is a popular trend in fashion design. The defining feature of a paperbag mini skirt is the gathered waistline, which creates a voluminous and cinched effect. This gathered waist is achieved through the use of excess fabric that is gathered and secured with a drawstring or elastic band. The excess fabric creates a pleated or ruched effect around the waistline, adding texture and visual interest to the skirt. The paperbag mini skirt is known for its versatility and can be styled in various ways for different occasions. It can be dressed up for a more formal look by pairing it with a blouse or a tailored jacket. Alternatively, it can be dressed down for a casual, everyday outfit by pairing it with a t-shirt or a cropped top. In terms of fabric choice, the paperbag mini skirt is commonly made from lightweight materials such as cotton, linen, or polyester, as these fabrics drape well and contribute to the relaxed and breezy aesthetic of the skirt. However, it can also be found in more structured and luxurious materials such as silk or satin, which can elevate the skirt's overall look. The paperbag mini skirt is a popular choice for its ability to accentuate the waistline and create a flattering silhouette. The gathered waistline creates the illusion of a smaller waist, while the short length showcases the legs. This combination makes it a go-to option for those looking to emphasize their curves. Overall, the paperbag mini skirt is a versatile and fashionable piece that adds a touch of flair and style to any outfit. Its unique gathered waistline and short length make it a standout piece in the world of fashion design.

Paperbag Pants

Paperbag pants are a style of pants that feature a distinct gathered waistband that creates a voluminous and pleated effect around the waist. The name "paperbag" comes from how the waistband resembles the cinching of a paper bag. These pants are typically high-waisted and have a loose fit around the hips and legs, often tapering towards the ankles. The gathered waistband is usually elasticated, allowing for a comfortable fit and easy movement. It is common for paperbag pants to also have a belt or a fabric tie that can be used to further cinch the waist and add definition. The unique waistband of paperbag pants adds a touch of femininity and sophistication to the overall look. It creates a flattering silhouette by accentuating the waist and providing a bit of structure to the pants. The gathered fabric adds volume and visual interest, making paperbag pants a popular choice for those looking to add some drama to their outfit. These pants can be made from a variety of materials, including lightweight fabrics like cotton and linen for a more casual and relaxed look, or more structured fabrics like wool or tweed for a formal or professional appearance. They can also come in different lengths, from full-length trousers to cropped styles. When it comes to styling paperbag pants, they are versatile and can be dressed up or down depending on the occasion. For a casual look, they can be paired with a tucked-in T-shirt or blouse and sneakers or sandals. To create a more polished and chic outfit, they can be worn with a fitted top, heels, and statement accessories. Overall, paperbag pants are a trendy and fashionable choice for those who want to experiment with different silhouettes and add a touch of uniqueness to their outfit. They offer a comfortable fit, flattering shape, and endless styling possibilities, making them a must-have piece in any fashion-forward wardrobe.

Paperbag Shorts

Paperbag shorts refer to a style of shorts that feature a high waistline and a gathered or ruffled waistband that resembles the top of a paper bag when cinched. This unique design element adds volume and interest to the waistline, creating a fashion-forward and flattering silhouette. These shorts typically have a loose and relaxed fit, making them comfortable and ideal for casual wear. They are often made from lightweight and breathable fabrics such as cotton or linen, which further enhance their comfort and versatility.

Paperbag Waist Pants

Paperbag waist pants are a type of pants that feature a high, gathered waistband that resembles the top part of a paper bag. This design detail gives the pants a unique and distinctive look that is both stylish and fashion-forward. The paperbag waistband is typically created by folding and scrunching the fabric at the waist to create volume and a gathered effect. This is often achieved by adding pleats or elastic to the waistband, which helps to create the desired shape and fit. The result is a cinched-in waistline that creates a flattering silhouette and adds visual interest to the pants.

Pareo

A pareo is a versatile piece of fabric that is commonly used in fashion design. It originated from the Pacific Islands, specifically Polynesia, and has become popular all around the world. The pareo is a rectangular-shaped cloth that can be tied, draped, or wrapped around the body in various ways to create different styles and looks. The pareo is often made from lightweight and breathable materials such as cotton, rayon, or silk, making it perfect for warm weather or beachwear. It can come in a wide range of colors, patterns, and prints, allowing for endless possibilities in terms of design and styling.

Parka

A parka is a type of outerwear garment that is designed to provide warmth and protection from cold weather conditions. It is a versatile and practical piece of clothing that is commonly used in outdoor and winter activities. Typically, a parka is made from durable materials such as cotton, polyester, or nylon, and is insulated with down or synthetic fibers to provide insulation and retain body heat. It features a long length, reaching below the hips or even down to the knees, and often has a hood with a fur or faux-fur trim to provide additional warmth and protection for the head and face.

Pattern Cardboard Cutters

Pattern cardboard cutters are tools used in fashion design to create accurate paper patterns for garments. They are typically made of durable cardboard material and come in various shapes and sizes to accommodate different pattern cutting needs. These cutters provide a convenient and efficient way for fashion designers to transfer their designs onto paper, which can then be used to create patterns for the actual garment construction. The primary purpose of pattern cardboard cutters is to ensure precision and consistency in pattern making. They are used to trace and cut out pattern pieces from paper or cardboard, allowing designers to replicate their designs with accuracy. By using these cutters, fashion designers can save time and effort compared to manual cutting methods, such as scissors or utility knives. The clean and smooth edges produced by pattern cardboard cutters also contribute to a more professional and polished appearance of the final garment.

Pattern Cardboard

Pattern cardboard refers to a stiff and rigid material that is commonly used in the field of fashion design. It is a key tool in the process of creating and refining garment patterns. In fashion design, pattern cardboard is primarily used to transfer and trace patterns onto fabric. It provides a stable and sturdy surface for designers to work on, ensuring accuracy and precision during the pattern-making process. The stiffness of the cardboard prevents the fabric from slipping or stretching, allowing for clean and precise pattern lines.

Pattern Cutting Tools

Pattern cutting tools are essential instruments used in the field of fashion design for creating patterns and templates that serve as guides for producing garments. These tools are designed to assist designers in achieving accurate and precise measurements, shapes, and sizes when drafting patterns. One common type of pattern cutting tool is the pattern ruler. Also known as a fashion ruler, this instrument features a variety of straight and curved edges, guides, and measurements. Pattern rulers help designers create straight lines, smooth curves, and accurate angles when drawing pattern pieces. They are typically made from transparent plastic to allow for easy visibility and alignment with existing pattern markings.

Pattern Digitizers

A pattern digitizer is an essential tool used in the fashion design industry to convert physical patterns into digital format. It is a device or software that captures the intricate details and measurements of a paper pattern and translates them into a digital image or file. The process of digitizing patterns is crucial for various reasons. Firstly, it allows for easy storage and retrieval of pattern data. Instead of relying on physical storage space for bulky paper patterns, digitized files can be organized and accessed digitally, saving time and space for designers. Additionally, digital patterns can be easily duplicated, modified, and shared, enabling efficient collaboration with other members of the design team or manufacturers. Pattern digitizers are commonly used alongside digitizing tablets or pen-based input devices, which allow designers to manually trace the lines and curves of a pattern. These tablets capture the movement and pressure of the stylus, accurately recreating the shape and details of the pattern on the computer screen. The digitizer software then converts these captured images into a digital format, often using CAD (Computer-Aided Design) software. Accuracy is a crucial aspect of pattern digitization. Designers rely on digitizers to accurately measure and capture every detail of the pattern, including curve shapes, notches, and seam allowances. The precision of the digitizer greatly impacts the quality of the final digital pattern, ensuring that the garment created from it will fit as intended. In addition to converting physical patterns into digital files, some pattern digitizers also offer advanced features. These features may include the ability to grade patterns (resize them for different sizes), add seam allowances or other annotations, and even simulate how a garment will drape and fit on a virtual model. These advanced functionalities further enhance the design process and enable designers to visualize and refine their ideas before actual production.

Pattern Digitizing Stylus

A pattern digitizing stylus is a tool used in the field of fashion design to convert physical garment patterns into digital format. It is a handheld device with a fine-point tip that allows designers to trace the lines of a pattern on paper or fabric, capturing the intricate details and measurements. By using the pattern digitizing stylus, designers can create precise and accurate digital versions of their patterns, which can be easily manipulated and modified using computer software. This digital representation of the pattern can then be utilized for various purposes, such as grading, resizing, and sharing with manufacturers or collaborators.

Pattern Digitizing Tablets

Pattern Digitizing Tablets are advanced technological devices used in the field of fashion design to convert hand-drawn or physical patterns into digital form. These tablets, also referred to as digitizers, offer fashion designers a more efficient and accurate method of transferring their designs into the digital realm. Pattern digitizing is an essential step in the modern fashion design process as it enables designers to easily modify and manipulate patterns on computer software. With a pattern digitizing tablet, designers can eliminate the need for manual measuring and drafting by digitally capturing their designs directly onto the tablet's surface. This allows for a faster and more precise creation of digital patterns. One of the key features of pattern digitizing tablets is their pressure-sensitive surface, similar to that of a graphic design tablet. This surface detects the pressure applied by the designer's hand, capturing every stroke or mark accurately. This feature allows for a natural and seamless transition from traditional sketching to digital pattern creation. Pattern digitizing tablets often come with specialized software that allows designers to further edit and refine their digital patterns. This software may include tools for resizing, rotating, and manipulating patterns, as well as options for adding details such as notches, seam allowances, and grain lines. In addition to their efficiency and accuracy, pattern digitizing tablets also offer designers the advantage of easy storage and accessibility. Once a pattern is digitized, it can be saved in various file formats and stored electronically. This eliminates the need for physical storage and allows designers to easily retrieve and share their patterns with others. Overall, pattern digitizing tablets have revolutionized the way fashion designers create and work with patterns. They provide a seamless transition from traditional to digital methods, offering increased efficiency, accuracy, and flexibility in the design process. These tablets have become an indispensable tool for fashion designers who strive to modernize their practices and keep up with the ever-evolving fashion industry.

Pattern Drafting Books

A pattern drafting book in the context of fashion design is a comprehensive reference guide that provides step-by-step instructions and templates for creating custom clothing patterns. These books are essential tools for fashion designers, pattern makers, and dressmakers, as they help in understanding the concepts and techniques of pattern drafting. The primary purpose of a pattern drafting book is to teach the process of creating precise patterns that accurately fit a specific body shape or size. These books typically cover various aspects of pattern making, such as taking measurements, understanding body proportions, and converting those measurements into a basic pattern. They also elaborate on the principles of pattern manipulation, allowing designers to modify existing patterns or create entirely new ones.

Pattern Drafting Kits

Pattern Drafting Kits are essential tools used in the field of fashion design. These kits consist of various instruments and supplies that are used to create pattern drafts, which serve as the blueprint for the construction of garments. The primary purpose of a pattern drafting kit is to enable fashion designers to create custom-made patterns that are precise and tailored to individual measurements. This process is crucial in the creation of well-fitted and visually appealing garments. The kits typically include a range of tools and materials such as rulers, French curves, hip curves, tape measures, tracing paper, and pattern hooks.

Pattern Drafting Machines

A pattern drafting machine is a mechanical tool used in the field of fashion design to create the basic pattern for a garment. It is a device that assists designers in the process of transforming their design ideas into actual patterns that can be used for cutting and sewing fabric. The machine consists of a drafting board, which is typically made of a smooth, flat surface such as wood or metal. The board is marked with a grid pattern of lines and measurement markings, which help guide the designer in creating accurate patterns. Alongside the drafting board, there is a system of rulers, guides, and templates that can be adjusted and manipulated to create various shapes and sizes for different parts of the garment. Designers use the pattern drafting machine to accurately reproduce their designs in multiple sizes. They start by placing a sheet of paper or fabric on the drafting board and secure it in place with weights or pins. They then use the rulers and guides to measure and mark the key points and lines of the design. This process helps ensure that each size of the pattern is consistent and proportionate. The pattern drafting machine enables designers to save time and effort by automating the process of creating patterns. It helps them to achieve precise measurements and shapes, which are crucial in the construction of garments. With this tool, designers can easily make adjustments to the pattern, such as adding or subtracting seam allowances, altering darts, or modifying the length or width of the garment. In addition to saving time and ensuring accuracy, pattern drafting machines also allow for greater efficiency in the production process. Once the pattern is created, it can be easily transferred onto a computer or saved for future reference, thereby minimizing the need for manual re-drafting. This is particularly advantageous in the fashion industry, where patterns need to be quickly replicated and scaled for mass production.

Pattern Drafting Mannequins

Pattern Drafting Paper

A pattern drafting paper is an essential tool used in fashion design to create and modify patterns for garments. It is a specialized type of paper that is specifically designed for pattern making and is widely used by professional and aspiring fashion designers. The pattern drafting paper typically comes in large rolls or sheets with grids and markings that assist in creating accurate and symmetrical patterns. The grids are typically made up of small squares, which help in measuring and drawing precise lines and angles for various pattern components.

Pattern Drafting Rulers

Pattern drafting rulers are specialized tools used in fashion design to create precise and accurate patterns for clothing. These rulers are made with specific markings and measurements that allow designers to create individual pieces that fit together perfectly when assembled. Pattern drafting rulers typically come in various shapes and sizes, each with different markings and uses. Common types include straight rulers, French curves, and L-squares. Straight rulers are used for drawing straight lines and measuring straight distances, while French curves and L-squares are used for drawing curved lines and shaping pattern pieces. These rulers are usually made of plastic or transparent materials, allowing designers to see through them and accurately place markings on fabric. The markings on pattern drafting rulers are designed to help designers accurately measure lengths, angles, and curves. They may include measurements in inches, centimeters, or both, as well as special markings for common design elements such as darts, pleats, and seam allowances. Some rulers may also have grids or grids with dots, which help designers create patterns with precise symmetry and alignment. When using pattern drafting rulers, designers typically start by taking measurements of the person or mannequin they are designing for. They then use the rulers to draw the basic shape of the garment, following the measurements and adjusting for ease and desired fit. The rulers make it easier to create accurate and consistent patterns, reducing the need for trial and error when constructing the final garment. In conclusion, pattern drafting rulers are essential tools for fashion designers. They allow designers to create patterns with precise measurements and shapes, ensuring a proper fit and professional finish. By using pattern drafting rulers, designers can save time and effort in the design and construction process, resulting in high-quality garments that meet the expectations of both the designer and the wearer.

Pattern Drafting Software

Pattern drafting software is a specialized computer program used in the field of fashion design to create precise and accurate patterns for garments. It allows designers to easily transform their ideas into tangible patterns that can be used for garment production. The software provides designers with a digital platform to draft, modify, and manipulate patterns with precision and efficiency. It eliminates the need for traditional manual pattern drafting techniques, such as using paper, rulers, and sewing tools. Instead, designers can utilize various tools and functions within the software to create patterns directly on their computer screens. Pattern drafting software typically includes features such as measurement input, shape drawing, line editing, and grading. Designers can input the measurements of a model or customer to create custom-fit patterns, which can be adjusted and modified as needed. They can draw and manipulate shapes, lines, and curves to create the desired pattern pieces for different garment components. The software also enables designers to edit and modify pattern lines, angles, and proportions with ease. Furthermore, pattern drafting software allows for the efficient grading of patterns. Grading involves systematically increasing or decreasing the pattern size to fit different body measurements or to create different sizes of the same garment. With the software's grading functionality, designers can easily scale patterns up or down and generate multiple sizes without the need for manual calculations or re-drafting. In addition to these core features, pattern drafting software often includes advanced capabilities such as pattern layout, 3D simulation, and integration with CAD (Computer-Aided Design) systems. These features allow designers to visualize how the pattern pieces will be laid out on the fabric, simulate how the garment will look on a virtual model, and seamlessly transition their patterns to other design software for further detailing and prototyping. Overall, pattern drafting software revolutionizes the fashion design process by providing designers with a powerful tool to create accurate patterns efficiently and effectively. It combines precision, flexibility, and convenience, enabling designers to bring their creative visions to life with ease.

Pattern Draping Accessories

Pattern draping accessories are essential tools used in the process of fashion design. These accessories are used specifically during the draping stage, where designers drape fabric directly onto a dress form to create the initial shape and structure of a garment. Pattern draping accessories include a variety of tools that aid in achieving the desired draping effect. These tools commonly include pins, weights, tape measures, rulers, and fabric marking tools. Each of these accessories serves a specific purpose in the draping process, helping to ensure accurate and precise results.

Pattern Draping Fabrics

Pattern draping fabrics in the context of fashion design refers to the process of laying and shaping fabric directly onto a dress form or model to create three-dimensional designs. This technique allows designers to visualize and develop their ideas before cutting and sewing the actual garment. Pattern draping fabrics involves using various types of fabrics that possess specific qualities to achieve desired design elements. The choice of fabric significantly affects the outcome of the draped pattern, as different textiles drape and behave differently when manipulated. The fabric's weight, stretch, texture, and fluidity all contribute to the overall look and structure of the draped design.

Pattern Draping Forms

Pattern draping forms are essential tools used by fashion designers to create and develop clothing designs. They are three-dimensional figures that mimic the shape and proportions of the human body. These forms, often made of dressmaker's mannequins or adjustable dress forms, provide a solid base upon which patterns can be draped and fitted. Draping is a technique used in fashion design where fabric is manipulated directly on the form to create a garment. It allows designers to experiment with different shapes, silhouettes, and styles without the need for flat pattern making. Pattern draping forms play a crucial role in this process as they serve as a realistic representation of the human body, enabling designers to visualize how the fabric will hang and drape on a real person. Using a pattern draping form, a designer starts by pinning muslin or another lightweight fabric onto the form to create the basic shape of the garment. They then manipulate and sculpt the fabric, using their artistic skills and understanding of the body's curves and proportions, to refine the design. This involves understanding how fabric drapes around the curves of the form, how to create pleats or gathers for volume, and how different fabrics behave when manipulated. Pattern draping forms also allow for fittings and adjustments during the design process. The fabric can be pinned or marked to indicate changes that need to be made, such as altering the drape, adjusting the length, or refining the fit. Designers can also experiment with different closures, collars, sleeves, and other design elements to enhance the overall aesthetic of the garment. Once the designer is satisfied with the draped pattern, it is carefully removed from the form and transformed into a flat pattern. This flat pattern can then be used to create multiple garments of the same design or scaled up for production. Pattern draping forms are indispensable tools for fashion designers, as they enable the creative exploration, development, and refinement of designs. They allow designers to visualize and manipulate fabric directly on a three-dimensional figure, providing them with invaluable insights into how the garment will look and fit on a real body. Without pattern draping forms, the process of creating unique and well-fitted designs would be much more challenging and less accurate.

Pattern Draping Stands

Pattern draping stands, also known as dress forms or mannequins, are essential tools used in the field of fashion design. These stands are three-dimensional representations of the human body, allowing designers to drape fabric directly onto them to create and refine garment patterns. The primary purpose of pattern draping stands is to help fashion designers visualize and manipulate their designs in real life. They serve as a practical and tactile way to experiment with fabric, shapes, and proportions. By draping fabric onto the stand, designers can see how the fabric falls and drapes on a three-dimensional figure, allowing them to perfect the fit and drape of their designs.

Pattern Draping Tape

Pattern draping tape is a tool used in the field of fashion design to create accurate and precise patterns for garments. It is a flexible and adhesive tape that is specifically designed to drape and conform to the body, allowing designers to visualize and create garment patterns directly on a dress form or a live model. When designing garments, fashion designers rely on pattern draping tape to accurately transfer their ideas and designs onto a three-dimensional form. The draping tape is typically made from a cloth-like material that possesses a certain amount of stretch and flexibility, which allows it to conform to the curves and contours of the body. This enables designers to achieve a more realistic and accurate representation of how the finished garment will fit and look.

Pattern Files

A pattern file, in the context of fashion design, refers to a set of digital files or physical templates that are used in the creation of garments. These files contain the measurements, shapes, and details necessary for producing the various parts of a garment, including the body, sleeves, collars, and other components. To create a garment, a fashion designer or pattern maker starts by developing a pattern. This involves taking the desired design and translating it into a set of precise measurements and geometrical shapes. The pattern file serves as a blueprint for the construction of the garment, providing the necessary guidelines for cutting the fabric and assembling the pieces. Pattern files can be created using different software applications or manually drawn and stored as physical templates. In digital form, these files are often saved in standard formats such as Adobe Illustrator (.ai) or AutoCAD (.dwg), which can be easily shared, modified, or scaled as per the specific requirements. Pattern files play a crucial role in the fashion design process. They enable designers to accurately reproduce a design in different sizes, ensuring consistency and precision in the final product. These files are also essential for communication between designers, pattern makers, and manufacturers. They provide a common reference point, allowing everyone involved in the production process to understand and execute the design accurately. Furthermore, pattern files can be reused and modified for creating different variations of a design or for developing new garments. They serve as a valuable resource for designers to build upon previous works and experiment with different design elements. In conclusion, pattern files are an integral part of fashion design, serving as the foundation for garment construction. Whether in digital or physical form, these files provide the necessary guidelines, measurements, and shapes for creating garments with precision and consistency.

Pattern Grading Rulers

A pattern grading ruler, in the context of fashion design, is a specialized tool used in the process of scaling or increasing the size of a pattern. It is commonly used in the garment industry to grade patterns to different sizes, ensuring that the proportions and fit of the garment are maintained across various sizes. The pattern grading ruler typically consists of a long, straight ruler with evenly spaced markings or increments along its length. These markings represent the desired size variations for each specific pattern piece. The ruler may have different measurements on each side, allowing for grading up or down in size.

Pattern Grading Software

Pattern Grading Software is a technological tool used in the field of fashion design to change the sizes of pre-designed patterns, while ensuring proportional and accurate scaling. It automates the process of grading patterns by eliminating the need for manual calculations and reducing human error, thus increasing efficiency and productivity in the garment manufacturing process. Designed for fashion designers, pattern makers, and manufacturers, Pattern Grading Software simplifies the process of creating patterns in different sizes, enabling the production of ready-to-wear garments in various measurements, including petite, regular, and plus sizes. It offers a user-friendly interface with a range of tools and features, allowing designers to easily modify patterns based on specific size requirements. With Pattern Grading Software, the designer input the original pattern and defines the desired size range. The software then calculates the necessary measurements for each pattern piece, adjusting them proportionally to maintain the overall design aesthetics. This includes resizing not only the main body parts but also other elements, such as sleeves, collars, and pockets, ensuring they remain consistent throughout the size range. Pattern Grading Software also provides the option to grade patterns in a single step or incrementally, depending on the desired outcome. It allows for customization by considering factors such as fit preferences, fabric characteristics, and manufacturing limitations. Once the grading process is complete, the software generates the resized pattern pieces along with the corresponding measurements for each size, which can be printed or exported for further use. In addition to saving time and effort, Pattern Grading Software offers accuracy and consistency in pattern resizing, contributing to improved garment fit and reduced production costs. It eliminates the need for manual pattern grading, which can be labor-intensive, time-consuming, and prone to errors. The software also facilitates collaboration between designers and manufacturers, as patterns can be easily shared and revised without compromising their integrity. In conclusion, Pattern Grading Software is a valuable tool in the fashion industry, streamlining the process of resizing patterns and enabling the production of garments in various sizes. Its automation capabilities, user-friendly interface, and accuracy contribute to increased efficiency, better fit, and enhanced collaboration between designers and manufacturers.

Pattern Grading Tools

Pattern grading tools refer to a set of instruments and techniques used in the field of fashion design to systematically and accurately enlarge or reduce the size of a pattern while maintaining its original proportions. This process is essential for creating garments that fit various body sizes and shapes without compromising the overall design and aesthetics. The main purpose of pattern grading tools is to streamline the process of scaling a pattern up or down, saving time and effort for designers and manufacturers. These tools are often used in conjunction with pattern drafting systems, which involve creating the initial pattern from scratch or modifying an existing one to meet specific design requirements.

Pattern Hooks

Pattern hooks, in the context of fashion design, refer to the specific elements or details added to garments in order to enhance their aesthetic appeal, create visual interest, or provide functional purposes. These hooks can take various forms, such as decorative embellishments, unique stitching, contrasting colors or fabrics, or specialized closures. They are often strategically placed on different parts of the garment to highlight or accentuate certain features, add texture or dimension, or create focal points. Pattern hooks play a crucial role in fashion design as they contribute to the overall design concept, help create a cohesive look, and can even communicate the brand's identity or style. They allow designers to showcase their creativity, innovation, and attention to detail, while also serving practical purposes. For example, pattern hooks can be used to create intricate embroidery or beading on a gown, adding a luxurious and glamorous touch. They can also be utilized in tailored jackets or coats, where unique buttons or closures add sophistication and individuality to the design. Similarly, pattern hooks can be employed in sportswear or activewear to improve functionality, like the use of zipper pockets or adjustable straps. The choice of pattern hooks depends on the designer's vision and the garment's intended purpose. They can be inspired by various sources, such as nature, art, history, or cultural influences, and can range from bold and eye-catching to subtle and understated. Ultimately, pattern hooks contribute to the overall aesthetic and appeal of a garment, making it unique, visually engaging, and desirable.

Pattern Making Kits

A pattern making kit in the context of fashion design refers to a set of tools and materials that are used to create patterns for garments. These kits provide essential resources for fashion designers and pattern makers to develop templates that accurately represent the shape and structure of each garment piece. Pattern making is an integral part of the fashion design process, as it involves translating a designer's vision into tangible patterns that can be used to construct garments. Pattern making kits typically include tools such as rulers, measuring tapes, tracing paper, pencils, scissors, and curve rulers. Each tool has a specific purpose and is essential for creating precise and accurate patterns. Rulers and measuring tapes are used to take precise measurements of the body or mannequin, ensuring that the patterns created will fit properly. Tracing paper is often used to transfer the measurements onto paper, allowing the designer to manipulate and alter the patterns as needed. Pencils are used to mark the measurements and make adjustments to the patterns. Scissors are necessary for cutting out the final patterns, while curve rulers help in drawing smooth and symmetrical curves. Pattern making kits can also include additional tools such as pattern notches, tracers, and awls, which aid in creating pattern details and markings. Pattern notches are small cuts made on the paper patterns to indicate specific points of alignment and assembly. Tracers are used to transfer pattern details onto fabric, ensuring accurate placement during garment construction. Awls are helpful in making small holes or marks on the fabric for pattern adjustments or for inserting fasteners. These kits typically come with instructions or guides on how to use the tools and materials effectively. They may also include basic pattern making templates or slopers, which are pre-made patterns for common garment components like bodices, sleeves, and skirts. These templates provide a starting point for designers and can be modified to create unique and customized designs. In summary, a pattern making kit in fashion design is a collection of tools and materials that are used to create accurate patterns for garments. These kits are essential for fashion designers and pattern makers, providing them with the necessary resources to bring their designs to life.

Pattern Making Pencils

A pattern making pencil is a tool used in the field of fashion design to create accurate and precise patterns for garments. It is a specialized pencil specifically designed for pattern making purposes. The pattern making pencil is typically made of high-quality graphite or lead, ensuring a smooth and consistent line when drawing patterns on paper or fabric. It is also designed to be sharpened to a fine point, allowing for intricate details and precise markings. One of the key features of a pattern making pencil is its ability to create straight and curved lines. The pencil is designed with a long, thin, and slightly flexible tip, allowing the designer to easily maneuver and control the shape and angle of the lines. This is particularly important when drawing sewing lines, darts, notches, and other details that determine the shape and fit of the garment. Additionally, pattern making pencils often have different colored lead or graphite to differentiate between various markings on the pattern. For example, red or blue lead may be used to indicate notches or symbols, while black or grey lead may be used for sewing lines or grain lines. This color-coding system helps the designer quickly identify and interpret the different elements of the pattern. Pattern making pencils are an essential tool for fashion designers, as they allow for accurate and precise pattern creation. By using a pattern making pencil, designers can ensure that their patterns are consistent, well-proportioned, and easy to follow for the construction of the garment. It is a versatile and reliable tool that aids in the overall production process, from initial pattern drafting to the final stage of garment construction.

Pattern Making Racks

Pattern Making Software

Pattern making software is a computer application specifically designed for the fashion industry, used by fashion designers and pattern makers to create digital representations of clothing patterns. It is an essential tool for the design and production process of garments. Pattern making software allows designers to create and customize patterns using various tools and features provided by the software. These tools typically include options for creating basic pattern blocks, grading patterns to different sizes, adding seam allowances, and making alterations to the pattern. The software also allows users to input specific measurements and generate patterns that are tailored to individual body sizes and proportions.

Pattern Making Tablets

A pattern making tablet, in the context of fashion design, refers to a digital device or tablet specifically designed for the creation and modification of patterns used in garment production. It offers a more efficient and convenient alternative to traditional manual pattern drafting methods. Pattern making tablets typically come with specialized software that allows fashion designers to digitize their pattern templates and make edits directly on the digital interface. The tablet's touchscreen or stylus input enables designers to draw, manipulate, and refine patterns with precision and ease.

Pattern Making Wheels

Pattern making wheels are essential tools used in the field of fashion design. They are circular tools that are used to create patterns and designs onto fabric. These wheels are typically made of a durable material such as plastic or metal and have small teeth-like edges on the circumference of the wheel. The main function of pattern making wheels is to transfer a design or pattern onto fabric or paper. Fashion designers use these wheels to create intricate patterns and designs quickly and easily. They are particularly useful for creating repetitive patterns such as stripes or checks. The teeth on the wheel grip the fabric or paper, allowing the designer to roll the wheel along the surface to transfer the pattern.

Pattern Making

Pattern making in the context of fashion design refers to the process of creating the blueprint or template for a garment before it is constructed. It involves transforming a designer's concept or sketch into a 2D representation that can be used to cut and sew the fabric into the desired shape. Pattern making is a crucial step in the production of a garment, as it determines the fit, drape, and overall design of the finished product. During the pattern making process, precise measurements are taken from the human body or a dress form, and these measurements are used to create a series of interconnected lines and curves. These lines and curves form the pattern pieces, which are traced onto paper, cardboard, or digital platforms. Each pattern piece represents a specific part of the garment, such as a sleeve, bodice, or skirt. The pattern pieces are then cut out and used as templates to cut the fabric.

Pattern Notation Pens

Pattern Notation Pens refer to specialized marking tools used in fashion design to create accurate and precise pattern markings on fabric. These pens are designed with fine, pointed tips that allow fashion designers to draw lines, symbols, and notations on fabric with ease and accuracy. In the field of fashion design, patterns play a crucial role in garment construction. A pattern serves as a blueprint or template for creating a garment, outlining the various pieces that need to be cut and sewn together. Pattern Notation Pens enable designers to clearly mark these pattern pieces, seam lines, dart locations, grainlines, notches, and other important details directly onto the fabric, ensuring that the construction process is precise and error-free.

Pattern Notation Software

A pattern notation software is a program specifically designed for fashion designers to digitally create, manipulate, and document the patterns used in the construction of garments. It provides a digital representation of the pattern pieces, along with detailed information on their dimensions, markings, and sewing instructions. The primary purpose of pattern notation software is to streamline the pattern-making process and enhance the accuracy and efficiency of garment production. It allows designers to easily create and modify pattern pieces using digital tools such as drawing tools, measurement tools, and shape manipulation tools. The software provides a platform for designers to experiment with different pattern variations and explore creative design possibilities without the need to physically create multiple paper patterns. Pattern notation software also offers features for digitizing existing paper patterns, enabling designers to convert their existing physical patterns into digital format. This functionality simplifies pattern storage, organization, and sharing among team members. It also reduces the risk of losing or damaging valuable pattern archives. Additionally, pattern notation software includes tools and features for generating detailed pattern instructions and sewing guidelines. Designers can annotate pattern pieces with information on grain lines, fabric layouts, and seam allowances. They can also create sewing notations, such as dart placements, pleat markings, and zipper placements, to ensure accurate fabrication of the garment. These annotations help guide the pattern cutter and garment assemblers, ensuring that the final product matches the designer's vision. In summary, pattern notation software provides fashion designers with a digital platform to create, modify, and document garment patterns. It enhances the efficiency and accuracy of the pattern-making process, facilitates collaboration among team members, and enables designers to experiment with different design variations. By digitizing the pattern creation process, it offers a more sustainable and flexible approach to fashion design.

Pattern Notation Tablets

Pattern Notation Tablets are tools used in fashion design to document and communicate the intricate details of design patterns. They are electronic devices with specialized software that allows designers to create, edit, and store patterns digitally, eliminating the need for physical paper patterns. This technology has revolutionized the fashion industry by streamlining the pattern development process and increasing the accuracy and efficiency of pattern creation. Pattern Notation Tablets consist of a touchscreen display that allows designers to draw, sketch, and manipulate patterns directly on the device. The software provides a wide range of tools and features to assist designers in their creative process, such as line drawing, curve smoothing, and shape resizing. These tablets also offer options for adjusting pattern measurements, scaling, and grade rules to ensure precise pattern sizing and fit. The advantage of using Pattern Notation Tablets in fashion design is the ability to create, edit, and modify patterns in a digital format. This eliminates the need for traditional paper patterns, reducing waste and storage requirements. Additionally, the digital nature of these tablets enables designers to easily share patterns with team members, manufacturers, and clients, speeding up the design process and enhancing collaboration. Pattern Notation Tablets also offer features for pattern visualization, such as the ability to preview patterns in 3D and simulate fabric drape. This allows designers to assess the look and fit of a pattern before it is physically created, saving time and resources. Furthermore, these tablets can store and organize pattern libraries, making it easy for designers to access and reuse patterns for future projects. In conclusion, Pattern Notation Tablets are innovative tools in fashion design that provide a digital platform for creating, editing, and storing patterns. They offer a range of features and benefits that enhance the pattern development process, including precise measurement adjustments, efficient collaboration, and realistic pattern visualization. By adopting Pattern Notation Tablets, fashion designers can streamline their workflow, improve pattern accuracy, and contribute to the overall sustainability of the industry.

Pattern Notchers

Pattern notchers are essential tools used in fashion design to create precise marks on the paper patterns. They are small, handheld tools with sharp, V-shaped blades on one end. When designing a garment, fashion designers create mock-ups of the garment on paper patterns before cutting and sewing the fabric. These patterns are typically made of tissue paper or other thin materials. Pattern notchers are used to mark important points on these patterns, such as the placement of darts, pleats, pockets, and seams. The process of notching the pattern involves holding the pattern flat and aligned, then making a small cut or notch at the desired point. The V-shaped blade of the pattern notcher ensures that the notch is clean and precise, allowing for accurate alignment and matching of pattern pieces during the sewing process. Pattern notching is a crucial step in pattern making because it helps the fashion designer maintain accuracy and consistency throughout the construction process. By clearly marking the important points on the pattern, pattern notchers ensure that the garment will be assembled correctly, with all the design elements in their intended positions. Pattern notching also helps in identifying the front and back of a pattern piece, as well as distinguishing between different sizes or versions of the same pattern. By making specific notches in specific positions, fashion designers can easily match corresponding pieces during assembly, saving time and reducing sewing errors. In addition to paper patterns, pattern notchers can also be used on other materials like cardboard or plastic for more durable and long-lasting patterns. They are lightweight, portable, and easy to use, making them indispensable tools in the fashion designer's toolkit.

Pattern Notching Machines

A pattern notching machine is a specialized tool used in fashion design to create precise cuts or notches in pattern pieces. These notches serve as alignment markers, allowing pattern pieces to be easily matched up during the sewing process. The machine typically consists of a durable, flat surface with a notching blade attached. The blade is adjustable, allowing for different notch widths and depths to be created. The machine may also have a guide or ruler to ensure accurate placement of the notches.

Pattern Pounce Wheels

Pattern Pounce Wheels are a tool used in fashion design to transfer intricate patterns onto fabric or paper. They consist of a handle attached to a circular wheel with evenly spaced spikes or teeth. The spikes are somewhat similar to those found on a wheel for pouncing a pattern onto a surface, hence the name "Pattern Pounce Wheels." These wheels are commonly used by fashion designers to create accurate and precise patterns on their fabrics or paper templates. They are particularly useful when working with complex or intricate designs that require careful placement and alignment. By utilizing the pattern pounce wheels, designers can transfer their patterns with ease and accuracy, saving time and effort in the process.

Pattern Punches

In the context of fashion design, pattern punches refer to the tools or devices used to create patterns on fabric or other materials. These punches typically consist of a handle attached to a metal or plastic plate with a specific pattern design. Pattern punches can have various shapes and sizes, and they are often used to add decorative or ornamental elements to garments or accessories. Pattern punches are commonly used in the process of creating textile patterns, especially in industries that focus on mass production. They provide a quick and efficient way to apply repetitive patterns or motifs onto fabric. Pattern punches can be used on various types of fabrics, including cotton, silk, leather, and synthetic materials. To use a pattern punch, a designer or technician aligns the punch onto the fabric and applies pressure using the handle. The punch will cut or impress the desired pattern onto the material, leaving behind a decorative element. The resulting pattern can be a cutout design or an embossed impression, depending on the type of pattern punch used. The use of pattern punches allows designers to create unique and intricate patterns in a more efficient and consistent manner. These tools enable them to add texture and visual interest to their designs without the need for complex techniques or extensive handwork. Pattern punches can be used to create a wide range of patterns, from simple geometric shapes to complex floral or organic designs. Pattern punches are versatile tools that can be used in various areas of fashion design. They are commonly used in the creation of accessories such as belts, bags, and shoes, where decorative elements are often incorporated. Additionally, pattern punches can be used to create patterns on garment pieces, such as cuffs, collars, and waistbands, to enhance the overall design aesthetic. In conclusion, pattern punches are essential tools in the world of fashion design. They provide designers with the ability to quickly and efficiently add decorative patterns to fabric and other materials. Pattern punches are versatile and can be used in various aspects of fashion design, allowing for the creation of unique and intricate designs.

Pattern Punching Machines

A pattern punching machine is a specialized tool used in fashion design to create consistent and precise holes in patterns or templates. These holes are commonly used for various purposes such as marking key points, indicating construction lines, or facilitating fabric manipulation. The pattern punching machine operates by using a motorized mechanism to drive a needle or punch through the pattern material. The needle or punch is positioned based on the desired hole location, and when activated, it quickly and accurately creates the hole with the desired size and shape.

Pattern Storage Boxes

Pattern storage boxes are essential tools for fashion designers to keep their pattern collections organized and easily accessible. These boxes are specifically designed to store and protect various pattern pieces, allowing designers to efficiently manage their design process. Pattern storage boxes are typically made of sturdy materials such as cardboard or plastic to ensure durability and longevity. They often come in a rectangular shape with a hinged or removable lid, providing easy access to the patterns inside. The boxes are available in different sizes to accommodate patterns of various dimensions. Inside the pattern storage box, there are compartments or dividers that help separate individual pattern pieces, making it easier to locate specific patterns when needed. These compartments may be adjustable or fixed, depending on the design of the box. Some pattern storage boxes also come with additional features such as labeling areas or index cards to further enhance organization. The primary function of pattern storage boxes is to protect patterns from damage and deterioration. Patterns are delicate and can easily tear or be misplaced if not properly stored. By keeping patterns in a dedicated storage box, designers can minimize the risk of damage and ensure the longevity of their patterns. Pattern storage boxes also facilitate efficient workflow for fashion designers. By having all patterns neatly organized in one place, designers can quickly identify and retrieve the patterns they need for a specific project. This saves valuable time and allows designers to focus more on the creative aspects of their work. In addition to storing individual patterns, pattern storage boxes can also be used to store pattern books or magazines. These boxes provide a convenient and space-saving solution for keeping a collection of pattern resources in one place. In summary, pattern storage boxes are indispensable tools for fashion designers. They offer a practical and organized way to store and protect pattern pieces, enabling designers to streamline their design process and preserve their valuable patterns for future use.

Pattern Tracers

Pattern tracers or pattern makers, in the context of fashion design, refer to individuals who specialize in creating and modifying patterns for garments. They possess extensive knowledge and expertise in understanding garment construction, body measurements, and fabric properties. Pattern tracers play a crucial role in the fashion design process as they are responsible for transforming creative designs into tangible patterns that can be used for garment production. They work closely with fashion designers and use their technical skills to translate design concepts into accurate pattern templates. The primary task of a pattern tracer is to analyze fashion sketches or concept drawings and convert them into practical patterns. They carefully study the design details, such as silhouette, darts, seams, and pleats, to ensure that the pattern accurately reflects the intended garment. This involves taking accurate body measurements and making necessary adjustments to the pattern to achieve the desired fit and style. Pattern tracers utilize various tools and techniques to create and modify patterns. They may use specialized software applications or work manually using pattern drafting tools, such as rulers, curves, and pattern paper. They apply their knowledge of patternmaking principles and garment construction techniques to ensure that the patterns are well-proportioned, precise, and easy to follow during production. In addition to creating initial patterns, pattern tracers also play a role in pattern grading. Pattern grading involves creating patterns in different sizes to accommodate the diverse range of body sizes and proportions. They follow specific grading rules to ensure that the patterns maintain their design integrity and fit across various sizes. Pattern tracers often collaborate with garment technicians, sample makers, and production teams to ensure the accurate translation of patterns into finished garments. They provide technical guidance, clarification, and modifications during the sampling and production stages. Their expertise in patternmaking is essential in achieving the desired fit, functionality, and aesthetic appeal of the final garment. In conclusion, pattern tracers in fashion design are highly skilled professionals who are proficient in translating design concepts into accurate and wearable patterns. They possess a thorough understanding of garment construction, body measurements, and fabric properties. Their role is vital in ensuring that the designer's vision is effectively transformed into a well-fitting and stylish garment.

Pattern Weaving Accessories

A pattern weaving accessory refers to a fashion design element that is used to enhance textiles and garments through the incorporation of intricate patterns and weaves. These accessories play a crucial role in adding visual interest, texture, and dimension to the overall aesthetic of a fashion piece. Pattern weaving accessories come in various forms and can be created using different techniques, such as jacquard weaving, brocade weaving, or tapestry weaving. These techniques often involve the use of specialized looms and tools to create intricate patterns and designs on the fabric.

Pattern Weaving Looms

A pattern weaving loom is a tool used in fashion design to create intricately woven patterns and designs in fabrics. It is a device that holds and organizes the threads or yarns used in weaving, allowing the designer to manipulate them in specific patterns to create unique and visually appealing textile designs. The loom consists of several essential parts, including a frame or structure, a set of warp threads, and a weft thread. The frame or structure provides stability and support to the loom, allowing the designer to work with ease. The warp threads are the vertical threads that are attached to the frame and serve as the foundation of the fabric. The weft thread is the horizontal thread that is interlaced with the warp threads to create the desired pattern. Using a pattern weaving loom requires a certain level of skill and expertise. The designer must have a clear understanding of different weaving techniques, such as plain weave, twill weave, or satin weave, to create various design effects. They must also have a good sense of color combinations and thread placements to achieve the desired visual impact. Pattern weaving looms can be categorized into different types, including handlooms, table looms, and floor looms. Handlooms are small and portable, making them ideal for small-scale projects or for designers who work in limited spaces. Table looms are larger and more versatile, providing the designer with more flexibility in terms of the size and complexity of their designs. Floor looms are the largest and most robust type of loom, allowing for the creation of large-scale and intricate fabric designs. In fashion design, pattern weaving looms are used to create a wide range of fabric products, including clothing, accessories, and home décor items. They enable designers to add unique and personalized elements to their creations, enhancing the overall aesthetics and value of the final product. Pattern weaving looms are also widely used in textile art and weaving traditions, preserving and promoting cultural heritage and craftsmanship.

Pattern Weaving Tools

A pattern weaving tool in the context of fashion design refers to a device or implement used to create intricate and varied fabric patterns through the process of weaving. It is an essential tool for fashion designers who aim to incorporate unique and visually appealing patterns into their designs. Pattern weaving tools include a range of instruments and equipment, each serving a specific purpose in the creation of woven patterns. One such tool is the weaving loom, which provides the structure and framework for the weaving process. Looms come in various sizes and types, including handheld looms, table looms, and floor looms, allowing for different scales and complexities of patterns. The warp threads are an important component of pattern weaving, and tools like warp boards or warping mills are used to measure and prepare them. These tools help ensure that the warp threads are evenly spaced and properly tensioned, resulting in well-defined and consistent patterns. In addition to woven patterns created solely through the interlacing of warp and weft threads, pattern weaving tools also enable the incorporation of supplementary techniques. These techniques include jacquard weaving, where a mechanism known as a jacquard head is used to control the patterning of individual warp threads. Jacquard weaving allows for intricate designs, such as figures or detailed motifs, to be incorporated into the fabric. Pattern weaving tools are also used to create various texture effects within woven fabrics. This can be achieved through the use of textured yarns, such as chenille or bouclé, or by manipulating the weaving process itself. Tools like shuttle sticks or pick-up sticks are employed to create texture by selectively raising or lowering specific warp threads during the weaving process. In conclusion, pattern weaving tools are a crucial component of fashion design, enabling designers to create unique and visually appealing fabric patterns. These tools encompass a range of instruments and equipment, from looms to warp boards, jacquard heads to shuttle sticks, each serving a specific purpose in the creation of woven patterns. With the help of pattern weaving tools, fashion designers can bring their artistic vision to life, adding texture, complexity, and intricacy to their designs.

Pattern Weights

Pattern weights are small, flat objects that are used in fashion design to hold down patterns and fabric during the cutting and shaping process. They are essential tools that help to ensure accuracy and precision when creating garments. The primary purpose of pattern weights is to keep the pattern pieces in place while tracing or cutting them out from fabric. Unlike pins, which can create holes or distort the fabric, pattern weights provide a reliable and non-invasive method of securing the pattern to the fabric. This helps to maintain the integrity of the fabric and ensures that the final garment will have the correct proportions.

Peasant Blouse

The Peasant Blouse is a type of loose-fitting top that originated from traditional European peasant clothing. It is characterized by its loose, billowy silhouette, gathered or pleated bodice, and sometimes features embroidered details or lace trim. The blouse typically has a round neckline, often accompanied by a keyhole or tie closure, and loose-fitting sleeves that may be short, three-quarter, or full-length. The Peasant Blouse is a versatile garment in fashion design, suitable for both casual and semi-formal occasions. It can be made from a variety of fabrics, including lightweight cotton, linen, silk, or chiffon. The loose silhouette allows for easy movement and comfort, and its relaxed fit makes it flattering on different body types. This type of blouse is often associated with bohemian or folk-inspired fashion styles, as it exudes a carefree and effortless appeal. The relaxed nature of the Peasant Blouse makes it perfect for pairing with denim jeans or skirts for a casual, everyday look. It can also be dressed up by pairing it with tailored pants or a high-waisted skirt, accessorized with statement jewelry and heels for a more polished ensemble. The Peasant Blouse has become a staple in many fashion collections and is often reinvented by designers to incorporate contemporary elements. While the basic design remains constant, variations in fabric choice, sleeve length, and trims allow for individual style expression. Some contemporary versions may feature off-the-shoulder necklines, bell sleeves, or intricate patterns, while others may have a more minimalist and streamlined aesthetic. In recent years, the Peasant Blouse has also made a resurgence in the sustainable fashion movement. As it is typically loose-fitting and made from natural fibers, it aligns with the principles of conscious consumption and ethical production. Many brands now offer versions of the Peasant Blouse that are made from organic or recycled materials, further promoting sustainability in fashion. Overall, the Peasant Blouse is a timeless and versatile garment that has transcended traditional peasant clothing to become a staple in modern fashion design. Its loose-fitting silhouette, comfortable feel, and ability to be dressed up or down make it a popular choice for those seeking both style and comfort.

Peasant Dress

A peasant dress is a type of dress that is inspired by traditional peasant clothing. It is characterized by its loose and flowing silhouette, typically featuring a high waistline and billowy sleeves. The design of the peasant dress is often simple, with minimal embellishments and details. This style of dress is typically made from lightweight and breathable fabrics such as cotton or linen, making it comfortable to wear during warm weather. The loose and relaxed fit of the peasant dress allows for ease of movement and is often considered to be a more casual and relaxed dress option.

Pegged Leg Jeans

Pegged leg jeans refer to a style of jeans that have a tapered or narrow cut from the thigh down to the ankle. The term "pegged leg" comes from the way the legs of the jeans are shaped, similar to a peg or wooden dowel. This design feature creates a slimming effect and gives the jeans a more tailored and streamlined look. Pegged leg jeans are commonly found in both men's and women's fashion. They can be made from various materials such as denim, twill, or even stretchy fabrics. The jeans typically have a higher rise, sitting at or just above the natural waistline, and feature a fitted waistband that helps to accentuate the waist. The legs of the jeans gradually taper down from the hips to the ankle, hugging the legs for a sleek and flattering fit. Because of their narrower leg opening, pegged leg jeans are often paired with different footwear styles depending on the desired look. For a more casual and relaxed outfit, they can be worn with sneakers or flats. To create a more polished and sophisticated appearance, they can be paired with heels or ankle boots. The versatility of pegged leg jeans allows them to be dressed up or down depending on the occasion. When it comes to styling pegged leg jeans, they can be worn with a variety of tops. Tucking in a blouse or a button-down shirt can help create a more put-together ensemble, while wearing a loose-fitting top can give a more effortless and relaxed vibe. Layering with a blazer or a cardigan can add an extra touch of sophistication to the overall outfit. In conclusion, pegged leg jeans are a fashionable and versatile choice for those looking for a sleek and tailored fit. Their tapered leg design creates a flattering silhouette and can be easily dressed up or down depending on the occasion and personal style preferences.

Pegged Pants

Pegged pants, also known as tapered pants or peg leg trousers, are a style of pants in the field of fashion design that have a specific cut and fit. These pants are characterized by a gradually narrowing leg, starting with a wider waist and hip area and tapering down towards the ankle. The tapering can be achieved through the use of pleats, darts, or simply by altering the pattern to create a narrower silhouette. Pegged pants gained popularity in the 1950s and have since evolved and adapted to fit different fashion trends. They can be found in various fabrics and can be styled to suit different occasions, from casual to formal settings.

Pencil Dress

A pencil dress is a form-fitting garment that is typically knee-length and designed to hug the body, highlighting the curves of the wearer. This style of dress gets its name from its resemblance to a pencil, as it is narrow and straight from top to bottom, with a slim silhouette. Pencil dresses are typically made from fabrics that have some degree of stretch, such as cotton, polyester, or spandex blends, to ensure a comfortable fit while maintaining shape. The dress usually has darts or seams that help to contour the body and create a flattering fit. These seams often run vertically along the dress, accentuating the natural curves of the wearer.

Peplum Dress

A peplum dress is a style of dress that features a flared ruffle or overskirt attached at the waistline, creating a unique silhouette. The peplum is typically gathered or pleated, adding volume and dimension to the dress. This design element can be found on various types of dresses, including cocktail dresses, evening gowns, and even wedding dresses. The peplum dress became popular in the 1940s and 1950s, where it was often seen as a glamorous and feminine style. It was a favorite among Hollywood actresses, who embraced its elegant and sophisticated look. The peplum dress has since made a comeback in modern fashion, reinvented with contemporary designs and fabrics.

Peplum Shirt

A peplum shirt is a style of top that features a distinctive exaggerated frill or flounce that extends from the waist or hips. The term "peplum" derives from the Greek word for tunic, and this design element has been incorporated into various garments throughout history. In fashion design, the peplum shirt has gained popularity as a feminine and flattering silhouette. The flounce is typically attached to the bottom hem of the shirt, creating a distinct shape that emphasizes the waist and adds volume to the hips. This style can be seen in both casual and formal wear, offering versatility for different occasions.

Peplum Skirt

A peplum skirt is a garment in the field of fashion design that features a flared or ruffled extension at the waistline, creating a distinctive silhouette. This type of skirt is characterized by a short overskirt or flounce that is attached to the waistline, typically with a seam or gathering technique. The peplum detail can be found in various styles, lengths, and fabric choices, allowing for versatility in design. It can be incorporated into skirts of different lengths, including mini, midi, and maxi, providing options for different occasions and personal preferences. The peplum can also be created with varying degrees of volume, from subtle ruffles to more exaggerated flares, adding visual interest and a feminine touch to the overall outfit.

Peplum Top

A peplum top is a type of women's garment that features a flared ruffle or "peplum" sewn onto the waistline of a fitted top or blouse. This design detail creates a distinct silhouette that enhances and accentuates the waist, while adding a feminine and stylish touch to the overall look. The peplum itself is a gathered or pleated strip of fabric that flares out from the waist, typically in a subtle or exaggerated manner. It can be sewn directly onto the waistline of the top or attached as a separate layer, giving the illusion of an extra layer or skirt-like detail.

Peter Pan Collar Blouse

A Peter Pan collar blouse is a type of garment commonly found in women's fashion design. It features a distinct collar style that has a rounded, flat shape that sits close to the neck. This collar style is named after the character Peter Pan from J.M. Barrie's novel, as it resembles the collars typically worn by the character in stage and film adaptations. The Peter Pan collar blouse is typically made from lightweight fabrics such as cotton, silk, or chiffon. It is often designed with a button-down front and can be sleeveless, short-sleeved, or long-sleeved, depending on the desired style and season. The blouse is generally fitted at the waist and may include darts or pleats for a more feminine silhouette. The main defining feature of the Peter Pan collar blouse is its collar, which is usually attached to the neckline of the garment. The collar is rounded and flat, extending from the front of the blouse to the back, and typically sits close to the neck. It is often finished with a small, delicate edge or trim, adding a touch of femininity and elegance to the overall design. The Peter Pan collar blouse is considered a versatile and timeless piece in women's fashion. It can be worn for both casual and formal occasions, depending on the fabric, color, and styling. For a more casual look, it can be paired with jeans or a skirt. To create a more polished and sophisticated outfit, it can be styled with tailored pants or a high-waisted skirt. Throughout the years, the Peter Pan collar blouse has become a popular choice among fashion designers and enthusiasts alike. Its charming and youthful design adds a playful and nostalgic touch to any outfit. Whether it is worn as part of a vintage-inspired ensemble or as a contemporary fashion statement, the Peter Pan collar blouse continues to be a timeless and beloved piece in women's fashion.

Pin Cushions

A pin cushion is a small padded cushion typically used by fashion designers and seamstresses to hold and organize pins, needles, and other sharp sewing tools. It is a practical and essential tool for professionals or hobbyists who work with fabric and require quick and easy access to their pins while working on various sewing projects. The main purpose of a pin cushion is to keep pins and needles securely in place, ensuring they are easily accessible and minimizing the risk of losing or misplacing them while working. The cushion's soft padding allows the pins to be inserted and removed effortlessly, providing a convenient storage solution that keeps the workspace clean and safe.

Pinafore Dress

A pinafore dress, in the context of fashion design, refers to a sleeveless garment that is typically worn as an outer layer over a blouse or a t-shirt. It is characterized by its square neckline, often with straps or suspenders that cross over the shoulders and fasten at the back. The dress itself is loose-fitting and usually falls to the knee or mid-calf length, although variations in length can also be found. Pinafore dresses are versatile and can be designed in various styles, fabrics, and colors, making them suitable for a wide range of occasions. They can be crafted from lightweight materials such as cotton or linen for a casual and comfortable daytime look, or from more luxurious fabrics like silk or satin to create a dressier ensemble for evening events. The choice of fabric greatly influences the overall aesthetic and can determine whether the dress has a more structured or relaxed silhouette. The design of the pinafore dress allows for easy layering and styling. It is often worn over a blouse or a t-shirt, with the straps or suspenders adding a playful and vintage-inspired touch. The dress can be cinched at the waist with a belt to create definition and add a flattering silhouette. Additionally, it can be paired with accessories such as statement necklaces or scarves to further enhance the outfit. Pinafore dresses have a timeless appeal and draw inspiration from traditional workwear worn by women in the early 20th century. The style has evolved over time, with contemporary designs incorporating modern elements and innovative details. Today, pinafore dresses are a staple in many women's wardrobes, offering a nostalgic yet fashionable aesthetic that can be easily customized to suit individual tastes and personal style.

Pinking Machine Blades

A Pinking Machine Blade is a cutting tool used in the fashion design industry to create decorative edges on fabric. It is specifically designed to cut a zigzag pattern, creating a scalloped or serrated edge. The pinking blade is a long, narrow strip of metal with teeth along one edge. When designing garments or accessories, fashion designers often use pinking machine blades to finish the raw edges of fabric pieces. This decorative edge not only enhances the look of the garment but also prevents the fabric from fraying, as the zigzag pattern acts as a barrier to unraveling threads.

Pinking Machines

A pinking machine is a specialized tool used in fashion design to create decorative edges on fabric. It is particularly useful for preventing fraying and adding a professional touch to garments and accessories. The pinking machine consists of a set of serrated blades that cut delicate zigzag patterns along the fabric edges. These blades are typically made of hardened steel and are positioned in a rotating wheel or a stationary plate. When the fabric is fed through the machine, the blades make quick and precise cuts, creating evenly spaced serrated edges.

Pinking Shear Blades

Pinking shear blades are cutting tools used in fashion design that are specifically designed to create a zigzag or serrated edge on fabric. These blades are commonly used by fashion designers to add decorative edges to garments and sewing projects. The blades of pinking shears are shaped in a zigzag pattern, with one blade having triangular teeth and the other blade having corresponding V-shaped notches. When the blades come together, these teeth and notches interlock, allowing the fabric to be cut in a zigzag pattern instead of a straight line.

Pinking Shears

Pinking shears are a specialized cutting tool used in fashion design to create decorative edges on fabric. They are designed with serrated blades that feature a zigzag pattern, which allows for precise and clean cuts that prevent fraying. These shears are often used to add a decorative finish to seams, hems, and edges of garments and textiles. The primary function of pinking shears is to cut fabric in a way that minimizes the risk of fraying. The zigzag pattern of the blades creates small triangular cuts along the edge of the fabric, which helps to seal the fibers and prevent them from unraveling. This is particularly useful when working with delicate or loosely woven fabrics that are prone to fraying, such as silk, chiffon, or linen. Aside from their functional purpose, pinking shears are also used for aesthetic reasons in fashion design. The zigzag edge created by these shears adds a decorative and visually interesting element to garments and textiles. It can be used to create decorative trims, accents, or to add an interesting detail to the overall design. Additionally, the pinked edge can be particularly flattering when used around necklines, cuffs, or other areas of the garment that are more visible. Pinking shears are essential tools for fashion designers, pattern makers, and seamstresses. They offer a quick and efficient way to finish fabric edges, reducing the need for additional steps such as serging or zigzag stitching. The use of pinking shears can help to streamline the production process and save time during garment construction. When using pinking shears, it is important to choose the right pair for the task. The quality of the blades, the handle design, and the overall construction can vary between brands and models. It is advisable to look for shears that are made of durable materials and have a comfortable grip for prolonged use. Proper care and maintenance, such as regularly sharpening the blades, can also prolong the lifespan and effectiveness of the shears.

Pleated Pants

Pleated pants are a type of trousers that feature folds or pleats at the waistband, which create a distinctive draping effect on the fabric. These pleats are sewn in a way that allows the fabric to gather and fold, adding texture and volume to the pants. Pleated pants are commonly used in formal or dressy settings, and are often seen as a classic and traditional style in menswear. Traditionally, pleated pants were tailored with double or single pleats, each creating a different look and fit. Double pleats involve two inward folds on both sides of the waistband, while single pleats have only one fold on either side. This additional fabric from the pleats provides more room and comfort in the hip and thigh area, making pleated pants a popular choice for individuals seeking a looser fit. However, contemporary fashion trends have shifted towards a more slim and streamlined silhouette, resulting in a decline in popularity of pleated pants. Nevertheless, pleats still make occasional appearances in fashionable contexts, often used to achieve a more relaxed or vintage-inspired look. Additionally, designers have experimented with different pleat variations, such as diagonal or asymmetrical pleats, to add an element of modernity and uniqueness to this classic style. In terms of styling, pleated pants are generally worn with dressier outfits or in formal occasions. They are commonly paired with blazers, shirts, and ties in professional settings, creating a sophisticated and polished look. However, they can also be dressed down by pairing them with casual shirts or sweaters for a more laid-back aesthetic. Overall, while pleated pants have experienced shifts in popularity throughout the years, they remain a timeless element in menswear. Whether worn for business or formal events, they possess a certain elegant charm that adds character to any outfit.

Pleated Shorts

Pleated shorts are a type of bottom garment that features pleats, which are folds of fabric that are stitched or pressed into place. These shorts are designed to have extra fabric at the waist, which is then folded and sewn to create the pleats. The purpose of the pleats is to provide additional fullness and movement to the shorts, as well as to create a more polished and tailored look. Pleated shorts are commonly made from lightweight and breathable fabrics, such as cotton, linen, or polyester. They are available in various lengths, ranging from mid-thigh to just above the knee. The waistband of pleated shorts is usually fitted and sits at the natural waist or slightly below. Some styles may feature a belt loop for added functionality and an adjustable fit.

Pleated Skirt

A pleated skirt is a type of skirt that is characterized by the presence of pleats, which are folds of fabric that are pressed and stitched into place. Pleats typically extend from the waistband of the skirt down to the hem, creating a decorative and functional design element. Pleats can be found in various sizes and styles, adding visual interest and texture to the skirt. Common types of pleats include box pleats, knife pleats, and accordion pleats. The pleating technique used can also vary, with some skirts featuring permanently pressed pleats that maintain their shape even after washing and wearing, while others may have pleats that can be pressed and repressed as needed. Traditionally, pleated skirts were often associated with school uniforms or formal attire, but they have since become a versatile and fashionable wardrobe staple. Pleated skirts can be found in a wide range of lengths, from mini to maxi, and in various fabrics, including cotton, silk, chiffon, and polyester. When designing a pleated skirt, the type of pleats, fabric choice, and placement of the pleats are all important considerations. The width and spacing of the pleats can create different visual effects, with wider pleats providing a bolder and more structured look, while narrower pleats offer a more delicate and feminine appearance. The pleated skirt can be styled in numerous ways, making it a versatile choice for different occasions. It can be paired with a tucked-in blouse and heels for a polished and sophisticated look, or dressed down with a graphic tee and sneakers for a trendy and casual outfit. In summary, a pleated skirt is a garment that features folded and stitched fabric folds, known as pleats, which add visual interest and texture. It is a versatile piece that can be styled in various ways, making it a timeless and fashionable choice in the world of fashion design.

Polo Dress

A polo dress is a type of dress that is inspired by the classic polo shirt typically worn in the sport of polo. It features a collar, a button-up placket, and short sleeves, similar to the polo shirt. However, unlike the polo shirt, a polo dress is designed to be worn as a dress, typically reaching the mid-thigh or knee-length. The polo dress is known for its sporty yet feminine aesthetic. It combines the casual and relaxed look of a polo shirt with the versatility and elegance of a dress. This makes it a popular choice for various occasions, from casual outings to more formal events. The design of the polo dress can vary, with different lengths, cuts, and details, allowing for a wide range of styles and interpretations.

Polo Shirt

A polo shirt is a type of shirt that has a collar, typically a soft fold-over collar, and a short buttoned placket at the neck. It is usually made of comfortable and breathable fabric such as cotton or a cotton blend, making it suitable for casual and sporty occasions. Originally designed for and worn by athletes, particularly tennis players, in the late 19th and early 20th centuries, the polo shirt has become a staple in the world of fashion. Its timeless design and versatility make it a popular choice for both men and women.

Poncho Sweater

A poncho sweater is a type of garment that combines the style and comfort of a poncho with the warmth and versatility of a sweater. It is designed to be loose-fitting and usually made from soft, cozy fabrics such as wool or cashmere. The poncho sweater typically features a wide, oversized silhouette that drapes over the body, providing a relaxed and effortless look. The key characteristic of a poncho sweater is its unique construction. Unlike a traditional sweater that is fitted and has defined sleeves, the poncho sweater is sleeveless and open on the sides, resembling a poncho. This design allows for easy layering and provides maximum freedom of movement, making it a popular choice for those who value comfort and style.

Poncho

A poncho is a loose-fitting outer garment, typically made from a single piece of fabric, that is worn over the shoulders and covers the upper body. It is commonly associated with South American and Mexican culture, but has also become popular in many other parts of the world. The poncho is characterized by its wide, open front, which allows for easy movement and provides ample space to accommodate different body sizes and shapes. This versatile design makes it suitable for both men and women of all ages.

Press Cloths

Press cloths are an essential tool in the world of fashion design. They are thin, lightweight fabrics that are used to protect delicate fabrics during the ironing process. These cloths act as a barrier between the iron and the garment, preventing direct contact and potential damage. The primary purpose of press cloths is to prevent heat transfer and shine marks that can occur when ironing certain fabrics. Delicate materials such as silk, satin, velvet, and wool are particularly susceptible to damage from direct heat. By placing a press cloth over these fabrics, the heat is distributed more evenly, reducing the risk of scorching or burning. In addition, the cloth helps to disperse the pressure from the iron, minimizing the risk of leaving unwanted imprints or creases on the garments.

Presser Feet

Presser feet are attachments used in fashion design to aid in the sewing process. They are metal or plastic attachments that can be added to the sewing machine to provide additional support and control while sewing different types of fabric and performing various techniques. There are several types of presser feet available, each designed for a specific purpose. One common type is the standard presser foot, which is typically used for general sewing. It helps to feed the fabric evenly through the machine and maintain a consistent stitch length. Another commonly used presser foot is the zipper foot, which has a narrow design that allows for easy installation of zippers. It enables the sewer to stitch close to the zipper teeth without accidentally sewing over them. Presser feet can also be used for decorative purposes. For example, the applique foot is used to attach applique patches or decorative trims to fabric. It has a transparent design that allows for easy visibility of the stitching line. Other decorative presser feet include the hemming foot, which helps create even and precise hems, and the gathering foot, which assists in creating gathers or pleats in fabric. Some presser feet are specifically designed for handling challenging fabrics. The walking foot, also known as an even feed foot, is used when sewing multiple layers of fabric or working with slippery or easily stretched materials. It has built-in feed dogs that work in conjunction with the machine's feed dogs to ensure smooth and even fabric feeding. In addition to their functional purposes, presser feet can also aid in achieving professional-looking finishes. The edge-stitching foot, for instance, is used to create precise topstitching for garment construction, while the buttonhole foot is used for creating evenly spaced buttonholes. The blind hem foot, on the other hand, helps in creating nearly invisible hems on garments. Overall, presser feet are versatile accessories that enhance the capabilities of sewing machines in fashion design. Whether it's for basic stitching, decorative techniques, or handling challenging fabrics, these attachments provide the necessary support and control to achieve high-quality and professional results.

Presser Foot Shank Adapters

A presser foot shank adapter is a crucial tool in the world of fashion design. It is a small attachment that allows the use of different types of presser feet with a sewing machine. In fashion design, sewing machines are used extensively to create garments and other textile products. The presser foot is an essential component of a sewing machine as it holds the fabric in place during the sewing process. Different presser feet are used for various sewing techniques, such as zipper insertion, buttonhole making, and hemming. However, not all presser feet are compatible with every sewing machine. This is where the presser foot shank adapter comes into play. The adapter acts as a bridge between the sewing machine and the presser foot. It allows the attachment of presser feet that may not be specifically designed for a particular sewing machine model. The presser foot shank adapter is typically made of durable metal or plastic material. It has a slot or hole where the shank of the presser foot is inserted. The shank is then secured in place using a screw or a lever mechanism, depending on the type of adapter. Using a presser foot shank adapter offers fashion designers versatility and flexibility in their sewing projects. It allows them to experiment with different presser feet and explore various sewing techniques without purchasing multiple sewing machines or limiting their options to a specific set of presser feet. In conclusion, a presser foot shank adapter is a valuable tool that expands the capabilities of a sewing machine in the realm of fashion design. It enables the use of different presser feet, providing designers with more options and creative freedom in their sewing projects.

Princess Dress

A princess dress, in the context of fashion design, refers to a type of formal gown that is designed to make the wearer feel like royalty. It is characterized by its floor-length skirt, fitted bodice, and elegant detailing, which often includes lace, embroidery, or beading. The princess dress is known for its feminine and romantic silhouette. The skirt of the dress is typically full and voluminous, creating a dramatic and regal effect. This is achieved through the use of layers of tulle, organza, or other lightweight fabrics, which are often gathered or pleated to add depth and movement to the design. The fitted bodice accentuates the waist and provides structure to the dress, while also offering support to the wearer. It is typically adorned with intricate details, such as floral appliques, pearls, or sequins, to enhance its visual appeal. Princess dresses are often associated with formal events and special occasions, such as weddings, galas, or red carpet events. They are designed to evoke a sense of glamour and sophistication, and are often chosen by individuals who want to make a statement with their attire. The princess dress is commonly seen as a symbol of luxury and elegance, and is a popular choice among brides who wish to have a fairytale-like wedding. When creating a princess dress, fashion designers pay close attention to the choice of fabrics, as well as the construction and fit of the garment. The goal is to create a dress that not only looks beautiful, but also feels comfortable to wear. This involves careful pattern-making, draping, and tailoring techniques, as well as considering factors such as ease of movement and breathability. The princess dress is often made to measure, ensuring a perfect fit for the individual wearer.

Prym Eyelets

Prym Eyelets are small metal rings that are used in fashion design to reinforce and embellish various garments and accessories. These eyelets are typically made of durable and corrosion-resistant materials such as brass or stainless steel, ensuring their longevity and functionality. When it comes to the construction of garments, Prym Eyelets offer a practical solution for reinforcing areas that may be subject to strain or tearing, such as buttonholes, drawstring openings, or lacing details. By adding eyelets, fashion designers can enhance the overall durability and longevity of their creations, ensuring that the garments withstand regular wear and tear. In addition to their functional benefits, Prym Eyelets also serve as decorative elements in fashion design. They come in various shapes, sizes, and finishes, allowing designers to incorporate them as stylish accents and embellishments. These eyelets can be strategically placed along seams, hems, or other design elements to add visual interest and create a unique aesthetic appeal. When working with Prym Eyelets, fashion designers typically use specialized tools such as eyelet pliers or an eyelet punching machine to create precise and secure openings in the fabric. The eyelets are then inserted into these openings and secured in place, either by hammering them down or by using a specific tool designed for the purpose. This ensures that the eyelets are securely fastened and will not come loose during regular use. Prym Eyelets are not limited to a particular type of garment or accessory, making them a versatile choice for fashion designers. They can be incorporated into various styles such as casual wear, activewear, or even formal attire. The range of available finishes, including options like silver, gold, or black, allows designers to match the eyelets with the overall color palette and design concept of their creations. In conclusion, Prym Eyelets are small metal rings that serve both functional and decorative purposes in fashion design. By reinforcing garment openings and adding visual interest, these versatile elements offer designers an effective way to enhance the durability and aesthetics of their creations.

Prym Snaps

Prym Snaps is a type of fastening system commonly used in fashion design. It consists of two components: a male part and a female part, which are attached together to securely hold garments in place. The male part is typically a small metal or plastic stud with a protruding head, while the female part is a socket or receiver that fits snugly over the stud. The primary purpose of Prym Snaps is to provide a convenient and reliable closure method for various clothing items, such as shirts, jackets, trousers, and skirts. They allow garments to be easily opened and closed, providing functionality and ease of use for the wearer. Prym Snaps are often used in areas where there is a need for frequent attachment and detachment, such as the front of shirts or the waistbands of trousers. One of the key advantages of Prym Snaps is their versatility. They come in a wide range of sizes, styles, and finishes, allowing fashion designers to choose the most suitable option for their designs. The different sizes ensure that Prym Snaps can be used for garments of various thicknesses, ensuring a secure fit. Additionally, the various styles and finishes enable designers to match the snaps with the overall aesthetic of the garment, enhancing its visual appeal. In terms of application, Prym Snaps are relatively easy to attach and detach. They can be sewn onto fabric using a sewing machine or hand stitching, depending on the preference and requirements of the designer. Prym Snaps are known for their durability and strength, ensuring that they do not easily come undone during regular wear and tear. In conclusion, Prym Snaps are a popular choice in fashion design due to their functionality, versatility, and durability. They provide a practical and secure closure method for garments, allowing for easy opening and closing. With their wide range of sizes, styles, and finishes, Prym Snaps offer fashion designers the flexibility to incorporate them seamlessly into their designs. Whether it's for shirts, jackets, trousers, or skirts, Prym Snaps are a reliable fastening system that adds both functionality and aesthetic value to clothing.

Puff-Sleeve Top

A puff-sleeve top refers to a type of blouse or shirt that is characterized by its voluminous sleeves. The sleeves of a puff-sleeve top are designed with extra fabric, creating a distinctive puffed or gathered appearance. These tops are often crafted from lightweight materials such as silk, chiffon, or cotton, allowing the sleeves to maintain their exaggerated shape without weighing down the overall garment. The puff sleeves are typically gathered at the shoulder and gradually taper down towards the wrist, creating a playful and feminine look.

Pullover Sweater

A pullover sweater, in the context of fashion design, is a versatile and timeless garment that is typically made of knitted fabric. It is designed to be worn by both men and women and is characterized by its long sleeves and the absence of buttons or zippers for closure. It is known for its functionality, comfort, and effortless style. The main feature of a pullover sweater is its pullover design, which means that it is slipped over the head to be worn. This design element allows for easy dressing and undressing, making it a convenient option for everyday wear. Additionally, the absence of buttons or zippers lends a clean and streamlined look to the sweater, making it a popular choice in casual and formal settings. Pullover sweaters are available in a wide range of fabrics, including cotton, wool, cashmere, acrylic, and blends of these materials. Each fabric offers its own unique qualities, such as warmth, softness, and durability, allowing individuals to choose a sweater that suits their preferences and needs. Furthermore, different knitting techniques and patterns can be used to create interesting textures and designs on the surface of the sweater, adding visual interest and dimension to the overall aesthetic. The silhouette of a pullover sweater can vary, ranging from fitted and form-flattering to loose and oversized. This variety allows for versatility in styling, as individuals can choose a silhouette that complements their body shape and desired look. Pullover sweaters can be paired with various bottoms, such as jeans, trousers, skirts, and shorts, making them suitable for different occasions and seasons. In terms of color and pattern, pullover sweaters come in a multitude of options. They can be found in classic solid colors, such as black, white, navy, and gray, as well as in vibrant hues and playful patterns, including stripes, polka dots, and Fair Isle designs. This wide range of choices enables individuals to express their personal style and create various outfits by combining different colors and patterns.

Quilting Frames

Quilting frames are essential tools used in the process of fashion design that provide stability and support for quilting fabrics. These frames consist of a rigid structure that holds the quilt layers tautly in place, allowing the designer to have complete control over the stitching process. The main purpose of quilting frames in fashion design is to create a flat surface for quilting and ensure even tension throughout the fabric. The frames are typically made of durable materials such as metal or wood and come in a variety of sizes and designs to accommodate different quilting projects.

Quilting Hoop Stands

A quilting hoop stand is a functional tool used in fashion design to hold and support quilting hoops securely, allowing fashion designers to work with ease and precision. It is designed to provide a stable base for the quilter's hoop, maximizing comfort and reducing strain during extended periods of work. The quilting hoop stand typically consists of a sturdy base with adjustable legs or a stand, which can be positioned at various heights and angles according to the quilter's preferences. This provides the designer with the flexibility to work in their most comfortable position, whether sitting or standing. The stand is often made of lightweight yet durable materials such as metal or wood, ensuring both stability and portability.

Quilting Hoops

A quilting hoop is a circular frame used in fashion design to hold fabric taut while it is being quilted. It consists of two round wooden or plastic hoops that fit together, with the fabric sandwiched in between. The top hoop has a tightening mechanism, such as a screw or a latch, that can be adjusted to keep the fabric securely in place. Quilting hoops are an essential tool for fashion designers who work with quilting techniques, as they provide stability and even tension to the fabric. By keeping the fabric taut, quilting hoops help prevent wrinkles, puckering, and uneven stitching. They ensure that the fabric remains flat and smooth, allowing for precise and accurate quilting stitches.

Quilting Mats

Quilting mats are essential tools in the field of fashion design, particularly in the creation of quilted garments and accessories. These mats are specifically designed to provide a stable and supportive surface for the quilting process, allowing designers to create intricate and detailed quilted patterns on their pieces. The primary function of quilting mats is to protect the fabric and maintain its integrity during the quilting process. The mat acts as a cushioning layer underneath the fabric, preventing it from shifting or stretching while being worked on. This is crucial in ensuring that the quilted pattern remains consistent and uniform throughout the design. Quilting mats are typically made from high-quality materials that offer both durability and flexibility. The surface of the mat is often constructed with a non-slip texture, preventing the fabric from slipping or sliding during the quilting process. This feature allows designers to have better control over the needlework, resulting in more precise and accurate quilted patterns. In addition to providing stability, quilting mats also offer a convenient measuring tool for fashion designers. Many mats are marked with grid lines and measurements, allowing designers to easily align and measure their fabric as they work. This ensures that the quilted pattern is symmetrical and aligned correctly, resulting in a visually pleasing final product. The size and thickness of quilting mats can vary depending on the specific needs and preferences of the designer. While some mats are designed for smaller projects such as quilting patches, others are larger and more suitable for quilting full garments or accessories. Similarly, the thickness of the mat can vary, with thicker mats providing more cushioning and support for intricate quilted designs. In conclusion, quilting mats are essential tools in the world of fashion design, particularly in the creation of quilted garments and accessories. They provide stability, protection, and measuring capabilities, allowing designers to create intricate and precise quilted patterns. With their high-quality construction and non-slip surfaces, quilting mats are a valuable asset for any fashion designer looking to incorporate quilted elements into their designs.

Quilting Racks

A quilting rack is a tool used in fashion design to hold and organize quilting fabrics and materials. It consists of a sturdy frame or stand with horizontal bars or hooks where the fabrics can be hung or draped. Quilting racks are essential for fashion designers who work with quilting techniques or incorporate quilting elements into their designs. They provide a convenient and efficient way to store and access quilting fabrics, allowing designers to easily see and select the materials they need for their projects.

Quilting Rulers

A quilting ruler is a measuring tool used in the process of creating quilts in the field of fashion design. It is a straight, firm, and transparent ruler made from materials such as acrylic or plastic. The ruler typically features a variety of measurements and markings, including inches, centimeters, grid lines, and angles. Quilting rulers play a crucial role in fashion design by ensuring accuracy and precision during the cutting and piecing together of fabric pieces. They help designers achieve clean and straight lines, consistent shapes, and precise angles, ensuring that each quilt block fits together seamlessly.

Quilting Templates

A quilting template, in the context of fashion design, refers to a pattern or guide used by garment makers to create intricate quilting designs on fabric. These templates are typically made of durable materials, such as plastic or metal, and come in a variety of shapes and sizes. Quilting templates are essential tools for fashion designers, as they help create uniform and precise quilting patterns on garments, accessories, or other textile products. These templates can be customized to create various quilting designs, such as geometric shapes, flowers, or abstract patterns, allowing designers to add unique and creative elements to their designs.

Raglan Sleeve Top

A raglan sleeve top is a type of clothing design commonly used in fashion. It is characterized by a specific type of sleeve construction that runs from the collar, forming a diagonal seam to the underarm. The sleeve allows for a broader range of movement compared to traditional sleeves, making it a popular choice for activewear and sportswear. The raglan sleeve top is named after Lord Raglan, a British officer who lost his arm during the Battle of Waterloo. To accommodate his injury, his tailor designed a sleeve construction that allowed for greater mobility and ease of movement. This unique construction was later adapted into clothing design and became known as the raglan sleeve.

Rash Guard

A rash guard is a form of athletic or swimwear designed to protect the skin from irritations and abrasions caused by contact with rough surfaces, such as sand, coral reefs, or surfboards. It is typically made of a stretchy, lightweight fabric that provides both sun protection and quick drying properties. The design of a rash guard incorporates a tight-fitting silhouette, with long sleeves and a high neckline, providing maximum coverage to the upper body. The sleeves are intended to guard against scrapes and cuts caused by contact with the environment, while the high neckline offers additional protection to the neck and chest.

Ready-To-Wear

Ready-to-Wear, also known as prêt-à-porter, is a term used in the fashion industry to describe clothing that is mass-produced and available in standard sizes. It refers to garments that have been designed and manufactured for the general market, as opposed to made-to-measure or haute couture pieces that are custom-made for individual clients. Ready-to-Wear collections are produced by fashion designers and brands with the aim of offering fashionable and stylish clothing at a more affordable price point. These clothes are typically sold through retail stores, online platforms, or department stores, making them easily accessible to a wide range of consumers.

Retail Merchandising

Retail merchandising in the context of fashion design refers to the strategic planning and execution of various activities involved in presenting and selling fashion products to customers in physical retail stores. It involves creating visually appealing displays, organizing products effectively, and implementing marketing strategies to attract and engage shoppers. The main objective of retail merchandising in fashion design is to maximize sales and enhance the overall shopping experience for customers. This is achieved through careful product selection and placement, as well as by creating an environment that entices potential buyers to explore and make purchases.

Ribbon Burners

Ribbon burners are a type of decorative trim used in fashion design. These burners are typically made from narrow strips of fabric, usually ribbon, that are sewn or glued onto a garment to add embellishment. In the world of fashion, ribbon burners serve as an ornamental element that enhances the overall aesthetic of a garment. They can be used to create various effects, such as adding texture, color, and visual interest to plain or simple designs. Ribbon burners are often used on items such as dresses, skirts, jackets, and even accessories like bags and headbands.

Ribbon Cutter Tools

Ribbon cutter tools are essential instruments in the field of fashion design. They are specifically designed to efficiently and accurately cut ribbons and similar materials to desired lengths and shapes, ensuring clean and precise cuts every time. These tools are typically handheld devices, consisting of a sharp blade or cutting wheel attached to a handle. The blade or wheel is made of durable and high-quality materials such as stainless steel or tungsten carbide to maintain its sharpness and longevity.

Ripped Jeans

Ripped jeans, also known as distressed denim, are a type of denim garment that has intentional rips or tears on the fabric. They are a popular fashion trend and have been embraced by designers and consumers alike. Ripped jeans are typically made by either cutting or tearing the denim fabric at specific places. The rips can be created on different parts of the jeans, including the knees, thighs, or back pockets. The size and placement of the rips can vary, ranging from small and minimalistic to large and dramatic. The purpose of ripping jeans is to create a worn or edgy look. Ripped jeans are often associated with a rebellious or grunge style, and they can add a sense of casualness and informality to an outfit. They are commonly worn by both men and women and can be found in various styles, such as skinny, straight, or boyfriend fit. Ripped jeans can be made from different types of denim, including raw, washed, or distressed denim. The choice of denim fabric can affect the overall appearance and feel of the jeans. Raw denim is untreated and has a stiff texture, while washed denim has been pre-washed to achieve a softer and more flexible feel. Distressed denim, on the other hand, has undergone additional distressing techniques, such as sanding or acid washing, to achieve a worn-in look. Traditionally, ripped jeans were associated with manual wear and tear, as they were often worn by individuals engaged in physical work or activities. However, in the world of fashion, ripped jeans are created intentionally to mimic this worn-in look, without the need for actual wear and tear. They have become a staple in many modern wardrobes and are often used to add an element of coolness or street style to an outfit.

Rotary Cutter Blades

Rotary cutter blades in the context of fashion design refer to small, circular blades that are used to cut fabric with precision and accuracy. These blades are typically made of high-quality steel and are attached to a handle, allowing fashion designers to easily maneuver and control the cutting process. The primary purpose of rotary cutter blades is to create clean, smooth cuts on various types of fabrics, including cotton, silk, wool, and synthetic materials. The circular shape of the blade enables designers to make curved cuts with ease, making it an essential tool for intricate pattern-making and garment construction. One of the key advantages of using rotary cutter blades in fashion design is their ability to cut through multiple layers of fabric simultaneously. This significantly saves time and effort compared to using traditional scissors, especially when working on large projects or creating repetitive shapes. The clean cuts achieved by rotary cutter blades also help ensure that fabric pieces align accurately during the sewing process, resulting in a professional and high-quality finish. Another benefit of rotary cutter blades is their versatility. With a range of blade sizes available, fashion designers can choose the most appropriate blade diameter for their specific cutting needs. Smaller blades are ideal for detailed work, such as cutting notches or trimming seam allowances, while larger blades are more efficient for cutting long, straight lines. To maintain optimum cutting performance, it is essential to regularly change and sharpen rotary cutter blades. Dull or worn blades can result in jagged or uneven fabric edges, making it difficult to achieve precise construction when sewing garments. Additionally, using a blade that is not sharp enough can cause fabric to snag or pull, leading to unnecessary waste and potentially compromising the overall design. In summary, rotary cutter blades are indispensable tools in the world of fashion design. Their ability to create precise cuts, save time, and accommodate various fabric types makes them essential for pattern-making, garment construction, and overall design precision. By investing in high-quality blades and properly maintaining them, fashion designers can achieve impeccable results in their creations.

Rotary Cutters

A rotary cutter is a handheld cutting tool commonly used in fashion design to cut fabric and other materials with precision and ease. Designed with a circular blade that rotates as it is pushed along the material, rotary cutters allow fashion designers to make clean, straight cuts without the need for scissors or shears. The blade is typically made of high-quality steel, ensuring durability and sharpness over time.

Rotary Cutting Blades

A rotary cutting blade is a versatile tool used in fashion design for cutting fabric with precision and efficiency. It consists of a circular blade attached to a handle or rotary cutter, which allows the blade to rotate freely while cutting through fabric layers. The primary function of a rotary cutting blade is to make clean, straight cuts through fabric, minimizing fraying and ensuring accurate pattern pieces. Fashion designers use these blades to cut various types of fabric, including but not limited to, cotton, silk, and wool. The sharpness and precision of the blade allow designers to achieve clean and professional-looking edges and shapes for their garments.

Ruffle Blouse

A ruffle blouse is a type of women's top that features decorative frills or gathers, known as ruffles, on the front, back, or sleeves. The ruffles are typically created by pleating or gathering excess fabric and sewing it in a way that creates a wavy or fluted effect. Ruffle blouses are a popular choice in fashion design as they add a feminine and romantic touch to an outfit. They can come in various styles, including long-sleeved, short-sleeved, or sleeveless, and can be made from different materials such as silk, chiffon, or cotton. The ruffles can range in size, from delicate and subtle to bold and voluminous, depending on the desired look. This style of blouse can be versatile, suitable for both casual and formal occasions. A ruffle blouse paired with jeans or tailored trousers can create a chic and fashionable daytime look, while a more elaborate ruffle blouse combined with a skirt or tailored pants can be appropriate for a formal event or office setting. The ruffles on a blouse can be strategically placed to accentuate certain areas of the body. For example, ruffles around the neckline can draw attention to the face, while ruffles around the waist can create the illusion of an hourglass figure. Additionally, ruffles can add volume and movement to the overall silhouette of the blouse, giving it a playful and dynamic appearance. Designers often use ruffle blouses to experiment with different textures and details. They may incorporate lace, embroidery, or pleating techniques to enhance the overall design. The placement and size of the ruffles can also vary, allowing for endless creative possibilities. In conclusion, a ruffle blouse is a feminine and decorative women's top that features frills or gathers, known as ruffles. It adds a romantic touch to an outfit and can be versatile for both casual and formal occasions. Designers use various techniques and materials to create unique and visually interesting ruffle blouses.

Ruffled Dress

A ruffled dress is a type of garment that features decorative or ornamental gathers or pleats of fabric, typically in horizontal layers, that create a wavy or frilly appearance. The ruffles are usually attached to the dress in a way that allows them to stand out and add visual interest and texture to the overall design. Ruffles can be found on various parts of the dress, including the neckline, sleeves, hemline, or throughout the entire garment. The size, shape, and placement of the ruffles can vary, giving designers the opportunity to create different effects and styles. Some ruffled dresses may have large, dramatic ruffles that make a bold statement, while others may feature smaller, more delicate ruffles for a subtler look.

Ruffled Jumpsuit

A ruffled jumpsuit is a fashionable garment designed for women that combines the comfort and versatility of a jumpsuit with the added detail of ruffles. It is a one-piece outfit that typically features a fitted bodice and wide-legged pants, creating a cohesive and visually appealing silhouette. The defining characteristic of a ruffled jumpsuit is the presence of ruffles, which are decorative strips or layers of fabric that add texture, volume, and movement to the garment. These ruffles can be located in various areas of the jumpsuit, such as the neckline, sleeves, waistline, or the pant legs. They can vary in size, shape, and arrangement, allowing for endless design possibilities and styles. Ruffles are commonly made from the same fabric as the jumpsuit or a contrasting fabric to create a bold and eye-catching effect. They may be created using techniques such as gathering, pleating, or folding, and can be sewn onto the jumpsuit or attached as removable embellishments. The placement and design of the ruffles can be strategically chosen to enhance certain areas of the wearer's body or to create a specific aesthetic. For example, a ruffled jumpsuit with vertical ruffles along the neckline can elongate the neck and draw attention to the face, while ruffles along the waistline can accentuate the curves of the body. Ruffled jumpsuits can be designed for various occasions and personal styles. They can range from casual and playful designs, featuring small and delicate ruffles, to more formal and elegant options, with larger and more dramatic ruffles. They are available in a wide range of colors, patterns, and fabrics, including lightweight and breathable materials for summer, or heavier fabrics for cooler seasons. When styling a ruffled jumpsuit, it is important to consider the overall balance of the outfit. Due to the intricate nature of the ruffles, it is usually best to keep the accessories and other elements of the outfit relatively simple. This allows the jumpsuit to be the focal point and showcases the unique design. Pairing it with minimal jewelry, neutral-colored shoes, and a sleek hairstyle can help create a polished and sophisticated look.

Runway Model

A runway model is a professional who showcases clothing and accessories on a catwalk or runway during a fashion show. They are hired by fashion designers, brands, or agencies to display new collections and trends to potential buyers, industry professionals, and the general public. The primary role of a runway model is to present garments in a way that captures the attention and interest of the audience. They use their physical appearance, poise, and unique walking style to bring life to the clothing they are wearing. Runway models must have excellent posture, a confident stride, and the ability to express the desired mood of the collection through their body language and facial expressions. They are trained to portray the personality and vision of the designer, ensuring that the audience understands the aesthetic and message behind the clothing. Runway models are typically tall and slender, with well-proportioned bodies that serve as a canvas for the clothes they wear. Their measurements are often referenced as standard sizes or industry norms. This allows designers to create garments that fit well and flatter the models, resulting in a cohesive and visually appealing presentation. While height and body type are important factors, diversity has become increasingly valued in the fashion industry, with a greater emphasis on inclusive representation of different ethnicities, body shapes, and ages. Prior to a fashion show, runway models undergo fittings where they try on various outfits to ensure the proper fit and style. They work closely with designers, stylists, and dressers who make any necessary adjustments to the garments. During the show, models follow a carefully choreographed order, timing their movements to music, lighting, and other technical aspects. The goal is to create a visually engaging and seamless presentation, highlighting each garment and its unique features. Beyond their physical appearance and walking abilities, runway models must possess professionalism, adaptability, and the ability to handle pressure and long hours. They often travel extensively, as fashion shows and events take place in different cities and countries. Being a runway model requires collaboration and the ability to work effectively in a team, as they interact with various individuals involved in the fashion show production process.

Runway Modeling

Runway modeling, in the context of fashion design, refers to the presentation of designer clothing and accessories on a raised platform known as the runway or catwalk. It is a crucial component of the fashion industry as it allows designers to showcase their creations to a wider audience, including industry professionals, buyers, and the general public. Runway models play a vital role in bringing the designer's vision to life and setting trends in the fashion world. During a runway show, models walk down the runway while wearing the designer's latest collections, showcasing their unique style, craftsmanship, and overall aesthetic. These shows often take place during fashion weeks or special events, and they serve as an important platform for designers to gain recognition and publicity.

Runway

A runway in fashion design refers to a long, narrow platform or pathway where models showcase various clothing designs during a fashion show or presentation. It serves as the central stage where designers exhibit their latest creations, allowing the audience to view and appreciate the garments from different angles. The runway holds great significance in the world of fashion as it not only provides a physical space for designers to showcase their work, but also sets the overall atmosphere and mood of the show. It acts as a visual backdrop that compliments and enhances the aesthetic of the clothing collection being presented. Runways are typically well-lit to ensure optimal visibility of the garments and to highlight their intricate details. The platform itself is often raised to ensure that all attendees have a clear view of the models as they walk, allowing for a more immersive and dynamic experience. Designers carefully coordinate the choreography of the models' movements on the runway, known as the "model walk" or "catwalk." They instruct the models on how to walk, pose, and present the garments in a way that effectively communicates the desired message or theme of the collection. This choreography adds a performative element to the presentation, making the fashion show a captivating spectacle for the audience. Furthermore, the design and decor of the runway are often tailored to complement the overall theme of the fashion show. This may include elaborate set designs, lighting effects, music, or even props, all of which contribute to creating a cohesive and immersive experience for the attendees. Overall, the runway plays a fundamental role in fashion design by providing a platform for designers to showcase their collections in a visually compelling and captivating manner. It serves as the bridge between the creative vision of the designer and the audience, allowing for the appreciation and interpretation of fashion as an art form.

Sailor Pants

Sailor Pants are a type of trousers that are characterized by their nautical-inspired design. They typically feature a high waistline, wide leg silhouette, and decorative buttons or embellishments along the front. The origins of Sailor Pants can be traced back to the early 20th century when they were initially designed for sailors in the navy. One of the defining features of Sailor Pants is their high waistline, which sits above the natural waist. This design element not only creates a flattering silhouette but also elongates the legs, making them appear longer. The wide leg silhouette of Sailor Pants further enhances this elongating effect, giving the wearer an elegant and sophisticated look. Sailor Pants often have decorative buttons or embellishments along the front, adding a touch of nautical charm to the design. These buttons are typically functional, allowing the pants to be fastened securely. However, they can also be purely decorative, adding visual interest to the garment. Traditionally, Sailor Pants were made from durable and sturdy fabrics such as cotton canvas or wool. These fabrics were chosen for their ability to withstand the harsh conditions at sea and provide the necessary protection for sailors. However, modern versions of Sailor Pants are now available in a wide range of materials, including lightweight fabrics such as linen and denim, making them suitable for various occasions and climates. Sailor Pants are versatile garments that can be dressed up or down depending on the desired look. They can be paired with a tucked-in blouse or shirt for a polished and sophisticated ensemble. Alternatively, they can be worn with a casual t-shirt or sweater for a more relaxed and effortless vibe. In conclusion, Sailor Pants are a stylish and timeless design in the realm of fashion. Their high waistline, wide leg silhouette, and decorative buttons make them a unique and eye-catching choice. Whether worn for a formal event or a casual outing, Sailor Pants add a touch of nautical flair to any outfit.

Sample Maker

A sample maker in the context of fashion design refers to an individual or a team responsible for creating prototypes or samples of various garment designs. They play a crucial role in bringing the designer's vision to life and ensuring the feasibility and functionality of the proposed designs. The primary task of a sample maker is to translate the designer's sketches or specifications into three-dimensional garments. They possess a deep understanding of garment construction techniques, fabric properties, and sewing methods. Using these skills, they meticulously cut, sew, and assemble the fabric pieces to create a sample that closely resembles the final product.

Sarong

A sarong is a versatile and stylish garment frequently used in fashion design. It is typically a large rectangular piece of fabric, often made from lightweight materials such as cotton or silk, that is wrapped around the waist to create a skirt-like garment. Sarongs are known for their vibrant colors, intricate patterns, and flowing drapes, making them a popular choice for resort wear, beach attire, and summer fashion. Sarongs originate from Southeast Asia, particularly Indonesia, Malaysia, and the Philippines, where they have been worn for centuries as traditional clothing. However, they have gained global popularity and are now embraced by fashion designers worldwide for their versatility and exotic aesthetic.

Sarouel Pants

Sarouel Pants, also known as harem pants or drop-crotch pants, are a unique style of trousers that originated in the Middle East and have become popular in fashion design. These pants have a distinct and relaxed silhouette, characterized by a baggy and voluminous fit in the upper leg area that tapers down towards the ankles or calves. Sarouel pants typically have a low-rise waistband that sits well below the natural waistline, emphasizing the drop-crotch design. This design feature creates extra fabric around the crotch area, resulting in a loose and draped fit. The waistband of these pants can be elasticated, drawstring, or have a combination of both for added comfort and adjustability. One of the defining features of Sarouel pants is the unique draping and pleating techniques used in their construction. These pleats are strategically placed to enhance the billowy and relaxed look of the pants while also adding texture and visual interest to the garment. The pleating can be concentrated in the front, back, or both, depending on the desired design aesthetic. Sarouel pants are often made from lightweight and flowing fabrics such as cotton, linen, rayon, or silk to enhance their drape and movement. However, they can also be crafted from heavier materials like denim or wool for a more structured and winter-appropriate style. These pants are available in a range of solid colors, prints, and patterns to cater to various fashion preferences. The versatility of Sarouel pants allows them to be styled in multiple ways. They can be worn casually with a basic t-shirt and sneakers for a relaxed and effortless look. Alternatively, they can be dressed up with a tailored blazer, blouse, and heels for a more sophisticated and chic ensemble. In recent years, Sarouel pants have gained popularity in the fashion industry as a gender-neutral and inclusive garment. Their loose fit and ease of movement make them a comfortable choice for people of all body shapes and sizes. Additionally, their cultural significance and historical roots add an element of global awareness and appreciation to contemporary fashion designs.

Scuba Suit

A scuba suit, also known as a wetsuit or dive suit, is a specialized garment designed specifically for underwater activities, particularly scuba diving. It is an essential piece of equipment that provides thermal insulation, protection, and comfort to divers in various aquatic environments. Typically made of neoprene, a synthetic rubber material, a scuba suit is designed to provide insulation by trapping a thin layer of water between the suit and the diver's skin. This layer of water is warmed by the diver's body heat, keeping them insulated from the colder water temperature. The neoprene material is stretchy, allowing for ease of movement and flexibility underwater. The main purpose of a scuba suit is to protect the diver from the elements and potential hazards while diving. It provides a barrier between the diver's skin and the surrounding water, preventing direct contact with potentially harmful marine life, sharp coral, and abrasive underwater surfaces. The thickness of the scuba suit can vary depending on the water temperature and diving conditions. Thicker suits are used in colder water to provide better insulation, while thinner suits are more suitable for warmer waters. In addition to insulation and protection, scuba suits are also designed with comfort in mind. They are typically form-fitting to minimize water flow and maximize heat retention. The suits often have reinforced knee and elbow pads for durability and protection during various underwater activities. Additionally, some scuba suits feature extra features such as hoods, boots, and gloves, providing additional insulation and protection to these exposed areas of the body. Scuba suits play a significant role in fashion within the diving community. They come in various colors and patterns, allowing divers to express their personal style and preferences. However, it is important to note that fashion considerations should never compromise the functionality and safety of the scuba suit. Proper fit and quality construction are crucial in ensuring the suit's effectiveness in protecting the diver and maintaining warmth underwater.

Seam Allowance Guide

A seam allowance is a specified measurement that is added to the pattern pieces of a garment during the cutting and construction process in fashion design. It refers to the fabric that extends beyond the seam line and is used to join two or more pieces together. The purpose of a seam allowance is to allow room for sewing and finishing techniques such as seam allowances, hems, and edge finishes. This additional fabric helps to ensure that the final garment has a clean and professional appearance, as well as providing durability and strength to the seams.

Seam Allowance Guides

A seam allowance guide in fashion design refers to a predetermined measurement added to the pattern pieces before cutting and sewing fabric together. It provides the necessary extra space between the stitched seam and the fabric edge, ensuring that the seam does not pull or pucker and allows for alterations if needed. Seam allowances are essential in garment construction as they help maintain the integrity of the design, provide flexibility for fitting adjustments, and facilitate proper finishing techniques. These allowances also allow for personalization and customization by enabling designers to modify the fit, style, and details of a garment.

Seam Guide Presser Feet

Seam Guide Presser Feet are essential tools used in fashion design for sewing purposes. These presser feet are attachments that are used in conjunction with sewing machines to guide the fabric accurately through the machine, ensuring precise and even seam allowances. Seam Guide Presser Feet come in various shapes and sizes, each designed to serve a specific purpose. They are typically made of durable metal, such as stainless steel, to withstand the pressure and abrasion of sewing. The feet are attached to the sewing machine's presser foot holder, which is located above the needle plate.

Seam Ripper

A seam ripper is a small, handheld tool used in fashion design to remove stitches and seams. It is an essential tool for both professional and amateur fashion designers as it allows for precise and efficient removal of unwanted stitches, allowing for alterations and adjustments to be made to garments. The design of a seam ripper typically consists of a handle, usually made of plastic or wood, and a sharp, pointed blade. The blade is carefully positioned between the layers of fabric and used to cut and remove individual stitches without causing any damage to the fabric itself. The sharpness of the blade ensures clean and quick removal of stitches, making it a valuable tool for any fashion designer. Seam rippers are especially useful in a variety of fashion design tasks. They can be used to unpick mistakes or botched stitches, allowing for quick fixes and repairs. They are also used in the process of pattern making, where seams may need to be altered or adjusted to achieve the desired fit and silhouette. When working with delicate or intricate fabrics, such as lace or silk, a seam ripper is crucial to avoid causing any damage. The sharp blade allows for precision and control, enabling designers to remove stitches without creating snags or tears in the fabric. This is particularly important when making adjustments to high-end garments or couture pieces, where any damage to the fabric would be costly and time-consuming to repair. In addition to its practical uses, a seam ripper can also be seen as a symbol of precision and attention to detail in the fashion industry. It represents the dedication and care that designers put into their work, ensuring that every stitch is flawless and every garment is of the highest quality. It is a tool that embodies the craftsmanship and artistry that goes into creating beautiful and well-fitting garments. In conclusion, a seam ripper is a small but indispensable tool in fashion design. Its sharp blade and ergonomic design make it an essential tool for removing stitches and seams with precision and ease. Whether used for alterations, repairs, or pattern making, a seam ripper plays a vital role in creating impeccable garments and showcasing the skill and expertise of fashion designers.

Seam Sealing Tape

Seam sealing tape, in the context of fashion design, refers to a narrow strip of specialized material that is used to waterproof the seams of garments. It is a crucial component in the production of high-quality outerwear, ensuring that the seams remain watertight and resistant to moisture penetration. The tape is typically made from a thin layer of thermoplastic material, such as polyurethane, that has been coated with a heat-activated adhesive on one side. This adhesive is activated when heat and pressure are applied to the tape during the garment construction process. Once activated, the adhesive bonds the tape to the fabric, creating a strong and durable seal.

Seamstress

A seamstress in the context of fashion design refers to a skilled individual who specializes in sewing, altering, and repairing garments. They possess a deep understanding of various fabrics, patterns, and sewing techniques to create high-quality clothing pieces. Seamstresses play an essential role in the fashion industry, contributing to the creation of custom-made clothing, as well as the production of ready-to-wear garments. The primary responsibility of a seamstress is to bring a designer's vision to life by creating well-fitting and visually appealing garments. They meticulously follow patterns, which act as blueprints for each piece, and carefully cut and stitch fabrics together using sewing machines and hand sewing techniques. Seamstresses are skilled in creating a variety of garment types, such as dresses, blouses, pants, jackets, and skirts, with precision and attention to detail. Seamstresses are also proficient in performing alterations on garments to ensure a perfect fit. This involves modifying existing clothing items based on individual body measurements and preferences. They skillfully adjust seams, hems, and darts, and may even restructure portions of a garment to achieve the desired fit and silhouette. Seamstresses possess excellent problem-solving skills, as they must find creative solutions to overcome challenges presented during the alteration process. Additionally, the role of a seamstress extends to garment repair. They are trained to fix damaged clothing by replacing buttons, mending tears, repairing zippers, and adjusting loose or broken seams. Seamstresses possess the expertise to seamlessly integrate repairs into the original design of the garment, ensuring that the repaired area blends seamlessly with the rest of the piece. Becoming a proficient seamstress require years of practice and experience. It involves acquiring a deep knowledge of various sewing techniques, understanding the properties of different fabrics, and honing skills in precision cutting and stitching. Seamstresses often undergo formal training in fashion design or garment construction, and continuously improve their skills through practical work experience. In conclusion, a seamstress in the fashion design industry is a highly skilled individual who specializes in sewing, altering, and repairing garments. They possess expertise in various sewing techniques, fabric properties, and pattern interpretation. Seamstresses contribute significantly to the creation of custom-made clothing and the production of ready-to-wear garments, ensuring that each piece fits perfectly and adheres to the designer's vision.

Sequined Blouse

A sequined blouse is a fashionable garment designed for women, typically made of lightweight materials such as silk, chiffon, or satin, that is embellished with sequins. Sequins are small, shiny, disk-shaped beads that are sewn onto the fabric, creating a visually striking effect. The sequined blouse is a popular choice for evening wear and special occasions, as it adds a glamorous touch to any ensemble. The shimmering sequins catch the light, creating a dazzling and eye-catching effect that instantly enhances the overall look of the blouse.

Serger Machines

Serger machines, also known as overlock machines, are essential tools in the field of fashion design. These machines are specifically designed to create professional and high-quality finished edges on garments and other fabric items. Unlike regular sewing machines, which use only one thread to create seams, serger machines use multiple threads to sew, trim, and finish fabric edges all at once. This unique feature allows fashion designers to achieve clean and polished seams that prevent fraying and ensure durability.

Serpentine Threads

Serpentine threads refers to a type of decorative stitching technique commonly used in fashion design. It involves the use of curving, sinuous lines of thread to create intricate patterns and designs on garments and accessories. This technique is often executed using a sewing machine with a specialized serpentine stitch setting, which allows for precise and even stitching along the desired path. Alternatively, it can also be done by hand using a needle and thread, although this requires a high degree of skill and precision.

Sewing Cabinets

Sewing cabinets are essential pieces of furniture used in the field of fashion design. These specialized cabinets are specifically designed to provide a functional and organized workspace for fashion designers and seamstresses. These cabinets typically feature a sturdy and spacious top surface that serves as a cutting table, allowing designers to lay out and measure fabric accurately. The top surface may also include a gridded or marked layout, making it easier to create symmetrical and precise cuts. Underneath the top surface, sewing cabinets often have a recessed area or a removable insert that houses a sewing machine. This placement allows the machine to be at a convenient height for sewing tasks, reducing strain on the designer's back and neck. The recessed area may also include a hinged cover to protect the machine when not in use, keeping it free from dust and debris. Sewing cabinets are intelligently designed to provide ample storage for sewing supplies and accessories. They typically include drawers, shelves, and compartments, allowing designers to keep their tools, threads, buttons, and other materials neatly organized and easily accessible. Some cabinets even feature customized compartments for specific tools such as scissors or measuring tapes. In terms of functionality, sewing cabinets are designed with durability and stability in mind. They are made from high-quality materials such as solid wood or sturdy engineered wood, ensuring that they can withstand the weight of the sewing machine and provide a stable work surface. Additionally, sewing cabinets often incorporate thoughtful features that enhance the sewing experience. These may include built-in lighting to illuminate the workspace, adjustable shelves and drawers to accommodate various sizes of sewing supplies, and ergonomic design elements to promote comfort during long hours of work. Overall, sewing cabinets are indispensable for fashion designers as they provide a dedicated, organized, and ergonomic workspace for various sewing tasks. They offer a convenient and efficient solution for storing and accessing sewing supplies while ensuring a stable and comfortable setup for sewing machines. These cabinets play a crucial role in facilitating the creative process and enabling designers to bring their fashion ideas to life.

Sewing Gauges

Sewing gauges are essential tools in the field of fashion design. They are small rulers or measuring devices that are used to ensure accuracy and precision in the sewing process. These gauges are typically made of metal or plastic and come in a variety of shapes and sizes. The main purpose of sewing gauges is to measure and mark fabric accurately. They are used for tasks such as hemming, seam allowance marking, buttonhole placement, and pleat and dart marking. By using a sewing gauge, fashion designers can ensure that their garments are sewn to the correct dimensions and that all elements are correctly aligned.

Sewing Machine Bobbin Cases

A sewing machine bobbin case is a small metal or plastic device that holds the bobbin in place within a sewing machine. It plays a crucial role in ensuring the smooth operation of the sewing machine and helps create even and consistent stitches. Bobbin cases are typically located beneath the needle plate of a sewing machine. They have different designs and mechanisms depending on the make and model of the sewing machine, but their essential function remains the same.

Sewing Machine Covers

A sewing machine cover is a protective textile accessory specifically designed to fit over a sewing machine when it is not in use. It serves the purpose of shielding the machine from dust, dirt, and other potential sources of damage, while also adding a decorative element to the sewing area. In the realm of fashion design, sewing machine covers are not merely functional objects; they also contribute to the overall aesthetic appeal of a sewing space. Fashion designers often invest considerable effort in creating a visually pleasing and inspiring workspace, and the choice of a sewing machine cover is an important aspect in achieving this goal.

Sewing Machine Extension Tables

A sewing machine extension table is a flat surface that is attached to the bed of a sewing machine. It provides extra space for manipulating and supporting fabric during the sewing process. The table is usually made of a durable material such as wood or acrylic and is designed to match the dimensions and shape of the sewing machine. Fashion designers often use sewing machine extension tables to enhance their workflow and create better results. The added surface area allows for easier manipulation of large or heavy fabrics, such as those used in couture garments or home décor projects. By providing a stable and level surface, the table helps prevent fabric from getting caught or pulled during sewing, resulting in more precise and professional-looking stitches.

Sewing Machine Lights

A sewing machine light is a small, built-in light fixture that is attached to a sewing machine to provide illumination while sewing. It is an essential tool for fashion designers as it allows for clear visibility of the fabric and sewing area, enabling precise and accurate stitching. The sewing machine light is typically positioned either above the needle or towards the bottom of the machine's body, illuminating the area where the fabric is being fed through and the stitching is taking place. This ensures that designers can easily follow the designated sewing lines, patterns, or markings on the fabric, resulting in neat and professional-looking garments.

Sewing Machine Oil

Sewing machine oil is a lubricant specifically designed for use with sewing machines in the fashion design industry. It is a clear, odorless liquid that is used to reduce friction and keep the moving parts of the sewing machine running smoothly. The use of sewing machine oil is essential in maintaining the longevity and efficiency of sewing machines used in fashion design. The constant movement and friction of the machine's parts can cause wear and tear, which can lead to the machine malfunctioning or breaking down. Sewing machine oil helps to prevent this by creating a thin layer of lubrication between the moving parts, reducing friction and preventing excessive heat buildup. One of the main benefits of using sewing machine oil is that it helps to prolong the life of the machine. By keeping the parts properly lubricated, the machine is less likely to experience mechanical issues and break down. This is especially important in the fashion design industry, where sewing machines are often used for long periods of time and are subject to heavy use. In addition to extending the life of the machine, using sewing machine oil also helps to maintain its efficiency. A well-lubricated sewing machine can operate smoothly and quietly, allowing for precise and accurate stitching. This is crucial in fashion design, where attention to detail is paramount. Sewing machine oil is easy to use and can be applied to the machine in small amounts. It is typically applied directly to the moving parts of the sewing machine, such as the needle bar, presser foot, and bobbin case. Regularly oiling the machine, following the manufacturer's guidelines, is recommended to ensure optimal performance. In conclusion, sewing machine oil is a vital component in the fashion design industry, as it helps to maintain the longevity and efficiency of sewing machines. By reducing friction and preventing excessive wear and tear, sewing machine oil ensures that the machine operates smoothly and accurately, allowing fashion designers to create high-quality garments with ease.

Sewing Machine Tables

A sewing machine table is a specialized piece of furniture designed to provide a stable and ergonomic working surface for fashion designers and other sewing enthusiasts. It is specifically designed to accommodate the unique needs and requirements of sewing machines, allowing users to work comfortably and efficiently. These tables typically feature a large flat surface area with a cutout or recessed section specifically designed to fit sewing machines. This allows the machine to sit flush with the table surface, providing an even and stable base for sewing. The table may also have adjustable height settings, allowing users to customize the working height to their preference or comfort level.

Sewing Machines

Sewing machines are mechanical or electronic devices designed to stitch fabric together with thread. They play a crucial role in the field of fashion design, allowing designers and seamstresses to create garments with precision and efficiency. Sewing machines consist of various components, including a needle, bobbin, and feed dogs. The needle is used to pierce the fabric, while the bobbin holds the lower thread that interlocks with the upper thread to create stitches. The feed dogs are small teeth that guide the fabric through the machine as it is being stitched. One of the key features of sewing machines is the ability to adjust stitch length and width, which allows for versatility in creating different types of seams and decorative stitches. Fashion designers often utilize different stitch options, such as straight stitch, zigzag stitch, or decorative stitches, to achieve specific design elements or enhance the functionality of the garment. Additionally, sewing machines may have various built-in features that make the sewing process more efficient and convenient. This can include automatic thread cutting, needle threading systems, and adjustable presser foot pressure. These features help save time and allow designers to focus on the creative aspects of their work. In fashion design, sewing machines are utilized for a wide range of tasks, such as garment construction, hemming, attaching zippers, and creating intricate details like pleats and ruffles. The use of sewing machines enables designers to execute their ideas more quickly and accurately than traditional hand sewing methods. Furthermore, sewing machines contribute to the production of ready-to-wear clothing on a larger scale. Industrial sewing machines are used in manufacturing facilities to sew garments in bulk. These machines are typically faster and more specialized, allowing for increased productivity in the fashion industry. In conclusion, sewing machines are essential tools in the realm of fashion design, providing designers and seamstresses with the means to create garments with precision and efficiency. Their diverse features and functions allow for a wide range of creative possibilities, making sewing machines indispensable in the fashion industry.

Sewing Pins

Sewing pins are small, slender tools used in the craft of fashion design. They are typically made of metal, with a sharp and pointed end that allows them to easily penetrate fabric without causing damage. These pins are an essential tool for fashion designers, as they are used to hold fabric pieces together temporarily, allowing for precise and accurate sewing. When working on a fashion design project, it is common for designers to need to join multiple pieces of fabric together to create a garment. Sewing pins are used to hold these fabric pieces in place before they are sewn permanently. The pins are inserted through the fabric layers at strategic points, ensuring that they hold the fabric securely and prevent any shifting during the sewing process.

Sewing Table

A sewing table, in the context of fashion design, refers to a dedicated workspace designed specifically for the art of sewing and garment construction. It is an essential piece of furniture that provides a stable and organized area for designers and seamstresses to work on their projects with precision and efficiency. The main purpose of a sewing table is to offer a comfortable and ergonomic surface for cutting, pinning, and stitching fabrics. It typically consists of a flat tabletop, which serves as the primary workspace, and various additional features to enhance the sewing experience.

Shacket (Shirt Jacket)

A Shacket, short for Shirt Jacket, is a versatile garment that combines the elements of a shirt and a jacket into one stylish piece. It is a perfect blend of casual and formal wear, suitable for various occasions and weather conditions. The Shacket is typically constructed with lightweight materials, such as cotton, denim, or flannel, making it a comfortable option for layering. Its design resembles that of a shirt, featuring a button-down front, collar, and cuffs. However, it is slightly thicker and more structured, giving it the characteristics of a jacket.

Shawl Cardigan

A shawl cardigan is a type of sweater that combines the design elements of both a shawl and a cardigan. It is a versatile and stylish piece of clothing that is popular in the world of fashion design. The shawl cardigan typically features a shawl collar, which is a wide, turned-over collar that extends across the chest and back of the sweater. This collar adds a touch of elegance and sophistication to the garment, making it suitable for both formal and casual occasions. The shawl collar may be plain or adorned with decorative details such as ribbing or cables, depending on the designer's aesthetic vision.

Shawl Collar Sweater

A shawl collar sweater is a type of sweater that features a collar that extends down the front of the garment in a continuous line, resembling the shape and appearance of a shawl. The collar of a shawl collar sweater typically sits wide and flat against the shoulders and chest, with a distinct V-shaped or U-shaped notch at the front. This style of sweater is a classic and timeless design that originated from men's fashion but has evolved to be worn by both men and women. The shawl collar adds a touch of elegance and sophistication to the sweater, making it suitable for various occasions, from casual to formal settings.

Sheath Dress

A sheath dress is a form-fitting garment that follows the contours of the body, typically without any waistline seam. Also known as a straight or shift dress, it is a timeless and classic silhouette that is popular in fashion design. The sheath dress is characterized by its simplicity and elegance. It is designed to be sleek and sophisticated, often skimming the body from the neckline to the hemline. The dress is usually sleeveless, although it can also feature short or long sleeves. The key feature of a sheath dress is its slim fit. It is designed to accentuate the natural shape of the body, hugging the curves without being too tight. The dress typically has darts or seams that help create a tailored look and provide shaping around the waist and hips. Sheath dresses are commonly made from fabrics like cotton, silk, or wool, although they can be found in a variety of materials. The choice of fabric can determine the dress's overall look and feel. For example, a sheath dress made from silk may have a more luxurious and formal appearance, while a cotton sheath dress can be more casual and comfortable. Sheath dresses are versatile and can be worn for a range of occasions. They are often seen as a go-to option for office wear, as they are professional and polished. However, they can also be dressed up or down depending on the accessories and styling. Pairing a sheath dress with heels and statement jewelry can create a more formal and glamorous ensemble, while wearing it with flats and minimal accessories can result in a more relaxed and casual look. In conclusion, a sheath dress is a stylish and versatile garment that flatters the body's natural shape. Its slim fit and clean lines make it a classic choice for various occasions, from the office to special events. Whether it is made from silk or cotton, the sheath dress is a timeless silhouette in fashion design.

Shift Dress

A shift dress is a type of dress that is typically short in length and features a loose, relaxed fit. It is characterized by having a straight cut, without any defined waistline or shaping seams. The dress hangs straight down from the shoulders, creating a straight silhouette that skims over the body rather than hugging it. This style of dress originated in the 1920s as a reaction to the restrictive and corseted fashion of the previous decades. It was popularized by the fashion designer Coco Chanel, who believed in creating comfortable and practical clothing for women. The shift dress quickly gained popularity for its simplicity and ease of wear. The shift dress is known for its versatility and timeless appeal. It can be dressed up or down depending on the occasion and is suitable for both casual and formal events. The loose fit of the dress allows for ease of movement and comfort, making it a popular choice for everyday wear. Shift dresses are typically made from lightweight and flowy fabrics such as silk, chiffon, or cotton. They can come in a variety of colors, patterns, and textures, allowing for endless possibilities in terms of styling. Some shift dresses may also feature embellishments such as embroidery, beading, or lace to add visual interest. The lack of a defined waistline in the shift dress makes it a flattering choice for a wide range of body types. It can help to create a streamlined and elongated silhouette, while also providing comfort and ease of movement. The dress can be styled with accessories such as belts or scarves to add definition to the waist if desired. In summary, a shift dress is a versatile and timeless style of dress that features a loose and relaxed fit. It is known for its simplicity and comfort, making it a popular choice for both casual and formal occasions. The lack of a defined waistline and the use of lightweight fabrics contribute to its flattering and easy-to-wear nature.

Shirt Dress

A shirt dress is a type of dress that is designed to resemble a shirt in its structure and details. It combines the look of a button-up shirt with the length and shape of a dress, resulting in a versatile garment that can be worn for various occasions. The shirt dress typically features a collar, button front closure, and cuffed sleeves, similar to a traditional shirt. It may have a tailored fit or a relaxed, oversized silhouette, depending on the desired style. The length of the dress can range from above the knee to ankle-length, with different options available to suit different body types and personal preferences. Shirt dresses are often made from lightweight and breathable fabrics, such as cotton or linen, which allow for ease of movement and comfort. However, they can also be crafted from other materials like silk or satin for a more luxurious and formal look. The dress may be solid-colored or feature patterns such as stripes, checks, or floral prints, adding visual interest and versatility to the garment. One of the key features of a shirt dress is its ability to be styled in different ways. It can be worn as a standalone piece, paired with accessories like belts to cinch the waist and add definition. Alternatively, it can be layered over jeans or trousers for a more relaxed and casual outfit. The versatility of the shirt dress makes it suitable for both formal and informal occasions, allowing the wearer to effortlessly transition from day to night.

Shirt Sweater

A shirt sweater is a type of garment that combines the characteristics of both a classic shirt and a sweater. It is designed to provide the wearer with the comfort and warmth of a sweater, while maintaining the tailored and structured look of a shirt. In terms of its construction, a shirt sweater typically features a button-down front and a collar, similar to a traditional shirt. It is usually made from soft and cozy materials such as cotton, wool, or a blend of fibers, which provide insulation and ensure optimal comfort.

Shoe Design Software

Shoe Design Software refers to a specialized computer program that enables fashion designers to create, visualize, and refine designs for footwear. It offers a range of tools and features to assist designers in various stages of the design process, from sketching initial ideas to producing detailed technical drawings. This software provides designers with an intuitive platform to explore their creativity and translate their visions into digital prototypes. It typically includes a vast library of pre-designed shoe components, such as soles, uppers, heels, and laces, which can be customized and combined to form unique designs. This allows designers to experiment with different styles, materials, colors, and patterns, enabling them to create a wide variety of shoe designs. Shoe design software also offers advanced rendering capabilities, allowing designers to view their creations in 3D. This feature gives them a realistic representation of how the shoes will look when produced and worn, helping them make informed decisions about elements such as proportions, textures, and finishes. It also facilitates communication and collaboration with manufacturers, as the 3D visualizations can be shared electronically, reducing the need for physical prototypes and minimizing production costs. In addition to visualizing designs, this software often includes tools for technical detailing and production planning. Designers can generate accurate and comprehensive technical drawings, specifying dimensions, materials, and construction methods. These drawings serve as blueprints for manufacturers, ensuring that the design is accurately reproduced during the production stage and minimizing errors or misunderstandings. Furthermore, shoe design software may integrate with other fashion design software or industry-specific tools, such as material sourcing databases or manufacturing workflow management systems. This integration streamlines the design-to-production workflow, enabling seamless data exchange and facilitating efficient collaboration among various stakeholders involved in the footwear production process. In summary, shoe design software is a powerful tool for fashion designers, providing them with the means to ideate, visualize, refine, and communicate their shoe designs effectively. By combining artistic creativity with technical precision, this software enhances the design process, reduces production costs, and ultimately contributes to the development of innovative and stylish footwear.

Shoe Lasts

Shoe Lasts Shoe lasts, in the context of fashion design, refer to the three-dimensional forms in the shape of a human foot around which shoes are constructed. They are typically made of wood, plastic, or metal, and play a crucial role in determining the fit, style, and overall comfort of shoes. Shoe lasts serve as a foundation for shoe manufacturing, guiding the design and construction process. They are used by shoemakers as a template to create shoes that will fit properly and comfortably on the wearer's foot. Lasts are created based on the specific measurements and characteristics of different foot shapes and sizes. The design of shoe lasts takes into account various factors such as width, length, arch height, and toe shape. These factors influence the overall fit and comfort of the shoe, ensuring proper support and ease of movement for the wearer. Lasts also help determine the overall aesthetic of the shoe, as they dictate the contours, curves, and angles of the design. Shoemakers and designers work closely with the lasts to create different shoe styles, such as sandals, heels, boots, and athletic shoes. They use the lasts as a guide to shape and mold the upper part of the shoe, as well as to determine the placement of closures, such as laces or straps. The use of shoe lasts is essential in achieving consistent sizing and fit across different shoe styles and sizes. By using standardized lasts, manufacturers can ensure that shoes of the same size will have a similar fit, regardless of the design or material used. This helps consumers in selecting the right size when purchasing shoes. In addition, shoe lasts allow for customization and adaptation to individual foot characteristics. They can be modified or adjusted based on specific requirements, such as orthopedic needs or unique foot shapes. This flexibility in last design allows for the creation of shoes that cater to a wide range of foot types and preferences. In conclusion, shoe lasts are a fundamental component in fashion design, providing the structure and form around which shoes are built. They play a vital role in determining the fit, style, and comfort of shoes, ensuring that they are both aesthetically pleasing and functional.

Shoulder Pads

Shoulder pads are structural elements used in fashion design to enhance the silhouette and shape of garments, particularly in the upper body area. They are designed to be inserted into the shoulders of jackets, blazers, coats, and other garments to create a more defined and structured look. Shoulder pads are typically made from materials such as foam, polyester, or cotton, and come in various shapes and sizes. They are often covered with a layer of fabric that matches the garment they are intended for, creating a seamless integration. The thickness and density of shoulder pads can vary, allowing designers to achieve different levels of volume and emphasis on the shoulders.

Shrug

Shrug is a type of clothing accessory commonly used in fashion design. It is designed to be worn over the shoulders and upper back, covering only a portion of the upper body. The shrug typically consists of two small fabric panels that are connected at the back, leaving the front open. It is often made from lightweight materials such as lace, chiffon, or knit fabric. The purpose of a shrug is to add a stylish and fashionable touch to an outfit while providing some degree of warmth or coverage to the shoulders. It is a versatile piece that can be worn on various occasions, such as formal events, casual outings, or even as part of a wedding ensemble. The open front of the shrug allows it to be easily draped over the arms and shoulders, creating a layered look that enhances the overall appearance of the outfit.

Ski Suit

A ski suit is a type of clothing designed specifically for skiing or snowboarding. It is typically a one-piece garment that offers protection from cold weather and snow, while also providing flexibility and freedom of movement for the wearer. One of the key features of a ski suit is its insulation. To withstand the extreme temperatures and wind chill experienced in ski resorts, ski suits are often made with high-quality materials such as down or synthetic insulation. This helps to trap heat and keep the wearer warm, even in freezing conditions. Ski suits also feature a waterproof and breathable outer shell. This is important to protect against moisture from snow or rain, while also allowing perspiration to escape. The outer shell is typically made with a durable and water-resistant fabric, such as nylon or Gore-Tex, to ensure the wearer stays dry and comfortable. In addition to insulation and weatherproofing, ski suits also prioritize functionality and comfort. They often include adjustable cuffs, hoods, and waistbands to ensure a good fit and prevent cold air or snow from entering. Many ski suits also have reinforced knees and seat areas for added durability and protection in high-wear areas. When it comes to design, ski suits are available in a wide range of colors and patterns, allowing individuals to express their personal style on the slopes. Some ski suits may also feature reflective elements for increased visibility in low light conditions. Overall, a ski suit is a fundamental piece of clothing for any skier or snowboarder. It combines insulation, weatherproofing, and practical design elements to provide the wearer with comfort, protection, and freedom of movement while enjoying winter sports.

Skinny Jeans

Skinny jeans are a popular style of pants in the fashion industry, characterized by their tight fit and slimming effect. They are typically made from a stretchy denim fabric that hugs the wearer's body, especially around the legs and hips. These jeans are designed to have a skinny silhouette, creating a sleek and streamlined look. Skinny jeans are versatile and can be worn by both men and women. They often feature a mid or high-rise waist, sitting above the hips to elongate the legs. The narrow leg openings are designed to taper towards the ankles, accentuating the shape of the legs. This tight fit can give the illusion of longer, leaner legs, making them a popular choice among fashion-conscious individuals.

Skirted Shorts

Skirted shorts, also known as skorts, are a hybrid garment that combines the design elements of a skirt with the practicality and functionality of shorts. They are a popular choice in women's fashion, providing the look of a skirt with the comfort and ease of wearing shorts. Skirted shorts typically feature a skirt-like fabric overlay that is stitched onto a pair of shorts, creating the illusion of a skirt while offering the coverage and mobility of shorts. The design of skirted shorts varies widely, offering different lengths, styles, and materials to suit various fashion preferences and occasions. They can be found in mini, midi, or maxi lengths, allowing wearers to choose a style that best complements their body shape and desired level of coverage. Some skirted shorts feature a wrapped or asymmetrical front panel, adding an element of visual interest and creating a more feminine aesthetic. Others may have pleats, ruffles, or decorative details to enhance the skirt-like appearance. Skirted shorts can be made from a wide range of fabrics, including cotton, denim, linen, and various synthetic blends.

Skorts

Skorts, in the context of fashion design, refer to a hybrid garment that combines the appearance of a skirt with the functionality of shorts. The term "skort" is a portmanteau of the words "skirt" and "shorts," reflecting its dual nature and design elements. Skorts typically feature a skirt-like front panel that extends to a certain length, providing the illusion of a skirt. However, skorts also have a pair of shorts or built-in shorts underneath the front panel, which are concealed from the front view. These shorts provide comfort, flexibility, and modesty to the wearer while maintaining the appearance of a skirt from the front.

Sleeve Board

A sleeve board is a small, portable, and specialized tool used in fashion design for pressing and manipulating sleeves during the garment construction process. It is primarily designed to provide stability and support to the narrow and curved shape of sleeves, allowing for efficient and precise pressing without damaging or distorting the fabric. The sleeve board typically consists of a flat, elongated surface that is padded and covered with a heat-resistant fabric, such as cotton or wool. Its dimensions are smaller compared to a traditional ironing board, making it more suitable for handling sleeves and other smaller garment parts. The surface of the sleeve board is often tapered or curved to mimic the shape of a sleeve and accommodate different sleeve sizes and styles.

Sleeve Ironing Board

A sleeve ironing board is a specialized ironing board designed specifically for ironing sleeves and other smaller garments. It is a small, narrow board that is shaped to fit inside a sleeve or pants leg, allowing for easier and more efficient ironing of these items. Unlike a regular ironing board, which is large and flat, a sleeve ironing board is designed to be compact and portable. It is typically made of a heat-resistant material, such as metal or silicone, and may have a padded surface to provide a smooth and even ironing surface.

Slip Playsuit

A slip playsuit is a garment designed for women, typically made of lightweight and flowy materials, that combines the style of a slip dress and a playsuit. It is a one-piece outfit that features a fitted bodice with spaghetti straps and a loose-fitting, shorts-style bottom. The slip playsuit draws inspiration from the slip dress, which was popularized in the 1990s as an undergarment but has since evolved into a stylish and versatile fashion piece. The slip dress is characterized by its sleek and minimalist design, often made of silky or satin-like fabrics, and is designed to loosely skim the body. It became a staple in the wardrobes of many fashion-forward women for its effortless yet sexy appeal. The slip playsuit takes the silhouette of the slip dress and incorporates it into a playsuit, which is a one-piece garment that combines a top and shorts. This fusion of styles creates a unique and modern look that is both feminine and playful. The bodice of the slip playsuit is typically fitted to accentuate the waist and the upper body, while the bottom features loose-fitting shorts that provide comfort and ease of movement. The slip playsuit can be styled in various ways to suit different occasions. It can be dressed up with heels, statement jewelry, and a clutch for a night out or a special event. Alternatively, it can be dressed down with flat sandals, a denim jacket, and a crossbody bag for a casual and relaxed look. The versatility of the slip playsuit makes it a go-to option for many women who want to look effortlessly chic.

Slouchy Pants

Slouchy pants are a type of trousers characterized by their relaxed and loose fit, typically with a dropped crotch, and a low-rise waist. This style of pants is often associated with a casual and laid-back aesthetic, offering both comfort and style. Slouchy pants first gained popularity in the early 1990s and have since become a staple in contemporary fashion. They are especially popular in streetwear and urban fashion, but they can also be found in high-end designer collections.

Slow Fashion

Slow fashion is an approach to fashion design that prioritizes sustainability and ethical practices throughout the entire fashion production process. It focuses on creating high-quality, timeless garments that are made to last, rather than following the fast-paced trends that dominate the fashion industry. Unlike fast fashion, which produces cheap, disposable clothing at a rapid rate, slow fashion emphasizes the importance of craftsmanship and quality. This means using sustainable materials, such as organic cotton and recycled fabrics, and taking the time to create well-constructed pieces that can withstand the test of time. Another key aspect of slow fashion is a commitment to fair labor practices. This means ensuring that workers are paid a living wage, working in safe conditions, and are not subjected to exploitation or abuse. Slow fashion brands prioritize transparency and traceability in their supply chains, allowing consumers to make informed choices about the clothes they buy. In addition to focusing on the production process, slow fashion also encourages a more thoughtful and conscious approach to consumption. It promotes the idea of buying fewer, but higher-quality garments, and encourages consumers to think about the long-term value and versatility of the clothing they purchase. Slow fashion also challenges the notion that clothing has an expiration date. Instead of following seasonal trends and constantly discarding and replacing clothes, slow fashion encourages consumers to invest in pieces that can be worn year-round and can be easily styled in different ways. Overall, slow fashion aims to create a more sustainable and ethical fashion industry by prioritizing quality, transparency, and conscious consumption. It is a movement that encourages designers, brands, and consumers to rethink their approach to fashion and make choices that have a positive impact on both people and the planet.

Smock Dress

A smock dress is a type of dress that is characterized by its loose and relaxed fit. It typically has a straight or slightly A-line silhouette and is often made from lightweight and flowy fabrics. The main feature of a smock dress is its smocking detail, which is a sewing technique that creates a gathered or pleated effect on the fabric. The smocking detail is usually found on the bodice or neckline of the dress, creating a decorative and textured element. This technique adds dimension and visual interest to the dress, making it stand out from other styles. Smocking can be done using various patterns, such as diamond, floral, or geometric designs, further enhancing the overall look of the dress. A smock dress is typically designed with comfort in mind. The loose fit allows for ease of movement, making it suitable for casual and informal occasions. It is often considered a versatile wardrobe staple that can be dressed up or down depending on the styling and accessories. Smock dresses are popular in warm weather climates or during the summer months due to their lightweight and breathable fabrics. They are commonly made from materials such as cotton, linen, or chiffon, which provide comfort and allow air circulation. The loose fit also helps to keep the body cool in hot weather. When it comes to styling a smock dress, it can be paired with various accessories to create different looks. It can be worn with sandals or flats for a laid-back and casual vibe, or dressed up with heels and statement jewelry for a more formal occasion. Layering the dress with a denim jacket or cardigan can also add a stylish and trendy touch. In conclusion, a smock dress is a loose-fitting dress with a smocking detail on the bodice or neckline. It is made from lightweight fabrics and is designed for comfort. This type of dress is versatile and can be styled in different ways depending on the occasion.

Snap Fastener Kit

A snap fastener kit is a set of tools and materials used in fashion design to create closures on garments or accessories. It consists of various components, including the snaps themselves, along with tools for attaching and securing them to fabric. The snaps in a snap fastener kit are small, round or square pieces made of metal or plastic, with a protruding stem or post on one side and a socket or cap on the other. These snaps are designed to interlock when pressed firmly together, creating a secure closure. They can be easily opened by pulling or prying them apart, allowing for convenient fastening and unfastening of garments or accessories.

Speedo

A Speedo is a type of high-cut, form-fitting swimsuit designed for competitive swimming and other water sports. It is a popular choice among athletes and recreational swimmers for its sleek and streamlined design, which allows for maximum freedom of movement in the water. Originally introduced in the 1920s, Speedo revolutionized the world of swimwear by introducing a more minimalistic and functional design compared to the traditional loose-fitting one-piece swimsuits of that time. The key characteristics of a Speedo include a low-cut waist, high-cut hips, and a snug fit that hugs the body's contours.

Spool Pins

Spool pins in the context of fashion design refer to small, cylindrical structures used to secure and fasten fabric layers together during the construction process. These pins are typically made of metal, although they may also be made of plastic or other materials depending on the designer's preference. Spool pins are commonly used in sewing and garment construction to hold fabric layers in place before they are stitched or sewn together. They are especially useful when working with delicate or slippery fabrics that tend to shift or move during the sewing process. By securely holding the fabric layers in place, spool pins help to ensure more accurate and precise stitching, resulting in a neater and better-finished garment.

Steam Presses

Steam presses are an essential tool in the field of fashion design, used to ensure that fabrics are pressed and creased with precision and finesse. As the name suggests, these presses utilize steam to facilitate the process. Steam presses consist of a large flat surface, often made of durable metal or heat-resistant materials, that is heated and moistened with steam. The steam is generated either by a built-in boiler or by an external steam generator, depending on the design and specifications of the press. The fabric to be pressed is placed on the surface of the press, and the steam is applied directly to the fabric. The combination of heat and moisture helps to relax the fibers of the fabric, allowing any wrinkles or creases to be smoothed out easily. The press surface may also have additional features, such as vacuum suction or padding, to further enhance the pressing process. Steam presses offer several advantages over traditional ironing methods. Firstly, they can provide a larger pressing area, allowing for the successful pressing of larger pieces of fabric or multiple garment sections at once. This can significantly increase efficiency and save time for fashion designers who need to press numerous pieces during the construction process. Additionally, steam presses can produce more consistent and professional results compared to handheld irons. The steam helps to evenly distribute heat and moisture, ensuring that the fabric is pressed uniformly and without any unsightly marks or lines. This is particularly important when working with delicate fabrics that require extra care. Furthermore, steam presses are often equipped with adjustable temperature and steam settings, allowing fashion designers to tailor the pressing process to the specific requirements of the fabric being used. This versatility is crucial in maintaining the integrity of different fabric types, including delicate silks, heavy woolens, or synthetic blends. In conclusion, steam presses are indispensable tools for fashion designers, enabling precise and efficient fabric pressing. By combining heat and steam, these presses help to eliminate wrinkles and creases, providing professional and consistent results. Their larger pressing area and adjustable settings make them ideal for working with a variety of fabric types, ensuring garments are well-pressed and ready for the runway or the retail rack.

Stitching Techniques

Stitching techniques in fashion design refer to the various methods and styles used to join fabric pieces together to create a garment or accessory. These techniques include both hand-sewing and machine-sewing methods, each with its own unique characteristics and applications. Hand-sewing techniques involve using a needle and thread to manually join fabric pieces. These techniques require skill and precision, as each stitch is carefully executed by the designer or seamstress. Common hand-sewing techniques include basting, backstitching, slipstitching, and blanket stitch. Basting involves temporary stitches used to hold fabric pieces in place before permanent sewing. Backstitching creates strong and secure seams by overlapping stitches. Slipstitching is a nearly invisible stitch used for hemming and finishing edges. Blanket stitch is a decorative stitch often used for appliqué or to finish raw edges. Machine-sewing techniques, on the other hand, involve using a sewing machine to quickly and efficiently join fabric pieces. These techniques are commonly used in mass production and require less manual dexterity than hand-sewing. Popular machine-sewing techniques include straight stitching, zigzag stitching, and overlock stitching. Straight stitching is used for basic seams and topstitching, creating a clean and straight line. Zigzag stitching is a versatile stitch used for finishing edges, adding elasticity, and decorative purposes. Overlock stitching is commonly seen in sergers and creates a strong and professional finish for seams. Stitching techniques are an essential part of fashion design, as they determine the durability, strength, and overall quality of a garment or accessory. Designers must consider the fabric type, desired aesthetic, and functionality when selecting and applying stitching techniques. Each technique has its own unique characteristics and applications, allowing designers to achieve different effects and finishes. Mastering various stitching techniques enables fashion designers to bring their creative visions to life and create garments that are both aesthetically pleasing and structurally sound.

Straight-Leg Jeans

Straight-leg jeans are a classic style of pants that are characterized by their straight, narrow silhouette from the waist to the hem. They are a staple in fashion and are known for their timeless and versatile design. Straight-leg jeans are typically made from denim fabric, which is a durable and sturdy material that has been a popular choice for jeans since its invention in the late 1800s. The fabric is woven in a twill weave, which gives it a diagonal pattern and adds to its strength. This makes straight-leg jeans a durable and long-lasting option for everyday wear. One of the defining features of straight-leg jeans is their straight and narrow leg opening. Unlike other styles of jeans, such as bootcut or flare, straight-leg jeans do not have any significant tapering or widening towards the hem. This creates a streamlined and tailored look that can be easily dressed up or down depending on the occasion. Straight-leg jeans are known for their versatility and can be styled in various ways to suit different fashion preferences and trends. They can be paired with a tucked-in blouse or a tailored blazer for a polished and sophisticated look. Alternatively, they can be worn with a casual t-shirt or a sweater for a more relaxed and effortless outfit. In terms of fit, straight-leg jeans are designed to sit at the natural waist or slightly below. They typically feature a traditional five-pocket design, with two front pockets, two back pockets, and a small coin pocket. This classic design adds to the timeless appeal of straight-leg jeans and makes them a wardrobe staple for both men and women. Straight-leg jeans are a go-to choice for those seeking a versatile and timeless denim option. With their straight, narrow silhouette and classic design, they offer a flattering and stylish choice for any occasion.

Strapless Bodysuit

A strapless bodysuit is a stylish garment designed for fashion-forward individuals who want to show off their shoulders and create a sleek, streamlined silhouette. It is a one-piece garment that combines the functionality of a bodysuit with the trendy design of a strapless top. The strapless bodysuit is constructed with a stretchy, form-fitting fabric that hugs the body and accentuates its natural curves. The absence of straps allows for a smooth and seamless look, making it an ideal choice for fashion enthusiasts who want to avoid any visible lines or bulges from shoulder straps.

Strapless Playsuit

A strapless playsuit is a one-piece garment that is designed to be worn without any shoulder straps. It is typically made of lightweight and comfortable fabric, such as cotton or linen, and is popular for its versatility and ease of wear. The strapless playsuit is characterized by its bustier-style top, which is fitted to the body and features a straight or sweetheart neckline. It may have boning or padding to provide support and enhance the shape of the bust. The absence of shoulder straps allows for a bare-shoulder look, making it a stylish choice for warmer climates or summer seasons.

Surf Rashie

A surf rashie is a type of garment that is specifically designed for individuals engaged in water sports such as surfing, paddleboarding, and kayaking. The term "rashie" is derived from the word "rash," as its primary function is to protect the wearer's skin from abrasions, irritations, and rashes that may occur as a result of prolonged exposure to water, sand, and surfboard wax. Typically, a surf rashie is made from a lightweight and quick-drying fabric such as nylon or polyester. The fabric is specifically chosen for its ability to wick away moisture, allowing the wearer to stay comfortable and dry even when in constant contact with water. Additionally, the fabric provides a level of UV protection, shielding the skin from harmful sun rays that can lead to sunburn and long-term skin damage. One of the key features of a surf rashie is its snug and form-fitting design. The garment is usually crafted with the intention of reducing friction between the wearer's skin and the surfboard or other equipment, minimizing the risk of painful chafing and friction burns. The close fit also prevents the rashie from impeding the wearer's movement, allowing them to perform various water sports activities with ease. Surf rashies are available in a variety of styles and designs to cater to different preferences and needs. Some may feature short sleeves, while others may have long sleeves for added protection against the sun. Additionally, surf rashies may come in various colors and patterns, enabling individuals to express their personal style while staying safe in the water. In terms of care, surf rashies are generally easy to clean and maintain. Most can be machine washed and dried, making them convenient for regular use. Due to their moisture-wicking properties, they also tend to dry quickly, ensuring that they are ready for the next water sports adventure in no time. In summary, a surf rashie is a specialized garment designed to protect the skin and enhance comfort for individuals engaged in water sports. With its lightweight, quick-drying fabric and snug fit, it provides protection against abrasions, irritations, and harmful sun rays. Whether it's for surfing, paddleboarding, or kayaking, a surf rashie is a practical and stylish choice for water sports enthusiasts.

Surf Shorts

Surf shorts, also known as board shorts or swim trunks, are a type of shorts specifically designed for water sports and activities, particularly surfing. They are a staple in the world of fashion and are widely popular among surfers and beachgoers alike. Surf shorts are typically made from quick-drying and lightweight materials, such as nylon or polyester. These fabrics allow for maximum comfort and flexibility when participating in water sports, as they do not become heavy or clingy when wet. The use of synthetic materials also ensures durability and resistance to wear and tear, making them suitable for the rough conditions often encountered while surfing. One of the distinguishing features of surf shorts is their longer length compared to traditional shorts. They usually extend below the knee, providing ample coverage and protection from the sun and potential irritants, such as saltwater and sand. The longer length also allows for greater freedom of movement, essential for activities like paddling and maneuvering on the surfboard. Surf shorts typically feature an elastic waistband or drawstring closure, allowing for easy adjustability and ensuring a secure fit during intense physical activity. Some designs also incorporate a Velcro fly for added convenience. Many surf shorts also have a small pocket on the back or side, ideal for storing small essentials like keys or wax for the surfboard. In terms of style, surf shorts come in a wide variety of vibrant colors, patterns, and prints. These designs often reflect the beach and surf culture, featuring tropical motifs, floral patterns, or bold graphics. The versatility of surf shorts allows individuals to express their personal style while enjoying the functionality and comfort they offer. Overall, surf shorts combine functionality, durability, and style to meet the specific demands of water sports, particularly surfing. While originally designed for surfers, they have become a popular choice for anyone seeking comfortable and stylish swimwear for beach-related activities. Whether hitting the waves or simply lounging by the shore, surf shorts are a go-to option for those looking for both performance and fashion in their swimwear.

Sustainable Dyeing Techniques

Sustainable dyeing techniques in the context of fashion design refer to the use of methods and processes that minimize the negative impact on the environment and human health, while still achieving desired colors and effects on textiles. These techniques prioritize the reduction of water consumption, energy use, and the release of toxic chemicals during the dyeing process. They also focus on the responsible sourcing and use of natural dyes and pigments, as well as the recycling and reuse of water and dye materials.

Sustainable Fashion Brands

Sustainable fashion brands are fashion design companies that prioritize environmental and social responsibility throughout their production processes. These brands strive to minimize the negative impact of the fashion industry on the environment, while also promoting fair trade practices and supporting sustainable communities. In terms of environmental responsibility, sustainable fashion brands aim to reduce their carbon footprint by using eco-friendly materials and implementing sustainable production practices. This can include using organic or recycled fabrics, reducing water consumption, and implementing energy-efficient manufacturing processes. These brands also prioritize waste reduction and recycling, ensuring that their production and packaging materials are as sustainable as possible. At the same time, sustainable fashion brands are committed to promoting social responsibility within the fashion industry. They prioritize fair trade practices, ensuring that garment workers are paid fair wages and working in safe conditions. These brands also foster transparency and accountability, providing information about their supply chains and production processes to consumers. In addition to these environmental and social considerations, sustainable fashion brands also prioritize timeless designs and quality craftsmanship. By promoting garments that are durable and built to last, these brands encourage consumers to invest in pieces that will withstand the test of time, reducing the need for frequent replacement and minimizing waste. Overall, sustainable fashion brands aim to transform the fashion industry into a more sustainable and ethical system. Through their commitment to environmental and social responsibility, these brands not only create beautiful and timeless designs, but also contribute to a more sustainable future for the industry as a whole.

Sustainable Fashion Certification

Sustainable Fashion Certification is a formal recognition given to fashion designers or brands by recognized authorities or organizations to acknowledge their efforts in adopting sustainable and ethical practices in the fashion industry. It signifies that the certified designer or brand has successfully met and maintained certain environmental and social standards throughout their design and production processes. This certification serves as a means to promote and support sustainable fashion practices and to encourage the fashion industry as a whole to move towards more responsible and eco-friendly approaches. It also helps consumers in making informed choices by identifying and supporting brands that prioritize sustainability and ethical practices.

Sustainable Fashion

Sustainable fashion, also known as eco-fashion or ethical fashion, is a design philosophy and practice that aims to create clothing and accessories in an environmentally and socially responsible way. It involves considering the entire lifecycle of a garment, from the sourcing of materials to production, distribution, and disposal. In sustainable fashion, designers prioritize the use of sustainable materials, such as organic and recycled fibers, and avoid the use of harmful chemicals and dyes. They also focus on reducing waste and minimizing the carbon footprint of their creations. This includes using energy-efficient production methods, implementing recycling and upcycling strategies, and promoting a circular economy where garments can be repaired, reused, or recycled instead of ending up in landfills.

Sustainable Textile Innovation

Sustainable Textile Innovation refers to the use of innovative techniques, materials, and processes in the fashion industry that promote sustainability and minimize environmental impact. It involves the development and implementation of sustainable practices throughout the entire lifecycle of textile products, from production to disposal. Key elements of sustainable textile innovation include reducing the use of harmful chemicals and toxic dyes, minimizing water and energy consumption, implementing recycling and upcycling methods, and fostering a circular economy. It also involves incorporating eco-friendly materials, such as organic cotton, hemp, bamboo, and recycled fibers, into the design and manufacturing processes. Sustainable textile innovation aims to address and mitigate the negative environmental and social impacts of traditional textile production methods. It emphasizes the need for transparency and traceability in supply chains, ensuring fair and ethical treatment of workers, and reducing waste and pollution. By adopting sustainable practices, fashion designers can contribute to a more sustainable and responsible fashion industry. Moreover, sustainable textile innovation goes beyond the environmental aspects and extends its focus to social and economic sustainability. It involves collaborating with local communities and artisans, supporting fair trade practices, and promoting social empowerment within the fashion supply chain. Overall, sustainable textile innovation in fashion design is about challenging conventional practices and exploring new ways to create beautiful, functional, and sustainable textile products. It requires a holistic approach that considers the entire lifecycle of a garment, from the choice of raw materials to its eventual end-of-life disposal. By embracing sustainable textile innovation, fashion designers can contribute to a more sustainable and responsible industry that respects both people and the planet.

Sweater Dress

A sweater dress is a type of dress made from a knit fabric, typically wool or a wool blend, that resembles a sweater in its construction and design. It is characterized by its relaxed and comfortable fit, making it a popular choice for casual occasions. Unlike traditional dresses, which are usually made from woven fabrics and are structured and form-fitting, sweater dresses are looser and more flexible. They are often designed to have the same cozy and warm feel as a sweater, with a slightly oversized silhouette and a relaxed neckline.

Sweatshirt

A sweatshirt is a type of casual and comfortable garment that is typically made from a thick, warm, and soft fabric, such as cotton or fleece. It is designed to be worn over the upper body and covers the chest, back, and arms. With its relaxed fit and versatile style, the sweatshirt has become a staple in the world of fashion, known for its practicality and ease of wear. The design of a sweatshirt typically includes long sleeves, a crew neckline, and ribbed cuffs and hem. It is often adorned with various embellishments, such as logos, prints, or embroidery, which add a touch of individuality and aesthetic appeal. Sweatshirts can come in a variety of colors, patterns, and designs, making them suitable for different occasions and personal styles. Sweatshirts are commonly associated with sports and athletic activities, as they provide warmth during physical exertion and can be easily layered with other garments. They are also favored by individuals seeking a casual and relaxed look, as they can be paired with jeans, leggings, or skirts for a comfortable yet fashionable outfit. While sweatshirts are typically seen as casual wear, fashion designers have incorporated them into high-end collections, elevating their status in the fashion industry. By adding unique details, luxury fabrics, and experimental cuts, designers have transformed the humble sweatshirt into a fashion-forward and statement-making piece. In recent years, sweatshirts have also gained popularity as a form of self-expression and a canvas for artistic designs. Many individuals choose to wear sweatshirts featuring slogans, graphics, or pop culture references to convey their personal beliefs, interests, or sense of humor. Overall, sweatshirts are a versatile and enduring fashion item that bridges the gap between comfort and style. Whether worn for athletic purposes or as a fashion statement, they have become a wardrobe staple for people of all ages and backgrounds.

Swim Briefs

Swim briefs, also known as speedos, are a type of swimwear popularized in the world of fashion design. These snug-fitting garments are characterized by their minimal coverage, high-cut leg openings, and waistband that sits low on the hips. Designed for both men and women, swim briefs are typically crafted from lightweight and stretchy materials such as nylon or polyester. They offer a body-hugging fit that allows for ease of movement in the water, making them a popular choice for competitive swimmers. The streamlined design of swim briefs reduces drag, enabling swimmers to glide through the water more efficiently and enhance their performance.

Swim Cover-Up

A swim cover-up is a garment designed specifically for wearing over a swimsuit, providing coverage and style when transitioning between the pool or beach and other activities. It is typically made from lightweight and quick-drying fabric, allowing it to easily be worn over a wet swimsuit without becoming heavy or uncomfortable. Swim cover-ups come in a variety of styles and designs, ranging from simple and minimalist to more elaborate and ornate. The primary function of a swim cover-up is to provide modesty and coverage while still allowing the wearer to showcase their swimsuit underneath. It is often worn when transitioning from the water to a different location, such as going to a beachside café or walking around a resort. The design of a swim cover-up allows it to be easily slipped on and off over a swimsuit, providing a convenient and stylish option for beach or poolside activities.

Swim Jammers

Swim jammers refer to a specific style of swimwear that is commonly used by professional swimmers and individuals who engage in competitive swimming. This swimwear design is characterized by its form-fitting and sleek appearance, offering both comfort and performance during swimming activities. Swim jammers are typically made from a combination of Lycra, spandex, or other stretchable materials that easily conform to the body and provide a full range of motion. The fabric used in swim jammers is lightweight and quick-drying, ensuring that swimmers can move effortlessly through the water while still maintaining optimum hydrodynamics. The design of swim jammers focuses on reducing drag and resistance in the water, allowing swimmers to achieve faster lap times and improved performance. The tight fit of swim jammers helps to streamline the body by minimizing wrinkles and excess fabric that may create additional drag when swimming. The length of swim jammers typically extends from the waist to just above the knee, providing adequate coverage while still allowing free movement of the legs. Swim jammers are often preferred by professional swimmers due to their competitive advantages, as they provide better compression and support to the muscles, which can enhance performance and reduce muscle fatigue. The snug fit of swim jammers also aids in muscle recovery during and after training sessions. In terms of fashion, swim jammers are typically available in a variety of vibrant colors and patterns. While functionality remains the primary focus, swim jammers have evolved to incorporate stylish elements that cater to personal preferences and fashion trends. This allows swimmers to express their individuality and personal style while still benefiting from the functional aspects of swim jammers.

Swim Romper

A swim romper is a versatile one-piece garment designed for women to wear while swimming or engaging in other water activities. It combines the functionality of a swimsuit with the comfort and style of a romper, creating a unique and fashionable look. The swim romper typically features a one-piece construction with a fitted bodice and shorts or skirt bottom. It is made from swimwear fabric that is lightweight, stretchy, and quick-drying, allowing for ease of movement in the water. The fabric is also designed to withstand the harsh chemicals found in swimming pools and the damaging effects of sun exposure. One of the key features of a swim romper is its versatility. It can be worn not only as a swimsuit but also as a casual summer outfit. The design often includes adjustable straps, allowing for a customizable fit. Some swim rompers also feature built-in cups or padding for added support and shaping. The swim romper comes in a variety of styles and designs to suit different body types and personal preferences. It can be found in various lengths, from thigh-length shorts to knee-length skirts. The neckline may be V-neck, scoop-neck, halter, or off-shoulder, providing options for different levels of coverage and style. In terms of colors and patterns, the swim romper offers a wide range of choices. It can be found in solid colors such as black, white, or vibrant hues, as well as in bold prints and patterns such as stripes, florals, or tropical motifs. This allows women to express their personal style and make a fashion statement while enjoying outdoor activities. Overall, the swim romper is a fashionable and practical choice for women who want to look stylish and feel comfortable while swimming or participating in water-related activities. Its combination of swimwear functionality and romper style makes it a versatile addition to any summer wardrobe.

Swim Trunks

Swim trunks, also known as swimming shorts or boardshorts, are a type of garment designed specifically for swimming and other water-based activities. They are a popular choice for men and boys, offering both comfort and mobility in the water. Swim trunks are typically made from lightweight and quick-drying materials such as nylon or polyester. These fabrics are chosen for their ability to withstand constant exposure to water, as well as their durability and ease of maintenance. The use of synthetic fabrics also allows for a wide range of vibrant colors and unique patterns, enabling swim trunks to be a stylish and fashionable choice for beachgoers and swimmers. One distinguishing feature of swim trunks is their length. They typically extend from the waistline to above the knee, providing coverage without restricting movement. The loose and relaxed fit of swim trunks allows for easy leg movement in the water, making them a practical choice for swimming and various water sports. Swim trunks are designed with comfort in mind. They often feature an elasticized waistband with a drawstring, allowing for a secure and adjustable fit. The waistband ensures that the swim trunks stay in place during active water activities, preventing any potential wardrobe malfunctions. Another common feature of swim trunks is the presence of pockets. These pockets are often found on the sides or back of the garment and provide a convenient place to store small items such as keys or a wallet while swimming or lounging by the pool. In terms of style, swim trunks offer a wide variety of options. They can range from solid colors and simple designs to bold patterns and prints. Some swim trunks also incorporate logos or branding for added style and visibility. With the wide range of choices available, individuals can select swim trunks that reflect their personal taste and fashion preferences. In conclusion, swim trunks are a versatile and functional garment for swimming and water-based activities. They are designed with lightweight and quick-drying materials, feature a comfortable fit with an elasticized waistband, and often include pockets for added convenience. Swim trunks offer a wide selection of styles and designs, allowing individuals to express their personal style while enjoying their time in the water.

Tailor's Awl

A tailor's awl is a specialized tool used in fashion design to create precise markings and puncture holes in fabric. It is typically a small, handheld tool with a sharp, pointed tip and a handle. The tip of the awl is used to make small indentations or holes in the fabric, allowing for accurate placement of stitches, darts, or other design elements.

Tailor's Chalk

Tailor's chalk is a specialized tool used in fashion design to mark fabric before cutting and sewing. It is a soft, compressed chalk that is designed to easily transfer temporary markings onto various types of fabrics. Traditionally, tailor's chalk is made from a combination of powdered chalk and pigments, which are then compressed into a small, rectangular or triangular shape. It is commonly available in white, but can also be found in other colors such as blue, yellow, or red, allowing for greater visibility on different fabric colors.

Tailor's Clapper

A tailor's clapper is a traditional tool used in the field of fashion design. It is a rectangular piece of wood, usually made from hardwood, that is smooth and polished. The clapper is an essential tool for achieving crisp and well-defined seams and creases in garments. When used in conjunction with a steam iron, the tailor's clapper helps to set pleats, darts, and other details on the fabric. After applying steam from the iron onto the fabric, the clapper is placed over the area where the steam was applied, and then held firmly in place. The weight and pressure from the clapper helps to lock in the shape and set the seam or crease.

Tailor's Ham

A tailor's ham is a specialized tool used in the field of fashion design and tailoring. It is a compact, pillow-like object that is typically made of tightly stuffed fabric or sawdust, and it is used to help shape and press fabrics during the sewing process. The tailor's ham is an essential tool for fashion designers and dressmakers as it aids in achieving smooth and professional-looking garments. It is especially useful for shaping curved or rounded areas of clothing, such as darts, cuffs, collars, and sleeves. When working with fabrics, especially those that have more structure or are prone to wrinkling, the tailor's ham provides the necessary support and pressure to shape the fabric precisely. By using the ham, designers can mold the fabric to the desired shape and maintain control over the garment's overall structure and fit. To use a tailor's ham, the fabric is carefully placed over the rounded surface of the ham and pressed with a hot iron. The pressure and heat combined help to reshape the fabric and remove any wrinkles or creases. The tailor's ham is particularly effective for pressing curved seams or areas that are hard to reach with a regular ironing board or flat surface. In addition to shaping and pressing, the tailor's ham also serves as a valuable tool for preventing unwanted imprints or marks on delicate fabrics. By placing the fabric over the rounded surface of the ham, designers can avoid any direct contact with seams, hems, or other elements that may leave imprints on the fabric. Overall, the tailor's ham is an indispensable tool for fashion designers and tailors, enabling them to achieve precise shaping, professional finishing, and enhanced control over the fabric during the construction of garments. Its compact and versatile design makes it suitable for a wide range of clothing items and fabric types, ensuring that the final product meets the highest standards of quality and craftsmanship in the field of fashion design.

Tailor's Press Cloth

A tailor's press cloth is a piece of fabric that is used by fashion designers and tailors to protect delicate fabrics from damage during the pressing and steaming process. It acts as a barrier between the iron or steamer and the fabric, preventing direct contact that may result in unsightly marks or shine. Press cloths are typically made from lightweight, thin, and smooth materials such as muslin, silk organza, or cotton. These fabrics allow for heat and steam to pass through while providing a protective layer. The cloth is usually cut into a square or rectangular shape, although it can be customized to fit specific garment areas or curves.

Tailor's Press Mitt

The tailor's press mitt is an essential tool in the field of fashion design. It is a hand-held device that is used to press fabric and seams to create crisp and professional-looking finishes in garments. The press mitt is typically made of heat-resistant materials such as silicone, allowing it to withstand high temperatures without melting or deforming. When designing and constructing garments, it is crucial to ensure that each seam and edge is pressed properly. The press mitt provides a convenient and efficient way to achieve this. It is specifically shaped to fit the hand, allowing for easy and controlled manipulation of the fabric. The mitt is designed to be used in conjunction with an iron or steam press, enhancing the precision and effectiveness of the pressing process.

Tailor's Pressing Ham

A tailor's pressing ham is a specialized tool used in the field of fashion design. It is shaped like a ham and is typically made of tightly compacted sawdust or other heat-resistant materials, often covered in fabric. The purpose of the pressing ham is to provide a firm yet pliable surface for pressing and shaping fabrics during the construction of garments. This unique tool is used primarily for pressing curved areas of garments, such as darts, princess seams, and collars. The rounded shape of the pressing ham allows for better control and precision when pressing these curved areas. It helps to ensure that the fabric is evenly and properly pressed, resulting in a professional finish.

Tailor's Tacks

Tailor's tacks are temporary sewing marks used in fashion design to transfer pattern markings from pattern paper onto fabric. They are typically made by hand using contrasting thread and are easily removable once the garment is stitched together. Tailor's tacks serve multiple purposes in the construction of a garment. Firstly, they indicate specific points on the fabric where pattern markings such as darts, notches, pleats, or pockets should be placed. These markings are crucial for ensuring accurate and precise construction of the garment. To create tailor's tacks, a tailor or fashion designer threads a needle with a contrasting thread color and secures one end of the thread to the pattern paper. Then, the needle is inserted through the paper and fabric layers in the desired location, creating a loop of thread on top of the fabric. The needle is then reinserted through the same point, creating a double-ended tack. The two ends of the thread are then tied together to secure the tack in place. Tailor's tacks are often used instead of permanent markings because they can easily be removed without damaging the fabric or leaving any residual marks. Once the garment is stitched together, the tailor's tacks can be gently pulled out, leaving no trace behind. This ensures a clean and professional finish to the garment. In addition to their practical use, tailor's tacks can also aid in the fitting process. As the garment is constructed, the tailor or designer can use the tacks as reference points to ensure that the fabric is aligned correctly and that any shaping details are positioned accurately. This allows for adjustments to be made before final stitching, resulting in a better-fitting garment. Tailor's tacks are an essential tool in fashion design, allowing for precise and temporary markings on fabric. They provide both practical and aesthetic benefits, ensuring accurate construction and facilitating the fitting process. With their easy removal and versatility, tailor's tacks are a valuable technique used by fashion designers and tailors to create professional-quality garments.

Tambour Beads

Tambour beads refer to a specific type of decorative embellishments used in fashion design. These beads are typically applied to fabric using a tambour hook, a tool that allows for precise stitching and placement of beads onto the surface of the fabric. Tambour beads are often used to add texture, sparkle, and visual interest to garments, accessories, and other fashion items. They are commonly seen on evening gowns, wedding dresses, handbags, shoes, and jewelry. The intricate beadwork created with tambour beads can elevate the overall aesthetic of a design, making it more luxurious and elaborate.

Tambour Hooks

Tambour hooks are tools used in fashion design to create intricate and detailed embroidery and embellishments on fabrics. These hooks are specifically designed to be used with a tambour needle, which is a slender, pointed needle with a small hook at one end. The process of using tambour hooks involves creating a chain stitch on the fabric. The hook is inserted through the fabric from the backside, then caught on a thread or yarn on the front side. The hook is then pulled through the fabric, creating a loop. This loop is then secured by inserting the hook through it and pulling it tight. The process is repeated to create a continuous chain of stitches. Tambour hooks are commonly used in traditional embroidery techniques such as tambour beading and tambour lace. Tambour beading involves attaching beads and sequins to fabric using the chain stitch created with tambour hooks. Tambour lace, on the other hand, uses the hooks to create lacy, delicate designs on fabric. The design possibilities with tambour hooks are virtually endless. The hooks can be used to create intricate patterns, floral motifs, geometric designs, and more. They can be used on various types of fabrics, including silk, satin, velvet, and even delicate materials such as tulle and organza. When using tambour hooks, it is important to have a stable surface to work on, such as a tambour embroidery frame or a hoop. This helps to keep the fabric taut and prevents it from puckering or stretching while stitching. It is also helpful to have a tambour handle to hold the hook, as it provides better control and grip. Overall, tambour hooks are essential tools for fashion designers and embroiderers looking to add intricate and detailed embellishments to their creations. With their versatility and ability to create stunning designs, tambour hooks are a true asset in the world of fashion design.

Tank Swimsuit

A tank swimsuit, also known as a tankini, is a type of swimsuit that provides coverage and support while allowing for freedom of movement in the water. It is a versatile and fashionable option for women who prefer more modest swimwear or desire extra coverage for their midsection. The tank swimsuit typically consists of a fitted top with a higher neckline and wider shoulder straps, resembling a tank top. This design offers more coverage than traditional bikinis or one-piece swimsuits, making it a popular choice for those who want to feel comfortable and confident while swimming or engaging in water activities.

Tankini

A tankini is a type of swimsuit that combines the coverage and comfort of a tank top with the ease and functionality of a bikini. It is a popular choice for women who want a more modest swimsuit option without compromising on style or flexibility. The tankini typically consists of a tank top that extends to the waist or hips and a separate bottom piece, usually in the form of bikini bottoms. The tank top provides coverage for the midsection, making it a great option for those who want to hide any stomach imperfections or feel more comfortable and secure at the beach or poolside.

Tassel Makers

A tassel is a decorative element commonly used in fashion design, especially in clothing and accessories. It consists of a group of threads or cords that are gathered together at one end and secured with a knot or a decorative cap. Tassels can be made from various materials, such as silk, cotton, wool, or synthetic fibers, and they come in different shapes, sizes, and colors. Tassel makers are tools or devices specifically designed to create tassels. They are used by fashion designers, craftsmen, or hobbyists to efficiently produce tassels with consistent shape and length. Tassel makers typically consist of two parts – a base and a winding mechanism. The base of a tassel maker is a generally flat or rounded surface with a series of evenly spaced pins or hooks arranged in a specific pattern. These pins or hooks serve as anchor points for the threads or cords used to make the tassel. The pattern and spacing of the pins or hooks can vary depending on the desired tassel design or style. The winding mechanism of a tassel maker is used to wrap the threads or cords around the pins or hooks on the base. It usually consists of a central rod or spindle around which the threads are wound. This rod or spindle can be rotated manually or with the assistance of a mechanism, allowing for controlled winding and adjustment of the tassel length. To create a tassel using a tassel maker, the threads or cords are first secured to one of the anchor points on the base. The winding mechanism is then turned, causing the threads to wrap around the pins or hooks in a specific pattern. The tassel maker allows for easy adjustment of the thread tension, ensuring that the tassel is evenly wound and compact. Once the desired length is achieved, the threads are secured at the other end with a knot or by attaching a decorative cap. Tassel makers provide a convenient and efficient way to produce tassels in fashion design. They enable designers to create tassels of consistent quality and appearance, saving time and effort compared to manual tassel-making techniques. Tassel makers are versatile tools that can be used for various applications, from creating tassels on clothing and accessories to embellishing home decor items or crafting projects.

Tea-Length Dress

A tea-length dress is a type of dress that falls between the knee and the ankle. This dress style is typically characterized by its hemline which ends a few inches below the knee or calf. Tea-length dresses are commonly used for formal occasions such as weddings, cocktail parties, or evening events. The term "tea-length" originated in the 1950s and was inspired by the tea parties of that era, where women wore dresses that elegantly grazed their calves while sipping tea. The length of the dress was considered to be appropriate for such occasions as it provided a balance between formality and practicality. Tea-length dresses are known for their versatility and timeless elegance. They are often made from lightweight and flowing fabrics such as chiffon, silk, or tulle, which add to their graceful appearance. The silhouettes of tea-length dresses can vary, ranging from fitted styles to A-line or flared skirts, depending on the desired look. In terms of design elements, tea-length dresses can feature various necklines, including off-the-shoulder, sweetheart, or high necklines. They may also include details such as lace overlays, beading, or embroidery to enhance their aesthetic appeal. Additionally, tea-length dresses can be sleeveless, have short sleeves, or feature long sleeves for a more modest look. When styling a tea-length dress, it is common to pair it with heels or pumps to elongate the legs and maintain the dress's proportion. Accessories such as statement earrings, a clutch or handbag, and a delicate bracelet can complement the dress and elevate the overall ensemble. Overall, tea-length dresses continue to be a popular choice among fashion-savvy individuals due to their flattering length, timeless charm, and versatility for both formal and semi-formal occasions.

Textile Design

Textile Design is a specialized field within the realm of fashion design that encompasses the creation and manipulation of fabric patterns, motifs, and textures. It combines artistic creativity with technical expertise to produce unique and aesthetically pleasing cloth materials for use in various fashion applications. In the world of fashion design, textiles play a critical role as they are the base upon which garments and accessories are constructed. They not only determine the overall look and feel of a fashion piece but also impact its functionality and durability. Textile designers, therefore, hold the responsibility of developing innovative and original fabric designs that can enhance the appeal and value of the final product. Textile designers utilize a range of techniques to create their designs, including block printing, digital printing, screen printing, embroidery, and weaving. They often draw inspiration from diverse sources such as nature, architecture, historical eras, and cultural traditions. Through their designs, textile designers strive to convey a specific mood, theme, or concept, aligning their work with the overall creative vision of a fashion collection. To create a textile design, designers must possess a deep understanding of fabric construction, composition, and properties. They carefully consider factors such as fiber content, yarn type, weave structure, and finish to ensure that the fabric fulfills its intended purpose. Additionally, they must possess knowledge of color theory, as color selection is a crucial aspect of textile design. The harmonious combination of colors can significantly affect the visual impact of a fabric design. Once a textile design is finalized, it can be produced on a larger scale through industrial manufacturing processes or crafted individually by hand. Textile designers collaborate closely with manufacturers, ensuring that the production processes faithfully capture the essence and intricacies of their designs. They may also experiment with various printing techniques, dyes, and embellishments to add further dimension and interest to their fabric creations. Ultimately, textile design is a dynamic and evolving art form that continues to push the boundaries of fashion design. By fusing aesthetics with technical expertise, textile designers contribute to the creation of innovative and captivating fabric designs that enrich the world of fashion.

Textile Designer

A textile designer in the context of fashion design is an individual who combines creative and technical skills to create original fabric designs for garments, accessories, and other textile products. These designers typically draw inspiration from various sources such as nature, art, culture, and current trends, blending different elements together to develop unique and visually appealing patterns, prints, and motifs.

Textile Mill

A textile mill is a facility that specializes in the production and processing of textiles, which are materials made from fibers that can be woven, knitted, or otherwise manipulated to create fabrics. Textiles are an essential component of fashion design, as they form the foundation of garments and other fashion products. Within a textile mill, various stages of textile manufacturing take place, including spinning, weaving, dyeing, and finishing. Spinning refers to the process of transforming raw fibers, such as cotton or wool, into yarns that can be further processed. Weaving involves interlacing these yarns to create stable and durable fabrics, while dyeing adds color to the fabrics, enhancing their aesthetic appeal. Lastly, finishing encompasses several treatments that improve the overall quality and characteristics of the textile, such as softening, wrinkle resistance, or water repellency. In the context of fashion design, textile mills are crucial for providing designers with a vast array of fabric options. These mills can produce textiles in different colors, patterns, and textures, allowing designers to incorporate their creative vision into their collections. Additionally, textile mills play a vital role in the production of sustainable and eco-friendly fabrics, which are increasingly sought after within the fashion industry. Textile mills are often equipped with advanced machinery and technology that enable efficient and large-scale production. This machinery includes various types of looms, dyeing and printing machines, and finishing equipment. Skilled workers, such as textile engineers and technicians, operate these machines to ensure the quality and consistency of the produced textiles. Overall, textile mills are essential entities in the fashion design industry, as they provide designers with a wide range of textile options and facilitate the production of high-quality fabrics. Through their expertise and advanced technology, these mills contribute to the innovation and development of new textiles, which constantly push the boundaries of fashion design.

Thimble Guards

Thimble guards are small protective devices used in the field of fashion design to prevent injury and enhance precision during the sewing process. These guards are typically made of durable materials, such as metal or plastic, and are designed to fit snugly over the fingertip of the user. Thimble guards serve as a barrier between the needle and the designer's finger, acting as a shield against accidental punctures or cuts. They are especially useful when working with delicate or intricate fabrics that require careful handling and attention to detail. By wearing a thimble guard, fashion designers can maintain control over the needle while reducing the risk of injury. In addition to their protective function, thimble guards also enhance precision and improve the overall sewing experience. Their design allows for a greater degree of dexterity, enabling designers to maneuver the fabric and needle with increased accuracy. This is particularly beneficial when executing intricate stitches or working on intricate embellishments. Thimble guards come in various sizes and shapes to accommodate different finger sizes and sewing techniques. Some are adjustable and can be fitted to match the specific needs of the designer. They may also feature textured surfaces or grippy materials to enhance grip and prevent slippage during sewing. While primarily used in fashion design, thimble guards can also be helpful in other sewing applications, such as quilting, embroidery, and tailoring. Their versatility and practicality make them a valuable tool for any sewing enthusiast or professional.

Thimble Pads

A thimble pad is a small, round, finger-like accessory used in fashion design to protect the fingertips during the process of hand sewing and embroidery. It is typically made out of soft, flexible materials such as leather or silicone. Thimble pads serve as a substitute for traditional thimbles, which are typically made of metal or hard plastic and can be uncomfortable for some fashion designers to use. Thimble pads are designed to fit over the fingertip, providing a cushioned surface that allows the needle to go through the fabric smoothly without causing discomfort or pain.

Thimble Pincushions

A thimble pincushion is a small, functional accessory used in the field of fashion design. It is a specialized tool that combines the functionality of a thimble and a pincushion into a single item. The primary purpose of a thimble pincushion is to provide convenience and efficiency during the process of garment construction and sewing. It is designed to be worn on the finger like a regular thimble, protecting the finger from the sharp points of sewing needles while also serving as a storage space for pins and needles. Thimble pincushions are commonly made from a variety of materials such as metal, plastic, or fabric. The exterior material is often chosen based on its durability and ability to hold the pins and needles securely. The interior is filled with a soft, cushion-like material that allows the pins to be inserted easily and provides a stable surface for pinning fabrics. The compact size of thimble pincushions makes them easy to carry and store, making them an essential tool for fashion designers who need to have their sewing supplies readily available at all times. They can be easily slipped onto the finger when needed, allowing for quick and efficient pinning and sewing without the need to constantly reach for a separate pincushion. In fashion design, accuracy and precision are vital, and thimble pincushions aid in achieving these qualities. By having the pins and needles conveniently accessible on the finger, designers can work more efficiently, increasing productivity and minimizing the chance of misplaced or lost pins. Overall, thimble pincushions are a practical and essential tool for fashion designers. They provide the dual function of protecting the finger and providing a secure storage space for pins and needles, ultimately enhancing the sewing experience and improving the quality of garment construction.

Thimbles

A thimble, in the context of fashion design, is a small protective device that is worn on the finger while sewing or manipulating fabrics. It is typically made of metal, although there are also thimbles made of other materials such as plastic or leather. The primary purpose of a thimble in fashion design is to protect the finger from the sharp needle when sewing by hand. By wearing a thimble, the designer or seamstress can push the needle through the fabric without worrying about pricking their finger. This not only prevents injuries but also allows for greater control and precision when creating intricate stitches.

Thought Leadership In Fashion

Thought leadership in fashion design refers to the ability of a designer to consistently generate innovative and original ideas that shape and influence the industry. It is a demonstration of deep expertise, unique insights, and a forward-thinking approach that sets a designer apart from others in the field. Thought leaders in fashion design not only create beautiful and aesthetically pleasing garments, but also challenge existing norms, push boundaries, and inspire others by their vision and creativity. A thought leader in fashion design often uses research, experimentation, and exploration to develop new concepts and techniques. They employ their knowledge of trends, cultural influences, and consumer behavior to anticipate and respond to evolving needs and desires of their target audience. They are not limited by existing design conventions or current trends, but rather lead the way by introducing fresh ideas, unconventional aesthetics, and innovative materials. Thought leaders in fashion design often take risks, going beyond what is expected or ordinary. They challenge conventional notions of functionality, silhouette, and form, striving to create designs that provoke thought and evoke emotions. Their work has the power to start conversations, spark trends, and redefine the boundaries of what is considered stylish and fashionable. In addition to their creative skills, thought leaders in fashion design possess excellent communication abilities. They are able to articulate their ideas and concepts effectively, bridging the gap between their inspirations and the real world. They have the ability to create narratives around their collections, enabling consumers to connect with the story and vision behind the garments. Thought leadership in fashion design requires constant self-reflection and a commitment to lifelong learning. It is a process of continuously seeking inspiration, staying informed about industry developments, and staying open to new ideas and perspectives. It involves understanding the historical context of fashion, appreciating cultural diversity, and recognizing the influence of social, political, and environmental factors on design. Overall, thought leadership in fashion design goes beyond mere creativity and skills. It encompasses the ability to inspire, innovate, and shape the industry, while also having a deep understanding of the broader social and cultural context in which fashion operates.

Thread Clippers

Thread clippers, in the context of fashion design, refer to specialized tools used for cutting and trimming threads in garments and other textile products. They are an essential tool for designers and seamstresses, aiding in the creation of clean and professional finishes. Thread clippers are typically small, handheld scissors with very sharp and pointed blades. They are specifically designed for cutting threads close to the fabric without damaging the surrounding material. The blades are usually made from stainless steel or high-quality metal to ensure durability and precision. Some thread clippers may also have serrated edges for better grip and control while cutting. The primary purpose of thread clippers is to remove excess threads or loose ends after sewing or stitching. This includes trimming loose thread ends, removing basting stitches, cutting off seam allowances, and snipping small areas for precise details. Unlike regular scissors, thread clippers have a finer and narrower blade profile, enabling users to reach tight and intricate spaces, such as corners, curves, or delicate embellishments. Thread clippers are especially useful in garment construction, where multiple threads are used during the sewing process. They help in achieving a clean and professional finish by ensuring that no loose threads are left hanging. This attention to detail is crucial, as even minor imperfections can affect the overall quality and aesthetics of a garment. Moreover, thread clippers are also employed in the process of altering or repairing clothing. They aid in removing unwanted stitches or altering the length of hems, waistbands, or other garment components. By using thread clippers, designers and seamstresses can achieve precise and seamless alterations, maintaining the integrity and structure of the original garment. Overall, thread clippers are indispensable tools in the fashion design industry. Their ability to trim threads with precision and ease makes them a valuable asset during the garment construction and alteration processes. By ensuring clean finishes and meticulous attention to detail, thread clippers contribute to the overall quality and aesthetic appeal of fashion products.

Thread Cone Holders

Thread cone holders are essential tools used in the field of fashion design. These holders are specifically designed for organizing and storing thread cones, which are commonly used in sewing and embroidery projects. Thread cones, also known as thread spools, are large and cone-shaped cylinders that hold various types of threads used in garment construction and decorative stitching. These threads are typically thicker and more durable than regular sewing threads, making them suitable for heavy-duty stitching, decorative topstitching, and embellishments. Thread cone holders are specially designed to accommodate these larger cones and keep them organized and accessible during the design process.

Thread Holder Stands

A thread holder stand in the context of fashion design refers to a device or tool used to hold and organize thread spools during the process of garment construction or sewing. It is an essential accessory for fashion designers, seamstresses, and tailors as it provides convenience and efficiency in handling threads. The primary purpose of a thread holder stand is to keep the thread spools easily accessible and tangle-free. It typically features a vertical post or rod with multiple arms or prongs where the thread spools can be placed. The arms or prongs can be adjusted or rotated to accommodate different sizes of spools and allow for easy thread retrieval.

Thread Lint Brushes

Thread lint brushes are essential tools used in fashion design to remove lint and loose thread fibers from garments. These brushes are specifically designed to effectively and efficiently clean fabric surfaces, ensuring a neat and polished finish to the final product.Thread lint brushes typically consist of a handle and a brush head made of soft bristles. The bristles are typically made of materials like horsehair or synthetic fibers, chosen for their ability to attract and trap lint and fibers without damaging the fabric. The brush head may vary in size and shape, allowing for precise and versatile cleaning on different types of fabrics and garment areas.

Thread Lubricants

A thread lubricant in the context of fashion design is a substance used to reduce friction and improve the performance of the sewing process. It is applied to the thread before it is used in the sewing machine or by hand to ensure smoother and more efficient stitching. Thread lubricants are commonly used in fashion design to prevent static electricity buildup, reduce thread breakage, and improve stitch quality. By reducing friction, these lubricants make it easier for the thread to move through the fabric, resulting in neater and more consistent stitches.

Thread Nets

Thread nets are a crucial element in the realm of fashion design. They are slender, net-like structures made from fine threads that serve multiple purposes in garment construction. First and foremost, thread nets are used to protect delicate and lightweight fabrics from being damaged during the sewing process. When sewing with delicate fabrics such as silk, chiffon, or lace, the fabric can easily get caught in the feed dogs or presser foot of the sewing machine, causing snags or puckering. By placing a thread net over the fabric, it acts as a barrier, preventing direct contact between the fabric and the sewing machine's mechanisms. This ensures that the delicate fabric remains unharmed and maintains its smooth and flawless appearance. Additionally, thread nets are utilized in fashion design to control the movement of loose threads throughout a garment. Loose threads can be unappealing and can potentially unravel or snag on objects, compromising the integrity of the garment. By securing these loose threads with a thread net, they are neatly tucked away, preventing any unwanted visible threads and ensuring the longevity of the garment. Moreover, thread nets are employed to provide support and shape to specific areas of a garment. In intricate or tailored designs, certain areas may require additional reinforcement to maintain their structure and silhouette. By strategically placing thread nets in these areas, such as neckline edges, hems, or cuffs, they act as invisible support, enhancing the overall appearance and drape of the garment. In summary, thread nets are indispensable tools in the fashion design industry. They safeguard delicate fabrics during the sewing process, control loose threads, and provide support and shape to various areas of a garment. Fashion designers rely on thread nets to ensure the quality and durability of their creations, as well as maintain the aesthetic appeal of the final garment.

Thread Nippers

A thread nipper is a small, essential tool in fashion design that is used to trim and remove excess threads from fabric and clothing. It is specifically designed to easily cut threads close to the surface of the material without causing any damage. Thread nippers are typically lightweight and compact, allowing for easy maneuverability and precision. They are commonly made with sharp, stainless steel blades that are strong enough to easily cut through various types of threads, but small and delicate enough to avoid cutting the fabric itself. The blades are usually curved or angled, which helps to ensure a clean and smooth cut.

Thread Organizers

Thread organizers in the context of fashion design are tools or accessories that are used to neatly and efficiently store and arrange various types of threads. These organizers help designers and artisans keep their threads organized, preventing them from tangling or becoming disorganized during the design process or while working on sewing projects. The main purpose of thread organizers is to provide a systematic and easily accessible way to store different colors and types of threads. This allows designers to quickly find the specific thread they need for their project, saving time and reducing frustration. By having a well-organized thread collection, fashion designers can work more efficiently and focus on their creative process.

Thread Racks

Thread racks in the context of fashion design are tools used for organizing and storing sewing threads. They are designed to hold spools of threads in a way that allows easy access and visibility of the different colors and types of threads. Thread racks typically consist of a wooden or plastic frame with multiple rows and columns of pegs or hooks. The spools of thread are placed on these pegs, with each peg being able to accommodate one spool. The racks come in various sizes, ranging from small ones that can hold a few dozen spools to larger ones that can hold hundreds of spools.

Thread Snips

Thread Snips are essential tools used in fashion design to cut and trim threads during the garment construction process.They are small handheld cutting tools, typically made of stainless steel, that have sharp blades designed specifically for cutting threads. Thread snips are commonly used to remove excess thread, basting stitches, or loose threads from the fabric.Thread snips have a compact size and a comfortable grip, making them easy to maneuver and control. They have pointed and narrow blades, allowing fashion designers to make precise cuts without damaging the fabric or the surrounding stitches.Thread snips are particularly useful when working with delicate fabrics or intricate designs, as they enable designers to carefully remove unwanted threads without disturbing the rest of the garment. They can also be used to trim thread tails after sewing seams or attaching buttons.In addition to their functionality, thread snips are often designed to be aesthetically pleasing, with various colors and decorative handles available in the market. This makes them not only practical but also visually appealing for fashion designers.Overall, thread snips are indispensable tools in fashion design, offering precision and convenience in cutting and trimming threads. Their compact size and sharp blades make them an essential accessory for every fashion designer's toolbox, ensuring clean and professional finishes in garment construction.

Thread Spool Racks

A thread spool rack, in the context of fashion design, is a device used to organize and store spools of thread. It consists of a vertical or horizontal rack with multiple pegs or slots where thread spools can be placed. Thread spool racks are commonly used in fashion design studios or sewing rooms to ensure easy access and efficient storage of thread. They are particularly useful for fashion designers who work with a variety of colors and types of thread.

Thread Stands

A thread stand is a functional accessory used in fashion design and sewing. It is a device or structure designed to hold and organize spools of thread during the sewing process. Thread stands come in various forms and sizes, but their primary purpose is to enhance the efficiency and organization of the sewing process. Thread stands are typically made of durable materials such as metal or plastic. They can be freestanding structures or attached to a sewing machine, depending on the specific design. The main function of a thread stand is to provide a convenient and accessible location for the spools of thread that are essential in garment construction.

Tiered Dress

A tiered dress is a type of dress that features horizontal layers or tiers of fabric that create a cascading effect. These tiers are usually sewn onto a fitted bodice or waistband, creating a voluminous and structured silhouette. Tiered dresses can have a variety of designs and lengths, ranging from mini to maxi length. One of the key characteristics of a tiered dress is the use of different fabrics or textures for each layer or tier. This creates visual interest and adds dimension to the dress. Common fabrics used for tiered dresses include chiffon, organza, tulle, and lace. The choice of fabric can greatly affect the overall look and feel of the dress; sheer and lightweight fabrics create a dreamy and ethereal effect, while heavier fabrics can give the dress a more dramatic and formal appearance. Tiered dresses are versatile and can be worn for various occasions, from casual events to formal affairs. They are often popular choices for weddings, proms, and evening parties. The tiered design adds a touch of elegance and sophistication to the dress, making it a chic option for those who want to make a fashion statement. Styling a tiered dress can be done in different ways depending on the desired look. For a romantic and feminine look, pairing the dress with delicate jewelry, soft curls, and strappy heels can enhance its overall charm. On the other hand, for a more edgy and modern look, combining the dress with bold accessories, sleek hair, and statement shoes can create a unique and contemporary ensemble. In conclusion, a tiered dress is a fashionable garment that features horizontal layers or tiers of fabric, creating a cascading effect. With its variation in fabrics and versatile styling options, it is a popular choice for both casual and formal events.

Tiered Skirt

A tiered skirt is a type of skirt that is characterized by multiple layers or tiers of fabric that are stacked on top of each other. The layers or tiers are typically gathered at the waistband and create a voluminous and layered silhouette. The number of tiers can vary, ranging from two to several, and each tier is generally wider than the one above it, giving the skirt a cascading effect. Tiered skirts have been a popular fashion choice throughout history and have been seen in various styles and lengths. They can be found in both formal and casual wear, and their design can be adapted to suit different fashion preferences.

Tracing Film

Tracing film, in the context of fashion design, refers to a transparent sheet made of thin plastic or acetate material that allows fashion designers to create and refine their designs with ease and precision. It is commonly used as a tool for sketching, tracing, and modifying clothing patterns and garment details. The primary purpose of tracing film in fashion design is to facilitate the process of translating design concepts from ideation to final execution. Fashion designers often start by sketching their ideas on paper or using digital software. Once they have a rough idea of what they want to create, they use the tracing film to refine and tweak their designs. The transparent nature of the film allows them to overlay it on top of their existing sketches or templates, enabling them to make adjustments without losing the original concept. Tracing film has several advantages for fashion designers. Firstly, it enables them to experiment with different variations and iterations of their designs without starting from scratch each time. They can easily duplicate and modify existing patterns or details, making it an efficient tool for pattern-making and sample development. Additionally, the transparency of the film allows designers to see how different layers and elements of the garment interact with each other, aiding in the visualization and planning process. Another benefit of using tracing film is its durability. Unlike paper, it is resistant to tearing or wrinkling, providing designers with a long-lasting and reliable medium for their creative process. It also allows for easy erasing and correction, as marks made on the film can be easily wiped off with an eraser or cloth. This flexibility and ease of use make tracing film a valuable tool not only during the design phase but also in the communication of ideas between designers, pattern-makers, and manufacturers. In conclusion, tracing film plays a crucial role in the fashion design process as a versatile and durable tool for sketching, tracing, and refining garment details. Its transparency allows for easy overlaying and modification of designs, while its durability ensures longevity during the creative process. By enabling designers to experiment and visualize their ideas effectively, tracing film contributes to the overall efficiency and success of fashion design projects.

Tracing Wheels

Tracing wheels are commonly used tools in the field of fashion design. These small, handheld devices consist of a wheel with sharp teeth or pins that are designed to transfer markings onto fabric or paper. In fashion design, tracing wheels are primarily used during the pattern-making process. Pattern-making involves creating the blueprint or template for a garment, which will then be used to cut and sew the fabric. Tracing wheels play a crucial role in this process by allowing designers to transfer markings from existing patterns or templates onto a new piece of fabric. To use a tracing wheel, a designer would place the template or pattern on top of the fabric, ensuring that the markings align. The tracing wheel is then rolled along the edge of the template, causing the pins or teeth of the wheel to perforate the fabric and leave behind a series of indentations. These indentations serve as a guide for cutting and sewing the fabric, ensuring accuracy and precision in the final garment. There are different types of tracing wheels available, each with its own unique purpose. For example, some tracing wheels have pins that are closer together, creating fine, precise markings. These are commonly used for intricate or delicate designs. On the other hand, tracing wheels with widely spaced pins are ideal for creating bolder markings or for use on thicker fabrics. Tracing wheels are versatile tools that can be used on a variety of fabrics, including woven, knit, and even leather. They are particularly useful for transferring markings such as dart placements, seam lines, or pattern notches. By using a tracing wheel, designers can ensure consistency and accuracy in their patterns, resulting in garments that fit well and have professional finishes. In conclusion, tracing wheels are essential tools in the fashion design process. They enable designers to transfer markings from templates or patterns onto fabric, aiding in the creation of precise and accurate garments. With their versatility and ease of use, tracing wheels are a valuable asset to fashion designers, helping them bring their creative visions to life.

Track Pants

Track pants, also known as joggers or sweatpants, are a type of casual bottoms that are commonly worn for athletic or leisure activities. They are characterized by their loose and relaxed fit, elastic waistband, and sometimes tapered legs. Track pants were originally designed for athletes and were primarily used for track and field events or other sports activities. However, they have since evolved into a popular fashion trend and are now commonly seen as everyday clothing. The design of track pants typically includes lightweight and breathable materials such as cotton, polyester, or a blend of both. This allows for comfortable movement and reduces the risk of overheating during physical activities. The elastic waistband and drawstrings provide a secure and adjustable fit, ensuring that the pants stay in place even during rigorous exercise. Some track pants may also feature zippered or elasticated ankle cuffs, allowing for further customization and ease of wear.

Treggings

Treggings are a garment that combines the fit and silhouette of trousers with the comfort and stretch of leggings. They are a popular fashion choice for women, providing both style and practicality. Treggings typically have a similar design to skinny trousers, with a fitted waist, hips, and legs. They are often made from stretchy materials such as spandex or elastane, which allows for movement and flexibility. This stretchy fabric also provides a smooth and comfortable fit, similar to that of leggings. One of the key features of treggings is their versatility. They can be dressed up or down, making them suitable for a range of occasions. They can be worn with a tailored blouse and blazer for a professional look, or paired with a casual t-shirt and sneakers for a more relaxed outfit. Treggings are often chosen as an alternative to jeans or trousers, as they offer a more flexible and comfortable option. In terms of design, treggings can vary in length and detailing. Some may have ankle zippers or decorative stitching, while others may have a plain and simple design. They are commonly available in neutral colors such as black, navy, or gray, which allows for ease of pairing with other garments. When it comes to styling treggings, the most important aspect is to ensure a proper fit. They should be snug but not overly tight, as this will ensure comfort and a flattering silhouette. Treggings can be worn with both longline tops or tucked-in blouses, depending on personal preference and the desired look. In conclusion, treggings are a fashion-forward choice for women, combining the structure of trousers with the comfort of leggings. They offer versatility in styling and can be easily dressed up or down for any occasion. With their stretchy fabric and sleek design, treggings provide a fashionable and practical alternative to traditional trousers.

Trench Coat

A trench coat is a classic and timeless outerwear garment that originated from military attire and has become a staple in modern fashion design. It is characterized by its long length, typically reaching the wearer's knees, and its double-breasted front closure, featuring buttons or sometimes a belt. Trench coats are known for their versatility and ability to be worn in various weather conditions. They are typically made from a durable and water-resistant fabric, such as cotton gabardine or leather, which helps protect the wearer from rain and wind.

Trend Analysis

Trend analysis in the context of fashion design refers to the process of studying and predicting the aesthetic and design preferences that are likely to gain popularity in the industry. It involves analyzing current and past fashion trends, consumer behavior, cultural shifts, and market demands in order to anticipate future trends. Fashion designers use trend analysis as a valuable tool to stay informed and relevant in an ever-evolving industry. By monitoring and analyzing various sources of inspiration such as runway shows, street style, social media, and celebrity fashion, designers can identify emerging patterns, silhouettes, colors, and materials that are likely to be embraced by consumers.

Triathlon Suit

A triathlon suit, in the context of fashion design, is a specialized piece of clothing designed to optimize performance and comfort for athletes participating in triathlon events. It is a versatile and functional garment that combines the features of a swimsuit, cycling shorts, and a running singlet into a single, streamlined outfit. The primary purpose of a triathlon suit is to enhance the athlete's performance by reducing drag in the water, providing padding and support during the cycling portion, and offering freedom of movement during the running segment. To achieve this, the suit is constructed using technologically advanced fabrics and ergonomic design principles.

Triathlon Wetsuit

A triathlon wetsuit, in the context of fashion design, is a specialized garment specifically designed for athletes participating in triathlon events. It is made from a combination of neoprene and other technical materials to provide the wearer with optimal performance and comfort during swimming, cycling, and running. The primary purpose of a triathlon wetsuit is to enhance the athlete's hydrodynamics in the water. The thickness and buoyancy of the neoprene help to improve the swimmer's body position and reduce drag, allowing them to swim faster and more efficiently. The wetsuit also provides thermal insulation, keeping the athlete warm in cold water conditions. Furthermore, the design of a triathlon wetsuit takes into account the unique movements and needs of triathletes. The wetsuit features strategically placed panels and seams to allow for unrestricted arm and shoulder movement, enabling swimmers to achieve a more natural stroke. It also has a flexible and stretchable construction that allows for ease of movement during the cycling and running portions of the race. In addition to the functional aspects, the aesthetic design of a triathlon wetsuit also plays a role. It often incorporates bold colors, vibrant patterns, and sleek lines to create a visually appealing garment that reflects the energy and spirit of the triathlon sport. The use of contrasting colors and reflective elements may also enhance the visibility of the athletes in open water or low-light conditions. Overall, a triathlon wetsuit is a specialized fashion garment that combines performance, comfort, and style. It is designed to improve the athlete's hydrodynamics, provide thermal insulation, and allow for unrestricted movement during the different disciplines of a triathlon event. Its functional and aesthetic features make it a key piece of clothing for triathletes who strive for both speed and style.

Trousers

Trousers, also known as pants, are a popular and essential garment in the field of fashion design. They are designed to cover the lower body from the waist to the ankles, providing comfort, style, and functionality for both men and women. Trousers are typically made from various fabrics, including denim, cotton, wool, and synthetic materials. Their construction involves a waistband that sits around the waist, a fly at the front (for men's trousers), and two individual leg portions that extend down to the ankles. These leg portions are typically tailored with seams to provide shape and fit.

Trumpet Dress

A trumpet dress is a type of formal dress that is characterized by its flared skirt that resembles the shape of a trumpet or a mermaid tail. This dress style is a popular choice for formal occasions, such as weddings, proms, and red carpet events, as it creates an elegant and glamorous look. The defining feature of a trumpet dress is its fitted bodice, which hugs the body's curves and accentuates the waist, while gradually flaring out from the mid-thigh or knee. This design creates a flattering silhouette that elongates the figure and enhances the natural feminine shape. The flared skirt of the trumpet dress can vary in volume, with some styles featuring a more subtle flaring and others having a more dramatic, exaggerated trumpet shape.

Trunks

A trunks in fashion design refers to a type of garment that is typically worn as swimwear or underwear. It is characterized by its loose-fitting and comfortable nature, providing coverage and freedom of movement to the wearer. Trunks are commonly worn by both men and boys, and are available in a range of styles, fabrics, and patterns to suit different preferences and occasions. The design of trunks usually features a short length that extends to the upper thigh or just above the knee. This length allows for ease of movement and flexibility, making trunks a popular choice for activities such as swimming, sports, and lounging by the pool or beach. The loose fit of trunks provides a relaxed and casual aesthetic, making them suitable for casual outings and everyday wear as well. Trunks are typically crafted from lightweight and quick-drying fabrics such as polyester or nylon, ensuring comfort and practicality in water-based activities. They often feature an elasticated waistband with a drawstring or a hook-and-loop closure for easy adjustability and secure fit. Some trunks may also include a mesh lining for added support and breathability. Trunks come in a variety of styles and design details to cater to different fashion preferences. These can include various prints, patterns, and colors, ranging from solid shades to vibrant and bold designs. Some trunks may feature branding or logos on the waistband or leg, adding a touch of branding or designer flair. When it comes to styling, trunks are versatile and can be paired with a range of tops depending on the occasion. For swimming or beachwear, trunks are typically worn as the main garment, often paired with a simple t-shirt or tank top. In a more casual setting, trunks can be styled with a relaxed button-down shirt or a polo shirt for a laid-back yet put-together ensemble. In conclusion, trunks in fashion design are loose-fitting and comfortable garments primarily worn as swimwear or underwear. They are available in various styles, fabrics, and patterns, and are suitable for a variety of activities and occasions. Trunks offer a combination of functionality, comfort, and style, making them a staple in many men's and boys' wardrobes.

Tube Top

A tube top is a type of garment that is commonly worn by women and is characterized by its strapless design. It is typically made of a stretchy fabric that hugs the bust and torso, providing a snug fit. The tube top derives its name from its cylindrical shape, resembling a tube that covers the upper body. Tube tops are versatile and can be worn in various styles and settings. They are popular in warm weather or beach destinations due to their lightweight and breathable nature. The strapless design exposes the shoulders and arms, making it perfect for showcasing sun-kissed skin. Tube tops are often favored by individuals who desire a fashionable and trendy look.

Tulip Skirt

A tulip skirt is a type of skirt that is characterized by its shape, which resembles the petals of a tulip flower. It is a popular design in the world of fashion, particularly in women's clothing. The tulip skirt is known for its unique silhouette, featuring a fitted waistband and a flared shape that tapers in at the hem. This creates a flattering and feminine look that enhances the curves of the wearer's body. The skirt is typically made from a soft and lightweight fabric such as silk, cotton, or a blend of the two, which lends itself well to the flowy and draped design.

Tunic Blouse

A tunic blouse is a versatile and stylish garment that combines the length and fit of a tunic with the aesthetic and detailing of a blouse. This fashion design is characterized by its loose and flowy silhouette, typically reaching mid-thigh to knee length, and features details such as collars, cuffs, buttons, and different types of necklines. Tunic blouses are designed to be worn by women and can be easily incorporated into various outfits and styles, making them a popular choice among fashion-conscious individuals. They are often made from lightweight and breathable fabrics such as cotton, linen, chiffon, or silk, ensuring comfort and ease of movement.

Tunic Dress

A tunic dress is a type of garment that combines the features of a tunic and a dress, commonly worn by women. It is designed to be a loose-fitting and easy to wear piece, making it suitable for various occasions. The tunic dress typically has a relaxed and flowing silhouette, with a length that falls above or at the knee. It often features loose or bell-shaped sleeves, adding to its comfortable and effortless style. The neckline of a tunic dress can vary, ranging from scoop necks to V-necks, and even high necks for a more modest look.

Tunic Shirt

A tunic shirt is a type of loose-fitting clothing garment that falls just above or below the hip line. It is characterized by its long length, reaching at least to the mid-thigh or extending down to the knees. The design of a tunic shirt is inspired by traditional garments worn in various cultural contexts, such as the tunics worn in ancient Greece and Rome, as well as traditional garments in Asian cultures. Tunic shirts are commonly made from lightweight fabrics such as cotton, linen, silk, or rayon, which allow for ease of movement and breathability. The loose fit of the tunic shirt gives it a relaxed and comfortable feel, making it a versatile piece of clothing that can be worn in both casual and formal settings. The neckline of a tunic shirt can vary, ranging from a simple round neck to a V-neck or a boat neckline. Some tunic shirts may also feature collar designs, such as a mandarin collar or a shirt collar, adding a touch of sophistication to the garment. In terms of sleeve length, tunic shirts can have short sleeves, long sleeves, or even three-quarter sleeves, offering options for different seasons and personal preferences. Tunic shirts are known for their versatility and can be styled in various ways to create different looks. They can be paired with leggings, skinny jeans, or trousers for a casual and comfortable outfit. Tunic shirts can also be dressed up by pairing them with tailored pants or skirts, accessorized with statement jewelry, and worn with heels or dressy flats. In recent years, tunic shirts have gained popularity in the fashion industry due to their ability to flatter different body shapes and sizes. The loose and flowy silhouette of the tunic shirt provides a forgiving fit that can camouflage areas of the body that one may want to conceal. Additionally, the longer length of the tunic shirt can create a flattering elongating effect, making it a popular choice for individuals seeking a stylish and comfortable option.

Tunic Top

A tunic top is a loose-fitting garment that typically falls to the hips or mid-thighs. It is designed with a relaxed and flowing silhouette, allowing for comfortable movement and an effortlessly stylish look. Tunic tops can be made from a variety of fabrics, including cotton, silk, chiffon, and linen, offering versatility in terms of style and occasion. Tunic tops are characterized by their longer length compared to regular tops or blouses. They often feature a V-neck or round neckline, providing a flattering neckline that elongates the upper body. Tunic tops may also have different sleeve lengths, ranging from long sleeves to short sleeves or even sleeveless options for warmer weather. The loose fit of a tunic top makes it an ideal choice for all body types. It skims over curves and emphasizes the natural shape of the body without clinging to it. This makes tunic tops a popular choice for both casual and formal occasions, as they can easily be dressed up or down depending on the accessories and bottoms paired with them. Tunic tops can be worn with a variety of bottoms, such as jeans, leggings, or skirts, allowing for endless styling possibilities. They can be effortlessly dressed up with the addition of statement jewelry, heels, or a tailored blazer, making them suitable for more formal events. On the other hand, tunic tops can also be styled in a more casual way with flats, sandals, or sneakers for a relaxed and comfortable outfit. In terms of patterns and designs, tunic tops offer a wide range of options. They can be solid-colored, making them a versatile wardrobe staple that can easily be mixed and matched with other garments. Tunic tops can also feature various prints, such as florals, stripes, or abstract designs, adding visual interest and personality to an outfit. Overall, a tunic top is a chic and versatile garment that provides both comfort and style. Whether for a casual outing or a formal event, a tunic top offers endless possibilities for creating fashionable outfits that suit various body types and personal preferences.

Tunic Turtleneck

A tunic turtleneck is a type of garment that combines the features of a tunic and a turtleneck. It is designed to be a versatile and fashionable piece of clothing that can be worn in various settings and styled in different ways. The tunic turtleneck typically has a longer length than a traditional turtleneck and falls below the hips, resembling a tunic. This longer length adds to its versatility as it can be worn as a dress, paired with leggings or trousers, or even layered over other garments. The tunic turtleneck is often made from soft, comfortable fabrics such as knit or jersey, providing a cozy yet stylish option for colder seasons.

Turtleneck Sweater

A turtleneck sweater is a stylish and versatile garment in the realm of fashion design. It is characterized by its high, close-fitting collar that extends up to cover and protect the neck. The collar is typically ribbed or folded, adding an extra layer of texture and detail to the overall design of the sweater. Turtleneck sweaters are crafted using various materials, including but not limited to wool, cotton, cashmere, or synthetic blends. These different fabrics offer different levels of warmth, comfort, and breathability, allowing individuals to choose a turtleneck sweater that best suits their needs and preferences.

Tuxedo Dress

A tuxedo dress is a formal garment designed for women that combines elements of a tuxedo and a dress. It is typically made of high-quality fabrics and features tailored details commonly associated with men's formalwear, such as a structured jacket silhouette, buttons, lapels, and sometimes even a bow tie. The tuxedo dress is a versatile and elegant option for various formal occasions, including black-tie events, galas, and cocktail parties. It offers a stylish twist on traditional women's eveningwear, borrowing elements from men's tuxedos to create a unique and sophisticated look.

Tuxedo Pants

Tuxedo pants are a type of formal trousers that are typically worn as part of a tuxedo ensemble. They are designed to be worn with a tuxedo jacket and are made from high-quality fabrics such as wool or silk. The defining feature of tuxedo pants is their formal and tailored appearance. They are typically made with a high waist, which helps to elongate the wearer's legs and create a flattering silhouette. Tuxedo pants often have a flat front, with no pleats or visible pockets, to maintain a clean and sophisticated look.

Tweed Coat

A tweed coat is a type of outerwear garment that incorporates tweed fabric in its construction. Tweed is a sturdy, woolen fabric typically characterized by its intricate weave pattern, which produces a textured appearance. The coat may be single-breasted or double-breasted and can vary in length from a shorter bomber-style jacket to a longer overcoat. While tweed coats have historical roots in rural and hunting attire, they have evolved to become a timeless and versatile garment in the world of fashion design. Tweed coats offer a range of benefits that contribute to their enduring popularity. The fabric's durable nature makes it ideal for colder climates and outdoor activities, providing warmth and protection against the elements. Furthermore, tweed's distinct appearance adds a touch of sophistication and elegance to any outfit, making it suitable for both formal and casual occasions. Its versatility extends to various styles, as tweed coats can feature different cuts, lapel designs, and pocket styles, allowing for personalization and adaptation to individual tastes. In terms of color, tweed coats often showcase earthy tones such as browns, grays, and greens, which complement the natural aesthetic of the fabric. However, contemporary designs may also incorporate brighter hues or patterns, introducing a modern twist to traditional tweed. Additionally, the texture of tweed fabric lends itself to creating unique visual interest and depth, adding a tactile element to the coat's overall appearance. Tweed coats can be seamlessly integrated into both formal and casual outfits. For a formal ensemble, they can be paired with tailored trousers or a pencil skirt, complemented by a blouse or button-down shirt. Adding accessories like heels or loafers and statement jewelry completes the sophisticated look. For a more laid-back style, tweed coats can be combined with jeans or pants and a cozy sweater or a casual blouse. Accompanied by boots or sneakers and minimal accessories, this creates a comfortable yet fashionable outfit. In conclusion, a tweed coat is a timeless and versatile outerwear garment that utilizes tweed fabric in its construction. With its sturdy nature, distinct appearance, and adaptability to various styles, tweed coats offer both practicality and fashion-forward elegance. Whether worn for formal or casual occasions, they add a touch of sophistication and warmth, making them a staple piece in the world of fashion design.

Twin Set Sweater

A twin set sweater is a versatile and timeless garment in the fashion design industry. It is typically composed of two matching pieces, a cardigan and a pullover, that are designed to be worn together as a coordinated set. The cardigan, which is usually full-length or cropped, features a button-down front and long sleeves. It can be made from a variety of materials such as wool, cashmere, or cotton, depending on the desired level of warmth and comfort. The cardigan is often finished with ribbed cuffs, hem, and neckline to add structure and a polished touch to the overall design. The pullover, on the other hand, is a lightweight sweater that is worn underneath the cardigan. It is typically sleeveless or has short sleeves and is designed to hug the body for a form-fitting silhouette. Like the cardigan, the pullover can be made from various fabrics, with popular choices including lightweight knits, silk, or cotton blends. The twin set sweater provides a myriad of styling options for fashion enthusiasts. When worn together, the cardigan and pullover create a cohesive and polished look that can be suited for both casual and formal occasions. The set can be worn with skirts, trousers, or jeans to effortlessly elevate any outfit. Alternatively, each piece of the twin set sweater can be worn separately, offering versatility and versatility. The cardigan can be styled over a blouse or dress, adding a layer of warmth and sophistication to the ensemble. The pullover, when worn on its own, can be paired with high-waisted bottoms or layered with jackets for a more relaxed and contemporary look. Overall, the twin set sweater is a classic and enduring fashion staple that embodies elegance and versatility. Its two-piece design allows for various styling options, making it a practical and stylish addition to any wardrobe.

Twinset Cardigan

A twinset cardigan is a versatile piece of clothing in the world of fashion design that consists of a matching set of a cardigan and a top. The term "twinset" refers to the two garments that are designed to be worn together, creating a cohesive and fashionable look. The cardigan, in the context of fashion design, is a type of knitted sweater that is open in the front and typically has buttons or a zipper closure. It can be made from various materials such as wool, cashmere, or cotton, offering different levels of warmth and comfort. Cardigans are known for their versatility and ability to be styled in various ways, making them a staple in many wardrobes. When combined with the matching top, the twinset cardigan creates a put-together and effortlessly chic ensemble. The top is usually a short-sleeved or sleeveless blouse that complements the style and color of the cardigan. The set can also include a camisole or a tank top that can be worn underneath the cardigan for added comfort and layering options. Twinset cardigans are beloved by fashion designers and wearers alike for several reasons. Firstly, they provide a complete and coordinated outfit without the need for much additional styling or pairing. This makes them a convenient choice for those who want a polished look with minimal effort. Secondly, twinset cardigans offer versatility in terms of both style and occasion. They can be dressed up or down, depending on the choice of accessories, bottoms, and footwear. For example, pairing a twinset cardigan with tailored trousers and heels creates a sophisticated and professional look, while teaming it with jeans and sneakers gives off a casual and comfortable vibe. Furthermore, the individual pieces of a twinset cardigan can be mixed and matched with other items in one's wardrobe, extending their usability and providing endless styling possibilities. The cardigan can be worn separately over a dress or with a different top, while the top can be paired with skirts or pants for a more versatile outfit. In conclusion, a twinset cardigan is a fashion design term that refers to a matching set of a cardigan and a top. It offers convenience, versatility, and endless styling possibilities, making it a popular choice among fashion enthusiasts and designers.

Twinset Sweater

A twinset sweater is a type of coordinated knitwear that consists of two pieces: a matching cardigan and a sleeveless or short-sleeved top. It originated in the 1940s and has since become a classic staple in women's fashion. The cardigan component of a twinset sweater usually features a button-down front, a V-neck or round neckline, and long sleeves. It is designed to be worn unbuttoned or closed, depending on the desired look. The sleeveless or short-sleeved top, often called a shell or vest, is typically made of the same knit fabric as the cardigan and is meant to be worn underneath it. Traditionally, twinset sweaters were made of lightweight knit fabrics such as cotton, cashmere, or merino wool, making them suitable for both spring and autumn seasons. However, modern variations can be found in a wide range of materials, including synthetic blends and heavier knits for colder weather. One of the defining features of a twinset sweater is its versatility. The two pieces can be worn together as a set, or each item can be mixed and matched with other garments to create different outfits. The cardigan can be paired with jeans or trousers for a casual look, or worn over a dress or skirt for a more polished ensemble. The shell or vest can be worn on its own as a standalone top, layered under blazers or jackets, or combined with skirts and pants. Twinset sweaters are known for their timeless and feminine aesthetic. They often exude a classic elegance and can be dressed up or down depending on the occasion. They have remained popular throughout the years due to their versatility, comfort, and ability to elevate any outfit.

Unitard

A unitard is a one-piece garment that closely fits the body and covers both the torso and limbs. It is commonly used in fashion design, particularly in the context of dancewear and performance costumes. The term "unitard" is a combination of the words "unit" and "leotard," highlighting its single-piece construction and the influence of traditional leotards. Unitards are typically made from stretchy, form-fitting materials such as spandex or Lycra. This fabric choice allows for a snug yet flexible fit that allows freedom of movement while emphasizing the body's contours. The close fit of the unitard also accentuates the wearer's physique, making it a popular choice in dance and athletic performances.

Upcycling

Upcycling in the context of fashion design refers to the practice of transforming unwanted or unused materials, such as old clothing or fabric scraps, into new, high-quality, and fashionable products. Unlike recycling, which involves breaking down materials to create new ones, upcycling focuses on finding creative ways to repurpose existing materials without degrading their quality or value. The concept of upcycling emerged as a response to the fast fashion industry's negative environmental impact and excessive waste production. By upcycling, designers can reduce the demand for new resources, minimize landfill waste, and promote sustainability within the fashion industry.

Utility Jumpsuit

A utility jumpsuit is a one-piece garment that combines functionality and style, designed specifically for practical use in various fields, such as fashion, construction, and labor-intensive activities. It is characterized by its overall style, with long sleeves, full-length pants, and a front button or zipper closure. The jumpsuit is typically made from durable and sturdy materials, such as cotton, denim, or twill, to withstand heavy-duty tasks and provide protection against potential hazards. The utility jumpsuit has its roots in the early 20th century, where it was initially designed as a practical workwear garment for industrial workers, mechanics, and military personnel. Over time, the jumpsuit has evolved into a fashion statement, adopted by designers and trendsetters to create versatile and chic outfits for various occasions.

Utility Playsuit

A utility playsuit is a versatile and functional garment designed for women, typically made of durable materials such as denim or cotton. Inspired by workwear and military uniforms, this playsuit combines practicality with style, creating a fashionable and effortless look. Featuring a one-piece design, the utility playsuit often incorporates elements such as button or zip closures, multiple pockets, and waist cinching details. These design elements not only add visual interest to the playsuit but also enhance its functionality by providing ample storage space for small essentials. One of the key characteristics of a utility playsuit is its ability to be dressed up or down depending on the occasion. It can be worn with a pair of sneakers and a casual jacket for a laid-back, everyday look or paired with heels and statement accessories for a more dressed-up ensemble. The utility playsuit is known for its versatility, making it a popular choice among fashion enthusiasts. Its effortless style and practical design make it suitable for various settings, including casual outings, social events, or even the workplace in some cases. When it comes to choosing the right utility playsuit, factors such as fabric, fit, and details should be considered. Denim playsuits offer a classic and timeless appeal, while cotton playsuits provide comfort and breathability. The fit of the playsuit should be tailored to suit individual body types, ensuring a flattering silhouette. In terms of styling, the utility playsuit can be accessorized to enhance its overall look. Statement belts can be added to cinch the waist and create a more defined silhouette, while scarves or bandanas can be tied around the neck for a touch of personality. Layering with jackets, cardigans, or blazers can also elevate the playsuit, particularly during colder seasons.

V-Neck Sweater

A v-neck sweater is a type of knitted garment that is designed with a distinctive V-shaped neckline, typically at the front. This style of sweater is often considered a classic and versatile wardrobe staple in the realm of fashion design. Characterized by its gently sloping neckline, a v-neck sweater creates a flattering silhouette that elongates the neck and draws attention to the face. The V-shaped neckline is formed by two diagonal lines that meet at the center, creating an angular opening that can vary in depth. Typically made from various types of yarn such as wool, cashmere, or cotton blends, v-neck sweaters can be designed to suit different seasons and occasions. They are available in a range of weights, from lightweight and breathable options for warmer climates to chunkier knits for colder weather. In terms of design, v-neck sweaters can feature different knit patterns and textures, such as ribbed, cable, or plain stitches. They often come in a variety of colors, from classic neutral tones such as black, navy, and gray, to more vibrant hues like red, green, or purple. Some v-neck sweaters may also incorporate patterns or motifs on the front or sleeves for added visual interest. Due to their versatility, v-neck sweaters can be styled in various ways to create different looks. They can be worn casually with jeans or paired with tailored trousers or skirts for a more formal ensemble. Layering a v-neck sweater over a collared shirt or blouse can add a touch of sophistication to an outfit, while accessorizing with scarves or statement jewelry can further enhance the overall aesthetic. Overall, the v-neck sweater is a timeless garment that offers both style and practicality. Its timeless design, range of materials, and adaptability make it a go-to choice for individuals seeking a wardrobe essential that effortlessly combines comfort and fashion.

Velcro Tape

Velcro tape is a fastening material widely used in the fashion industry for its convenient and efficient nature. It consists of two components: hook and loop, which when pressed together form a secure and adjustable closure. This tape is made up of fabric strips, with one side containing small "hooks" and the other side featuring "loops" that interlock when pressed together. Due to its versatility and ease of use, Velcro tape has become an essential tool for fashion designers. It provides quick and efficient closures for garments, accessories, and shoes, eliminating the need for traditional buttons, zippers, or snaps. This makes it particularly useful for creating fastenings in garments that require frequent opening and closing, such as jackets, handbags, or shoes.

Victorian Blouse

A Victorian blouse, in the context of fashion design, refers to a type of blouse that incorporates design elements inspired by the Victorian era. The Victorian era, which spanned from the mid-19th century to the early 20th century, was a time of elegance, refinement, and strict societal norms. A Victorian blouse typically features unique details such as high collars, ruffles, lace trimmings, and puffed sleeves, all of which were popular during the Victorian era. The high collar, often referred to as a "stand-up" collar, adds a touch of formality and sophistication to the blouse. It was commonly made of lace or embellished with delicate embroidery. The ruffles, which can be found on the neckline, cuffs, or down the front of the blouse, serve to add a feminine and romantic touch. They may be created using fabric manipulation techniques such as pleating or gathering, giving the blouse a sense of volume and texture. In addition, Victorian blouses often incorporate puffed sleeves, which were fashionable during the time. These sleeves are characterized by their voluminous appearance, created by gathering fabric at the shoulder and cuff. Puffed sleeves were seen as a symbol of femininity and were often accentuated with extra adornments like lace or ribbons. Victorian blouses can be made from a variety of fabrics, including silk, cotton, and lace. The choice of fabric can greatly influence the overall appearance and formality of the blouse. While silk blouses are often associated with formal occasions, cotton or lace blouses can be more versatile and suitable for both casual and formal contexts. When it comes to styling, Victorian blouses can be paired with different types of bottoms, depending on the desired look. They can be worn with skirts for a more feminine and vintage-inspired ensemble, or with trousers or jeans for a modern twist. Accessorizing with delicate jewelry such as pearl earrings or a cameo brooch can further enhance the Victorian aesthetic. In conclusion, a Victorian blouse is a fashion design garment that draws inspiration from the elegance and refinement of the Victorian era. Characterized by high collars, ruffles, lace trimmings, and puffed sleeves, it offers a feminine and romantic look. The choice of fabric and styling options allow for versatility and adaptability to various occasions, making it a timeless and classic addition to any wardrobe.

Vintage Fashion

Vintage fashion refers to clothing, shoes, accessories, and styles that were popular and in vogue during a previous era, typically from the early 1920s to the late 1980s. It is a nostalgic and historical representation of fashion trends that have made a comeback and become desirable once again. Vintage fashion is characterized by its unique and timeless appeal. It often embodies the craftsmanship and quality of a bygone era, as well as the individuality and personality of the wearer. Vintage pieces are typically one-of-a-kind or limited edition, making them highly sought after by fashion enthusiasts and collectors.

Virtual Fashion Shows

Virtual Fashion Shows are digital presentations that showcase fashion designs and collections through virtual platforms, allowing designers and brands to reach a global audience without the need for physical events. Unlike traditional fashion shows, which require physical venues and audience attendance, virtual fashion shows take advantage of technology to create immersive and interactive experiences. They can be accessed online, through websites or social media platforms, allowing fashion enthusiasts from all around the world to participate in the event.

Visual Merchandising

Visual merchandising in the context of fashion design refers to the presentation and arrangement of clothing, accessories, and other fashion-related products in a retail environment. It involves creating visually appealing displays and layouts that attract customers and encourage them to make purchases. The main goal of visual merchandising is to effectively communicate the brand's image and the qualities of its products to customers, ultimately driving sales and enhancing the overall shopping experience. It is a strategic combination of art, design, and marketing techniques that aims to captivate and engage consumers by creating visually stimulating and cohesive displays. Visual merchandising encompasses various elements such as window displays, store layouts, signage, product placement, lighting, and overall store ambiance. These elements work together to create an inviting and enticing atmosphere that captures the attention of shoppers and effectively communicates the brand's desired message. Window displays are a crucial aspect of visual merchandising as they serve as the storefront's first impression. They should be eye-catching, innovative, and reflect the brand's identity to entice potential customers into entering the store. Once inside, the store layout should guide customers through a well-organized and aesthetically pleasing space, making it easy for them to navigate and browse the merchandise. Product placement is another key element of visual merchandising. Strategic placement of products can help highlight key items or collections, create focal points, and encourage customers to explore the store further. Grouping complementary items together or showcasing them in a visually appealing manner can also create a sense of cohesion and inspire customers to purchase multiple items. Lighting plays a crucial role in visual merchandising as it helps create the desired atmosphere and enhances the visibility of the products. Proper lighting can accentuate the colors, textures, and details of the merchandise, making them more appealing to customers. Additionally, the overall store ambiance, including the music, scents, and overall atmosphere, should align with the brand's image and enhance the shopping experience. In conclusion, visual merchandising in fashion design is the art of creating visually captivating displays and layouts that effectively communicate a brand's image and entice customers to make purchases. It involves various elements such as window displays, store layouts, product placement, lighting, and store ambiance, all working together to create an inviting and engaging shopping experience. By utilizing these techniques, fashion retailers can create a strong brand presence, increase customer satisfaction, and ultimately drive sales.

Wardrobe Consulting

Wardrobe consulting is a specialized service within the fashion design industry that involves providing expert advice and guidance on personal styling and outfit selection. The primary role of a wardrobe consultant is to assist individuals in creating a well-curated and functional wardrobe that aligns with their personal style, body type, and lifestyle. A wardrobe consultant is knowledgeable in current fashion trends, clothing styles, and brands, allowing them to effectively assess their client's existing wardrobe and provide recommendations for updating, organizing, and enhancing their clothing collection. They often work closely with their clients to understand their personal preferences, fashion goals, and specific needs, in order to create a tailored wardrobe that suits their individuality. During a wardrobe consultation session, the consultant will typically conduct an in-depth analysis of the client's current wardrobe. This can involve assessing the fit, condition, and versatility of each item, as well as its relevance to the client's personal style and lifestyle. Based on this analysis, the consultant will make recommendations on which pieces to keep, alter, donate, or discard. They may also suggest new clothing items or accessories to fill any gaps and create a cohesive and versatile wardrobe. In addition to analyzing the client's existing wardrobe, a wardrobe consultant may also offer personal shopping services. This involves accompanying the client to select stores or boutiques and assisting them in finding the perfect pieces that align with their desired style and fit. The consultant will provide guidance on fit, color choices, and styling options, while also considering the client's budget and preferences. Overall, wardrobe consulting serves as a valuable resource for individuals seeking to elevate their personal style and fashion choices. The expertise of a wardrobe consultant helps clients develop a better understanding of fashion, enabling them to make more confident and informed decisions when it comes to their wardrobe. Through personalized advice and guidance, wardrobe consultants empower individuals to curate a wardrobe that accurately represents their unique personality and showcases their individuality.

Wardrobe Stylist

A wardrobe stylist is a fashion professional who specializes in creating and curating outfits and ensembles for individuals or groups. They have a keen eye for fashion and trends, and are able to combine clothing, accessories, and personal style to create cohesive and visually appealing looks. Wardrobe stylists work closely with clients, whether it be for personal styling or for a specific project such as a photoshoot or fashion show. They begin by understanding the client's needs, preferences, and goals, and then use their expertise to select and assemble garments, shoes, and accessories that best suit the client's body type, personal style, and the occasion. As part of their role, wardrobe stylists stay up-to-date with the latest fashion trends, designers, and collections. They are knowledgeable about different fabrics, cuts, and silhouettes, and are able to make informed decisions about what will flatter their clients and make them feel confident and comfortable. They also have a strong understanding of color theory and can use this knowledge to create outfits that are visually appealing and harmonious. In addition to selecting garments, wardrobe stylists may also provide guidance on hair and makeup, as these elements play a crucial role in completing a look. They often work closely with makeup artists and hairstylists to ensure that the overall styling is cohesive and complements the client's outfit. Wardrobe stylists possess excellent communication and interpersonal skills, as they need to effectively communicate with clients, designers, photographers, and other professionals in the fashion industry. They must be able to translate a client's vision into a tangible reality and be open to feedback and adjustments. Overall, a wardrobe stylist plays a vital role in the fashion industry by helping individuals and groups express their personal style and create memorable and impactful looks. Through their knowledge, creativity, and attention to detail, they contribute to the visual storytelling and aesthetics of fashion and help their clients look and feel their best.

Wearable Tech

Wearable tech is a rapidly emerging field within fashion design that integrates advanced technology into garments and accessories. It involves incorporating electronic components, sensors, and connectivity capabilities into clothing items and accessories to enhance their functionality and aesthetics. This integration of technology and fashion brings forth a new level of innovation and opens up possibilities for creating smarter and more interactive clothing. By seamlessly incorporating technology into wearable items, designers can create products that not only serve their traditional purpose but also offer additional features and benefits that enhance the wearer's overall experience.

Wetsuit

A wetsuit is a type of garment designed for individuals engaging in water activities, particularly in colder temperatures. It is commonly used in water sports such as surfing, diving, and paddleboarding to provide thermal insulation and protection against the elements. The construction of a wetsuit typically involves using multiple layers of synthetic rubber, often neoprene, which is known for its excellent insulation properties. The neoprene material is highly flexible, allowing for freedom of movement while maintaining warmth in cold water. The wetsuit is designed to fit snugly to the body, reducing the amount of water that can enter and reducing heat loss through conduction. The primary purpose of a wetsuit is to keep the wearer warm in cold water conditions. When the body is immersed in water, it loses heat much faster than in air due to the higher thermal conductivity of water. The insulating properties of the wetsuit prevent this heat loss by trapping a thin layer of water between the suit and the skin. This layer of water is quickly warmed by the body's heat and acts as an effective barrier against the cold water outside the suit. In addition to providing thermal insulation, wetsuits also offer protection against abrasions, cuts, and stings from marine life. The thick neoprene material acts as a buffer between the wearer and potential hazards in the water, minimizing the risk of injury. The tight fit of the wetsuit also helps in reducing the impact of external forces, such as strong currents or waves, on the body. Wetsuits are available in various styles and thicknesses, catering to different water temperatures and activity levels. Full suits cover the entire body, including the arms and legs, providing maximum coverage and warmth. Shorty suits, on the other hand, have shorter sleeves and legs, offering more flexibility and freedom of movement. The thickness of the neoprene material can vary between wetsuits, with thicker suits providing better insulation in colder waters. Overall, wetsuits are an essential piece of equipment for water enthusiasts, enabling them to stay comfortable and protected in cold water conditions. Their design and functionality make them a staple in the world of fashion design for water sports, combining both style and practicality to enhance the wearer's experience in the water.

Wide-Leg Culottes

Wide-leg culottes are a type of women's pants that feature a wide and loose fit, resembling a skirt. They are designed to be cropped and typically fall between the calf and ankle. The term "culottes" originated from the French word for "breeches" and was traditionally used to describe knee-length pants worn by men in the 16th century. However, modern wide-leg culottes have undergone various adaptations to cater to the fashion preferences of women. Wide-leg culottes are characterized by their voluminous silhouette, which is achieved through the use of wide and flowing fabric that drapes loosely around the legs. They often have a high waistline, which helps to accentuate the waist and create a flattering silhouette. Wide-leg culottes can be made from a variety of fabrics, including cotton, linen, silk, and denim. The choice of fabric will determine the overall look and feel of the culottes, with lighter fabrics offering a more relaxed and airy aesthetic, while heavier fabrics provide a more structured and formal appearance.

Wide-Leg Jumpsuit

A wide-leg jumpsuit is a type of garment in fashion design that features a one-piece design with wide-leg trousers integrated with a top. It is a popular choice among fashion-conscious individuals, as it combines style, comfort, and versatility. The defining feature of a wide-leg jumpsuit is the wide-leg trousers, which provide a relaxed and flowing look. These trousers are wide from the waist to the hem, creating a loose and billowing silhouette. The wide-leg design offers a flattering fit for various body types, as it elongates the legs and provides a balanced and proportionate look. Wide-leg jumpsuits are available in various styles and designs, ranging from casual to formal. They can be made from various fabrics, including cotton, linen, silk, or polyester, each offering a unique texture and drape. The choice of fabric influences the overall aesthetic and drape of the jumpsuit, allowing for different levels of formality and versatility. In terms of top design, wide-leg jumpsuits can have different necklines, such as V-neck, square, boat, or halter necklines. The top can be fitted or loose, depending on the desired look and level of comfort. Some wide-leg jumpsuits may also feature sleeves, ranging from cap sleeves to long sleeves, or they can be sleeveless for a more summery and casual feel. Wide-leg jumpsuits can be styled in various ways to suit different occasions. For a casual and laid-back look, they can be paired with sandals or sneakers and accessorized with a belt or a statement necklace. To create a more formal and elegant ensemble, wide-leg jumpsuits can be paired with high heels and complemented with delicate jewelry. In conclusion, a wide-leg jumpsuit is a versatile and stylish garment that combines the comfort of trousers with the sophistication of a one-piece design. Its wide-leg silhouette offers a relaxed and flattering fit, catering to different body types and personal styles. With its range of styles, fabrics, and design options, the wide-leg jumpsuit is a timeless choice for both casual and formal occasions.

Wide-Leg Pants

Wide-leg pants, also referred to as wide-leg trousers or palazzo pants, are a style of pants characterized by their wide and loose fit throughout the leg. The width of the leg can vary, ranging from a slight flare to an exaggerated wide cut that drapes away from the body. Wide-leg pants have been a prominent fashion trend since the early 20th century and have experienced various iterations and reinterpretations throughout the years. This style of pants provides a relaxed and flowing silhouette, offering comfort and a sense of effortless glamour.

Wide-Leg Playsuit

A wide-leg playsuit is a style of clothing typically designed for women that combines the ease and comfort of a one-piece garment with wide-legged trousers. It is a versatile and fashionable option that can be worn for various occasions. The defining feature of a wide-leg playsuit is its loose-fitting silhouette, which flares out from the waist down. This relaxed fit allows for ease of movement and makes it a comfortable choice for everyday wear. The wide-leg design also gives the playsuit a chic and modern look.

Windbreaker

A windbreaker is a type of jacket designed to protect the wearer from strong winds, typically lightweight and made from a nylon or polyester fabric. It is a versatile outerwear piece commonly used in various outdoor activities and has become a popular fashion trend in recent years. Originally developed for sports and outdoor enthusiasts, windbreakers are now widely worn by people of all ages and genders. The primary function of a windbreaker is to shield the wearer from wind chill and light rain, making it an essential garment for unpredictable weather conditions. Windbreakers often feature a full front zipper or snap button closure, allowing the wearer to easily put on or take off the jacket. They also commonly have elasticized cuffs and hem to provide a snug fit and prevent cold air from entering the jacket. Additionally, many windbreakers come with a hood that can be adjusted or folded away when not in use, adding further protection against the elements. In terms of design, windbreakers can be found in a wide range of colors, patterns, and styles, making them a versatile choice for various outfits. They are often designed with a minimalist aesthetic, focusing on functionality rather than intricate details. However, fashion-forward windbreakers may include unique embellishments, such as contrast panels, branding, or reflective accents, to add visual interest. Due to their lightweight and packable nature, windbreakers are highly convenient for travel and outdoor activities. They are frequently favored for activities like hiking, cycling, running, and even as a layering piece during colder seasons. Moreover, the popularity of windbreakers in streetwear and athleisure fashion has made them a stylish choice for everyday wear, with many high-end fashion brands incorporating them into their collections. In conclusion, windbreakers are a practical and fashionable outerwear option designed to protect the wearer from wind and light rain. Their versatility, lightweight construction, and sporty aesthetic make them a popular choice for individuals seeking both functionality and style in their wardrobe.

Window Display

Window Display refers to the visual presentation of merchandise and fashion design concepts in the windows of retail stores. It is a key element of visual merchandising, aimed at attracting and engaging potential customers by showcasing products and creating a compelling and immersive shopping experience. Window displays play a significant role in the fashion industry as they serve multiple purposes. First and foremost, they act as a powerful marketing tool, effectively capturing the attention of passersby and enticing them to enter the store. By carefully curating and arranging merchandise, window displays can communicate the brand's aesthetic, values, and current fashion trends, helping to establish a strong brand identity and position in the market. A well-designed and thoughtfully executed window display has the potential to not only drive foot traffic but also increase sales by encouraging impulse purchases. Fashion designers and retail store owners use window displays as a means to highlight their latest collections, new arrivals, or limited edition items. Through imaginative and creative arrangements, they aim to present the merchandise in a visually appealing and aspirational way, inspiring customers to make a purchase and try out the featured styles. Window displays also provide an opportunity for fashion designers to showcase their artistic talents and creative vision. By incorporating elements of storytelling, they can evoke emotions and tell a story through their displays, transporting viewers into a different world or capturing the essence of a particular theme or concept. Whether it's a whimsical fairytale-inspired window or a minimalist, sleek arrangement, window displays allow fashion designers to express their unique style and create a memorable brand experience for customers. Furthermore, window displays serve as a platform for experimentation and innovation in fashion design. They enable designers to push boundaries, explore unconventional materials, and present their work in unconventional ways. By breaking free from the constraints of a traditional garment display, designers can use window displays to challenge norms and provoke thought, ultimately inviting engagement and dialogue among viewers. In conclusion, window displays are a crucial aspect of fashion design, serving as a powerful marketing tool, a platform for creativity and storytelling, and an opportunity for designers to showcase their work. By creating visually captivating and immersive displays, fashion designers can effectively attract and engage potential customers, ultimately contributing to the success of the brand and the overall shopping experience.

Wrap Cardigan

A wrap cardigan is a versatile and functional piece of clothing in fashion design. It is a cardigan that features a front closure that wraps around the body, providing protection and warmth. The design of the wrap cardigan allows for easy adjustment and styling, making it a popular choice for both casual and formal occasions. Typically made from knit or woven fabric, the wrap cardigan is known for its comfort and softness. It often has a loose fit, allowing for ease of movement and a relaxed silhouette. The front closure of the cardigan can be in the form of buttons, snaps, ties, or even hooks and eyes. The wrap design allows for different levels of coverage and customization, making it suitable for various body types and preferences.

Wrap Dress

A wrap dress is a style of dress that is characterized by its wrap-around design, usually secured by a tie or a belt at the waist. The dress typically consists of a V-neckline, which is created by the crossed fabric on the front of the dress. The skirt of the dress is also wrapped and may feature a tulip shape or a full skirt with pleats. Originally introduced in the 1970s by fashion designer Diane von Furstenberg, the wrap dress became an iconic symbol of women's liberation and empowerment. Its versatility and flattering silhouette have made it a timeless classic in the world of fashion.

Wrap Jumpsuit

A wrap jumpsuit is a type of garment that combines the style and functionality of both a wrap dress and a jumpsuit. It is designed to be a one-piece outfit that is easy to put on and wear, while also being fashionable and versatile. The wrap jumpsuit typically features a wrap-style bodice that wraps around the torso and secures at the waist with a tie or a button. This gives the garment a flattering and adjustable fit, as the wearer can tighten or loosen the wrap to their liking. The wrap bodice often has a V-neckline, which adds a touch of femininity and elegance to the overall design. One of the main characteristics of a wrap jumpsuit is its wide, flowy legs. Unlike traditional jumpsuits that have fitted or straight legs, the wrap jumpsuit has a more relaxed and billowing silhouette. This not only adds comfort to the garment but also creates movement and fluidity when the wearer walks or moves. In terms of materials, wrap jumpsuits can be made from a variety of fabrics, depending on the desired look and occasion. It can be made from lightweight and breathable fabrics such as cotton or silk for a casual or summer-ready ensemble. On the other hand, it can also be made from more structured fabrics like linen or twill for a more polished and formal look. The versatility of the wrap jumpsuit makes it a popular choice among fashion designers and consumers alike. It can be dressed up or down, depending on the styling and accessories. For a more formal or evening look, it can be paired with statement jewelry, high heels, and a clutch. For a more casual or daytime look, it can be styled with sandals, a straw hat, and a crossbody bag. All in all, the wrap jumpsuit is a stylish and practical garment that offers the best of both worlds. It combines the convenience and ease of a jumpsuit with the flattering and adjustable fit of a wrap dress. Its wide legs and flowy silhouette add a touch of elegance and movement to any outfit, making it a versatile choice for a variety of occasions.

Wrap Mini Skirt

A wrap mini skirt is a type of skirt that is designed to be wrapped around the waist and secured with ties or buttons. It is characterized by its short length, typically hitting above the knee. The wrap design allows for adjustable fit and styling options, making it a versatile choice for various occasions. When it comes to fashion design, the wrap mini skirt offers endless possibilities for creativity and expression. Designers can play with different fabrics, patterns, and textures to create unique and statement-making pieces. From lightweight summer materials like cotton and linen to luxurious options such as silk or velvet, the choice of fabric greatly influences the overall look and feel of the skirt.

Wrap Skirt

A wrap skirt is a type of skirt that wraps around the waist and is secured with a closure, such as a button or tie. It is a versatile and timeless piece in fashion design, offering a feminine and flattering silhouette. The wrap skirt typically features an overlapping front panel that can be adjusted to fit different waist sizes. This adjustability is achieved through the use of ties, buttons, or snaps, allowing the wearer to customize the fit and create various styles. For example, the skirt can be wrapped tightly for a more fitted look or loosely for a flowy and relaxed silhouette. One of the key design elements of a wrap skirt is its asymmetrical hemline. The front panel is usually longer than the back, creating an elegant and dynamic look. This asymmetry adds movement and visual interest to the skirt, making it a popular choice among fashion enthusiasts. Wrap skirts are available in various lengths, from mini to maxi, allowing for versatility in styling. Mini wrap skirts are perfect for a playful and flirtatious look, while midi and maxi lengths create a more sophisticated and elegant appearance. Additionally, the skirt can have different types of closures, such as buttons, ties, or even Velcro, offering even more flexibility in design. When it comes to fabric choices, wrap skirts can be made from a wide range of materials. Light and flowy fabrics, such as chiffon or silk, are commonly used to create a breezy and feminine look. On the other hand, heavier fabrics, like denim or wool, can add structure and warmth, making the skirt suitable for cooler weather. The beauty of a wrap skirt lies in its simplicity and versatility. It can be effortlessly dressed up or down, making it a staple in any wardrobe. Whether paired with a casual t-shirt and sandals for a day at the beach or with a blouse and heels for a night out, the wrap skirt offers endless options for creating stylish and fashionable outfits.

Wrap Sweater

A wrap sweater is a type of garment designed to be worn by individuals as a top layer in cool or cold weather. It is a versatile and stylish option that is popular in the world of fashion design. Characterized by its wrap-around design, a wrap sweater typically features a front closure that allows the wearer to wrap one side of the garment across the body and secure it with buttons, ties, or other fasteners. This closure creates a flattering and adjustable fit that can be customized to the wearer's preference.

Wrap Top

A wrap top is a type of garment that is designed to be wrapped around the upper body and secured using ties, buttons, or other fasteners. It typically consists of a front panel that overlaps with a back panel, creating a flattering V-neckline and a cinched waist. The wrap top is versatile and can be worn for both formal and casual occasions, making it a popular choice in women's fashion. One of the key design features of a wrap top is its adjustable fit. The front panel can be wrapped around the body as tightly or as loosely as desired, allowing for a customizable fit that flatters various body shapes and sizes. This versatility makes the wrap top a flattering option for a wide range of body types.

Yarn Winders

A yarn winder is a tool used in the fashion design industry to prepare yarn for use in creating garments and accessories. It is a mechanical device that winds yarn into neat and organized balls or cakes, making it easier to work with during the design process. The main purpose of a yarn winder is to transform skeins or hanks of yarn into more manageable forms. Skeins or hanks are long, twisted strands of yarn that are typically sold in this format by yarn manufacturers. However, these forms can be difficult to work with directly, as the yarn tends to tangle easily and can become tangled or knotted during the garment-making process. By using a yarn winder, a fashion designer can efficiently and neatly wind the yarn into a ball or cake shape. This helps to prevent tangling and ensures that the yarn is easily accessible while working on a design. The resulting wound yarn is also more compact and takes up less space, making it easier to store in the design studio. Yarn winders come in various sizes and designs, but they generally consist of a spinning mechanism and a central post. The skein or hank of yarn is attached to the central post, and as the mechanism spins, it winds the yarn around the post, creating the desired shape. Some yarn winders also have additional features, such as yarn guides or tensioners, which help to regulate the winding process. Using a yarn winder offers several benefits to fashion designers. Firstly, it saves time and effort by quickly transforming yarn into a usable form. Instead of manually winding the yarn, which can be a tedious and time-consuming task, designers can rely on the efficiency of a yarn winder. Furthermore, the neatly wound yarn ensures a consistent tension throughout the design process, resulting in more even and professional-looking stitches. In conclusion, a yarn winder is a valuable tool for fashion designers, allowing them to efficiently wind yarn into organized balls or cakes. By using a yarn winder, designers can save time, prevent tangling, and ensure consistent tension in their designs. This tool is a must-have for any fashion design studio.

Zero-Waste Fashion

Zero-Waste Fashion refers to a design and production approach in the fashion industry that aims to eliminate textile waste and minimize the environmental impact of clothing production. It is founded on the principle of utilizing all fabric resources efficiently, with the ultimate goal of creating garments with minimal or no leftover scraps. The concept of zero-waste fashion emerged as a response to the alarming amount of textile waste generated by the fashion industry. Traditional garment production methods often result in significant fabric waste, as patterns are cut from rectangular or square-shaped fabric pieces, leaving behind unused remnants. Additionally, the disposal of textile waste poses numerous environmental challenges, including water and air pollution, as well as increased landfill utilization. Zero-waste fashion design requires a shift in the design process itself. Designers must carefully consider and plan the pattern layout to ensure that all fabric is utilized efficiently, leaving no wasted scraps. This often involves creating patterns that can be strategically positioned to eliminate or minimize leftover fabric. Creative pattern cutting techniques such as draping, pleating, folding, and using modular elements are employed to optimize fabric use. The adoption of zero-waste principles extends beyond just pattern cutting. It encompasses considerations throughout the entire production process, including the sourcing of sustainable materials, responsible manufacturing practices, and mindful consumption. Putting an emphasis on using eco-friendly and biodegradable fabrics, such as organic cotton, hemp, or recycled materials, can further enhance the sustainability aspect of zero-waste fashion. Zero-waste fashion also encourages the reimagining and repurposing of existing garments and materials. Upcycling, or transforming discarded clothing or textiles into new pieces, is a favored method within the zero-waste fashion movement. It promotes resourcefulness and creativity, offering an alternative to the linear production and consumption model. By embracing the principles of zero-waste fashion, designers and manufacturers have the opportunity to contribute to a more sustainable and circular fashion industry. It challenges the conventional norms of fashion design, promoting innovation and eco-consciousness. Ultimately, zero-waste fashion advocates for a fundamental shift in the way clothing is created and consumed, prioritizing environmental responsibility and minimizing waste throughout the entire lifecycle of a garment.